Spirituality in
Nursing Practice

Doreen Westera, MscN, MEd, RN, obtained a master of nursing degree from the University of Toronto and a master of education (counseling) degree from Memorial University, St. John's, Newfoundland and Labrador, Canada. She taught nursing for more than 30 years at three different universities in Canada: University of Alberta, Edmonton, Alberta, Canada; Queen's University, Kingston, Ontario, Canada; and Memorial University (from which she retired in 2015). Her clinical practice experience includes participation in a crisis team in a large general hospital emergency room, working as a community health nurse in a large city, and working with a local counseling agency. She has developed and taught a course on the spiritual dimensions of practice at Memorial University for many years. She has also conducted workshops and presentations on spirituality in nursing and health care both nationally and internationally. She has developed 14 video programs—13 on spirituality in various clinical contexts, plus one on resilience, for which spirituality is a theme—that are being distributed nationally and internationally. She has also conducted research related to spirituality in nursing and health care. She conducts workshops on the topic of spirituality in nursing and health care practice for Nurses Christian Fellowship Canada.

Spirituality in Nursing Practice

THE BASICS AND BEYOND

Doreen A. Westera, MscN, MEd, RN

SPRINGER PUBLISHING COMPANY

NEW YORK

Springer Publishing Company, LLC
11 West 42nd Street
New York, NY 10036
www.springerpub.com

Acquisitions Editor: Joseph Morita
Senior Production Editor: Kris Parrish
Composition: Westchester Publishing Services

ISBN: 978-0-8261-2062-5
e-book ISBN: 978-0-8261-2063-2
Instructor's Manual ISBN: 978-0-8261-2139-4

Instructor's Materials: Qualified instructors may request supplements by e-mailing textbook@springerpub.com

16 17 18 19 20 / 5 4 3 2 1

The author and the publisher of this Work have made every effort to use sources believed to be reliable to provide information that is accurate and compatible with the standards generally accepted at the time of publication. Because medical science is continually advancing, our knowledge base continues to expand. Therefore, as new information becomes available, changes in procedures become necessary. We recommend that the reader always consult current research and specific institutional policies before performing any clinical procedure. The author and publisher shall not be liable for any special, consequential, or exemplary damages resulting, in whole or in part, from the readers' use of, or reliance on, the information contained in this book. The publisher has no responsibility for the persistence or accuracy of URLs for external or third-party Internet websites referred to in this publication and does not guarantee that any content on such websites is, or will remain, accurate or appropriate.

Library of Congress Cataloging-in-Publication Data

Names: Westera, Doreen, 1951– author.
Title: Spirituality in nursing practice : the basics and beyond / Doreen A. Westera.
Description: New York, NY : Springer Publishing Company, LLC, [2017] | Includes bibliographical
   references.
Identifiers: LCCN 2016028848 | ISBN 9780826120625 (print) | ISBN 9780826121394 (instructors manual) |
   ISBN 9780826120632 (e-book)
Subjects: | MESH: Spirituality | Nursing Care—psychology
Classification: LCC RT42 | NLM WY 87 | DDC 610.73—dc23 LC record available at https://lccn.loc
   .gov/2016028848

Printed in the United States of America by McNaughton & Gunn.

This book is dedicated to my parents, Frazer and Pearl Oakley, who provided a strong foundation for my spiritual development; to my husband, Nick, as well as to my children, Aaron and Rachel, who have nurtured my spirit in countless ways; and to God, who daily sustains me, giving me meaning and purpose, hope, joy, and peace.

Contents

Appendix A
**Boutell's Inventory for Identifying the Nurses' Assessment of Patients'
Spiritual Needs**   329

Appendix B
Wellness Spirituality Protocol   335

Index   339

Preface

I grew up in a culture that was infused with spirituality, both in terms of the broader culture and also with respect to various subcultures within that broader culture. Choosing a career in nursing arose out of my spiritual roots. My interest in spirituality in nursing began very early in my nursing career. Being acutely aware of the importance of spirituality and religion in my own life primed me to be curious and attentive to the place of spirituality/religion in the lives and situations of clients I have encountered throughout my nursing practice. While working on a crisis team in the emergency room of a large general hospital, I specifically asked to be assigned to clients for whom spiritual/religious issues were of concern. I increasingly incorporated spiritual assessment and care into my practice as a community health nurse and then did the same in my counseling practice in response to my clients' needs. As a nurse educator, I incorporated spirituality into the courses that I taught. I developed a complete course on the spiritual dimensions of practice to address what I perceived to be a gap in nursing education. As a nurse educator, I found myself to be constantly advocating for the inclusion of the spiritual dimension in nursing curricula through a variety of forums: faculty meetings, faculty/nursing education committee work, nursing education conferences, presentations focused on nursing education, and more. Many of the scholarly activities in which I have engaged by way of writing, research, and presentations at conferences have focused entirely, or in part, on spirituality in nursing/health care and/or counseling. I developed 13 videos focused on spirituality in various clinical contexts to allow the voices of clients and practicing health care professionals to be heard on the topic. While developing these videos, I was constantly amazed at how the comments of the people featured in the videos verified and corroborated much of what was written about the place of spirituality/religion in health and illness.

All of these professional experiences, and a host of personal life experiences, have transformed an initial interest in spirituality in nursing into a passion. This passion has developed a strong sense of the need to advocate for spirituality in the large context of nursing practice. Although my efforts to advocate in this area of practice have been fueled by many sources, they are driven primarily by my subjective experiences with clients and a realization of the potential for inclusion of spirituality in nursing care to result in better health outcomes for clients—and their families. This book is a tangible piece of this advocacy effort. I hope that it will not only inspire interest and passion for the inclusion of spirituality into nursing practice, but will also prepare nursing students and nurses to better attend to and provide spiritual assessment and care. As such, the overall goal is that truly holistic nursing practice, one of the key pillars of nursing, will be realized.

FORMAT OF THE BOOK

In terms of the overall focus of the book, the comments by Miner-Williams (2006) are very appropriate:

> Spirituality . . . must be understood as part of the holistic vision of the person's health, and not simply as just another "dimension" of the person. The ability to understand something, however, is sometimes limited when viewed only in its wholeness. If one can grasp an identity with smaller aspects of the whole, one can appreciate the whole better . . . we appreciate the phenomenon of spirituality by examining its inherent concepts, realizing that it is only by their "interrelatedness" [that we can] begin to understand the whole. It is seeing the picture of the puzzle by examining its pieces and putting them together. (p. 814)

Miner-Williams is writing about examining the general concept of spirituality. However, her comments are also true with respect to how spirituality in nursing practice is approached in this book. Aspects of spirituality in general and spirituality in the context of nursing practice are explored, examining all these aspects and interconnections "under a microscope" so as to better understand the whole. However, recognition of the client as a whole being and spiritual care as total care of the client should always be the lens through which each aspect of spirituality in nursing practice is viewed.

The title of this book, *Spirituality in Nursing Practice: The Basics and Beyond*, was chosen for a couple of reasons. First of all, no single work can contain everything there is to know about a given topic, including spirituality in nursing practice. This book attempts to provide the basics needed to attend to this dimension of care. Yet, throughout the book, there are directives to explore further—to go beyond the basics. This occurs through the many reflections interspersed throughout each chapter; through encouraging exploration of select literature resources/websites; through a wide range of suggested activities; and through exploring case studies. Additionally, the 14 video programs I have developed (including the 13 on spirituality, plus one on resilience, for which spirituality is a theme) can be accessed. Ten-minute preview segments from each of these videos can be viewed at www.ucs.mun.ca/~dwestera (the full length for each video is about 30 minutes). Facilitator's guides for each of the videos can also be obtained in an ancillary instructor's manual. ***Qualified instructors may obtain access to ancillary materials by e-mailing textbook@springerpub.com.***

The book consists of two parts: Part I," Spirituality in Nursing: The Basics," comprises the first six chapters, and it provides the basis from which to proceed to Part II. Part II, "Spiritual Assessment and Care in Various Clinical Contexts," comprises the last four chapters and focuses on the importance of spirituality in various clinical settings and contexts.

FEATURES OF THE BOOK

Several features in the book serve to expand knowledge and reflection about spirituality in nursing practice. Each of the chapters in the book contains a number of reflections scattered throughout. These reflections encourage the reader to engage personally (and professionally, in some cases) with the chapter material. This feature was included in recognition of the importance of self-reflection in learning about nursing practice, including spiritual care practice. Tables, illustrations, and boxes highlight various aspects of the discussion and provide examples. At the end of each chapter in Part I, there is a concise summary of major points related to the chapter focus ("The Bottom Line"). There are also a number of activities that can be undertaken individually or in groups ("Taking It Further"). Such activities should serve to further expand learning relevant to the chapter focus. Inclusion of these activities stems from my commitment as a nurse educator to experiential learning as being essential in the development of nursing practice. At the end of each chapter in Part II, information pertaining to case studies is included along with a list of questions pertaining to each case study. These case studies are focused on the clinical area of concentration for that particular chapter. The reader should access the references given for each case study in order to read the case study and to engage in the exploration that the questions stimulate. This method has been chosen in keeping with my philosophy of teaching, which is to be a catalyst for students and nurses who are assuming responsibility for their own learning. Case studies have been chosen because of their inherent value to learning by focusing on "real clients" and examining relevant issues related to spirituality/religion within that context. Accessing the case studies and engaging with them will further expand knowledge pertaining to the chapter material. It should also facilitate the transfer of that knowledge into actual practice.

Each chapter contains a reference list of literature resources that can be accessed for further information and examination. Although direction is provided throughout each chapter to explore specific references, the reader is encouraged to consult all of them—and to expand the reference list further as each topic is explored. There are thousands of references pertaining to spirituality in nursing and health care to explore. Continually reading in this area of practice will be key in developing a strong knowledge base for incorporating spirituality into nursing practice.

REFERENCE

Miner-Williams, D. (2006). Putting a puzzle together: Making spirituality meaningful for nursing using an evolving theoretical framework. *Journal of Clinical Nursing, 15*(7), 811–821. doi:10.1111/j.1365-2702.2006.01351.x

Acknowledgments

I would like to acknowledge and thank the many nurse scholars and nurse colleagues who, through their writing, research, and conversations, have substantially contributed to my interest and thoughts about the place of spirituality in nursing practice, education, and research. The clients in my clinical practice also deserve to be acknowledged as they have made much of the theoretical information about spirituality in health and illness "come alive" as they have discussed the place of spirituality/religion in their lives and situations. I have enjoyed each and every conversation with them about spiritual matters and concerns. Nursing students whom I have been privileged to teach have also encouraged me with their questions and comments about issues and concerns pertaining to the spiritual dimension in nursing practice.

I would also like to thank the editorial staff at Springer Publishing Company for their assistance in bringing this book into existence. A special thanks goes to Joseph Morita, Senior Acquisitions Editor, for his encouragement with developing the proposal for the book, and also for his ongoing encouragement during the writing of the book. Locally, I would also like to thank Jenna Flogeras, copy editor, for her assistance in the organization and formatting of the book.

Finally, a special thanks goes to my husband, Nick Westera. Not only has he provided encouragement and support during the genesis and development of this book, but he has also painstakingly read every word of the manuscript, providing invaluable editorial advice and help. Without his help, this book would not exist.

1

Spirituality in Nursing: The Basics

1

The Concept of Spirituality

The domain of spirituality is enormous with a literature that encompasses 4,000 years of oral and written tradition from every tribe and nation and from every language living and dead" (Pesut, Fowler, Reimer-Kirkham, Taylor, & Sawatzky, 2009, pp. 341–342). This chapter focuses on the very concept of spirituality. A full understanding of this concept is foundational to examining its place in nursing practice. Various definitions of spirituality are explored and themes inherent in those definitions of spirituality are identified. Metaphors are given to further illuminate the concept. How spirituality is expressed and nurtured is discussed; and brief comments about the connection between spirituality and culture, spiritual well-being, and spiritual development are made. It is anticipated that the ensuing discussion will provide not only a better understanding of the concept of spirituality, but also the motivation to delve more deeply into the literature focusing on this concept.

There is overwhelming evidence for the relevance of spirituality to nursing. More than 20 analyses of the concept of spirituality can be found in the nursing and health care literature, including Sessanna, Finnell, and Jezewski (2007), McBrien (2006), and Burkhardt (1989). Philosophical approaches to the study of spirituality have been discussed with exemplars of each approach provided (Tinley & Kinney, 2007). Attempts to clarify the concept of spirituality are plentiful, including Paley (2008) and Tanyi (2002). Analyses and debates about the concept of spirituality within the field of nursing abound in the literature, including Pesut and colleagues (2009), Clarke (2009), and McSherry and Draper (1998). Literature reviews of studies pertaining to spirituality in the health sciences, including nursing, have been conducted, including Clarke (2009) and Chiu, Emblen, van Hofwegen, Sawatzky, and Meyerhoff (2004). Scientific issues related to the study of spirituality have been discussed (MacDonald, 2011), including the analysis of the brain and its relationship with spirituality (Barnum, 2011). Models of spirituality for use in nursing theory development, research, and practice have been proposed, including Kreitzer (2012), MacDonald (2011), Smith (2006), and Buck (2006). Studies exploring nurses' perceptions of spirituality have been conducted in a diversity of cultures and contexts around the world, for example, in Iran (Markani, Yaghmaei, & Fard, 2013), the United Kingdom (McSherry & Jamieson, 2013), Turkey (Ozbasaran,

Ergul, Temel, Aslan, & Coban, 2011), Singapore (Tiew, Creedy, & Chan, 2013), and the United States (Salmon, Bruick-Sorge, Beckman, & Boxley-Harges, 2010). Nurses' views of spirituality and spiritual care in various clinical contexts have been explored: in palliative care (Taylor, 2013; Tiew, Kwee, Creedy, & Chan, 2013); in acute care (Deal & Grassley, 2012; Gallison, Xu, Yurgens, & Boyle, 2013; Ronaldson, Hayes, Aggar, Green, & Carey, 2012); and in maternal child care (Linhares, 2012). Nursing students have also been the focus of the study in Pesut (2002); and there are numerous articles in the nursing literature pertaining to the teaching of spiritual care in nursing curricula. The perspective of clients and their families about spirituality has also been elicited for a number of demographics, including Americans (Taylor & Brander, 2013), Chinese (Mok, Wong, & Wong, 2010), and Japanese (Shirahama & Inoue, 2001). There are also numerous articles on the concepts of spirituality and religion in nursing practice, including the nursing role in spiritual assessment, spiritual nursing diagnoses, spiritual care in various nursing contexts, and many more. Clearly, spirituality is a focus for debate and discussion within the nursing profession, and it is appropriate to consider this concept as it has captured the nursing world.

Reflection 1.1

This is a clustering exercise:

- Write the word "spirituality" in the center of a blank sheet of paper and circle it.
- Think about what the word "spirituality" means to you personally, and write any words and phrases that come to your mind in a circle around the word "spirituality" in the center. Circle these words and phrases.
- Think about the strength of the relationship between each word/phrase and your own spirituality. Draw a thick black line between the word/phrase and the center word "spirituality" to indicate a strong relationship; a dotted line to indicate a weak or distant relationship; a squiggly line to indicate a conflictual relationship; and a strong black line with a squiggly line drawn through it to indicate a strong but conflictual relationship. Your diagram should look something like this (Figure 1.1).
- Based on your reflection, write your own personal definition of the word "spirituality."
- Reflect on the process of completing this exercise. Was it easy for you? Why or why not? What feelings or emotions were you aware of? Where do these come from? What insights, if any, did you gain?
- Might you be able to use this exercise with clients; and if so, how might you do this?

Adapted from Rew (1989).

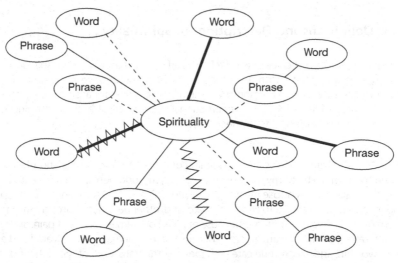

Figure 1.1 Personal concept of spirituality.

DEFINING SPIRITUALITY

There are many approaches to considering and understanding the concept of spirituality. For example, Coyle (2002) offers three such approaches (pp. 591–592):

- The structural-behaviorist approach, in which behaviors and practices associated with religion are key, providing meaning and purpose, hope, and a sense of connectedness

- The value guidance approach, in which spirituality is intricately connected to values that provide meaning and purpose in life

- The transcendent approach, in which transcendence is a key attribute; for example, transpersonal and intrapersonal transcendence. Such transcendence has a number of effects on the person, such as engendering a sense of peace and harmony, and being a resource in times of need

Spirituality comes from the Latin word *spiritus*, which means "breath" or "something which is within the body providing the life force" (Wasner, Longaker, Fegg, & Borasio, 2005, p. 100). Although these descriptions give some hint about what spirituality could mean, looking at some of the definitions of spirituality in the nursing and health care literature will be illuminating. It is important to remember that any definition that is offered is rooted in the philosophical view of the person(s) presenting the definition; each has its own implications for nursing practice. A sampling of definitions of spirituality from the nursing and health care literature is provided in Table 1.1. Included in this table is also a definition of "ecospirituality" because of its relevance for many indigenous people (Lincoln, 2000). An appropriate exercise for each definition is to seek to determine and identify the author's worldview—for example, Christian, postmodern, Eastern, humanistic, and so on.

Table 1.1 **Definitions and Descriptions of Spirituality**

[Spirituality is] "...a quality that goes beyond religious affiliation, that strives for inspiration, reverence, awe, meaning and purpose, even in those who do not believe in any good. The spiritual dimension tries to be in harmony with the universe, strives for answers about the infinite, and comes essentially into focus in times of emotional stress, physical (and mental) illness, loss, bereavement and death" (Murray & Zentner, 1989, p. 259).

[Spirituality is] "...who I am—unique and personally connected to God. That relationship with God is expressed through my body, my thinking, my feelings, my judgments, and my creativity. My spirituality motivates me to choose meaningful relationships and pursuits. Through my spirituality I give and receive love; I respond to and appreciate God, other people, a sunset, a symphony, and spring. I am driven forward, sometimes because of pain, sometimes in spite of pain. Spirituality allows me to reflect on myself. I am a person because of my spirituality—motivated and enabled to value, to worship, and to communicate with the holy, the transcendent" (Stoll, 1989, p. 9).

[Spirituality is] "...a belief or value system which permeates all of a person's life, giving life meaning in the context of six basic human relationships: 1) to God, or whomever or whatever is considered ultimate reality, 2) to self, 3) to others, 4) to the environment, 5) to the past, and 6) to the future" (Hoshiko, 1994, p. 5).

[Spirituality is] "...energy capable of producing internal harmony of body, mind and spirit.... Energy which can be focused internally fortifies and strengthens positive thinking, and can be used creatively to achieve harmony and mobilize or enhance internal defences, thereby facilitating well-being and inner healing" (Goddard, 1995, p. 813).

"Spirituality is the way in which a person understands and lives life in view of her or his ultimate meaning, beliefs, and values. It is the unifying and integrative aspect of the person's life and, when lived intentionally, is experienced as a process of growth and maturity. It integrates, unifies, and vivifies the whole of a person's narrative or story, embeds his or her core identity, establishes the fundamental basis for the individual's relationship with others and with society, includes a sense of the transcendent, and is the interpretive lens through which the person sees the world. It is the basis for community for it is in spirituality that we experience our co-partnership in the shared human condition. It may or may not be expressed, or experienced in religious categories" (Fowler, cited in Fowler & Peterson, 1997, p. 47).

"Ecospirituality is a manifestation of the spiritual interconnection between human beings and the environment.... Ecospirituality engages a relational view of person to planet, soul to soil, and the inner to outer landscape.... The concept of ecospirituality [supports] holistic nursing practice in the realm of self-care, care of others and care of the environment" (Lincoln, 2000, p. 228).

"Spirituality is the center or nucleus in human experience from which all other dimensions find ultimate meaning" (Seeber, Park, & Kimble, 2001, p. 76).

(continued)

Table 1.1 Definitions and Descriptions of Spirituality (*continued*)

"Spirituality encompasses a personal, interpersonal and transpersonal context of four interrelated domains: (a) higher power or universal intelligence—a belief in a higher power or universal intelligence that may or may not include formal religious practices; (b) self-discovery—the spirituality journey begins with inner reflection and a search for meaning and purpose . . . ; (c) relationships—an integral connection to others based on deep respect and reverence for life . . . ; and (d) eco-awareness—an integral connection to nature based on a deep respect and reverence for the environment and a belief that the Earth is sacred. The four domains of spirituality are conceptualized as interconnected and interdependent within a dynamic relationship" (Delaney, 2005, p. 152).

[Spirituality is]: " . . . that most human of experiences that seeks to transcend self and find meaning and purpose through connection with others, nature and/or a Supreme Being, which may or may not involve religious structures or traditions" (Buck, 2006, pp. 289–290).

"Spirituality has about it a sense of the transcendent. It deals with those values that reach beyond the material world and its self-serving goals. These are the values not merely espoused but deeply felt within by human . . . . Spirituality, then is experiential, existential, and touches the inner core of each human being, where he or she most truly lives" (Barnum, 2011, pp. 2–3).

Any or all of these descriptions and definitions of spirituality may seem confusing. These definitions frequently spark internal debates. Spirituality deals with such subjective perspectives that have led to the definition of spirituality being the subject of much debate and discussion in the nursing and health care literature. In fact, the lack of consensus with respect to the definition of spirituality is identified as one of the largest obstacles to focusing on spirituality in nursing practice and research (Cohen, Holley, Wengel, & Katzman, 2012). Additionally, Kevern (2012) maintains that spirituality is not an empirical concept that can be subjected to the same testing as for physical phenomena. Consequently, it may not be realistic to expect consensus on what constitutes spirituality.

Spirituality *is* hard to define, as demonstrated in Reflection 1.1. As Carson and Stoll (2008) confirm, "Spirituality is an elusive word to define . . . and we struggle to define it. Why? Most likely because spirituality represents 'heart' not 'head' knowledge, and 'heart' knowledge is difficult to encapsulate in words" (p. 4). In fact, O'Connor (2001) quotes one writer as saying that trying to formulate a definition of spirituality is as difficult as trying to nail jelly to a wall. Another apt description of the difficulty in defining spirituality is given by Paley (2008): "The concept of spirituality is under construction, so much so that the cranes and scaffolding are still visible" (p. 178). Paley goes on to describe the attempts of those who try to define spirituality as "bolting modules on to a structure that is still in the process of being built" (p. 179).

It is important in considering the extensive array of definitions to remember that not all definitions of spirituality are developed for use in nursing practice. For example, Reinhert and Koenig (2013) developed a definition focused on its applicability to nursing research. Examining those definitions that are most useful for practice will narrow the scope. If a particular description of spirituality is too broad and general, then it may be difficult to tease out the specific implications for spiritual care as opposed to psychosocial care. Contextualization of definitions is crucial (Clarke, 2009). Choosing a definition that fits a particular context or setting will ensure that it is more likely to be appropriately implemented in practice.

Reflection 1.2

- Think about each definition in Table 1.1. Which comes closest to your own definition of spirituality that you constructed in Reflection 1.1?
- Did any of the definitions evoke a reaction or any emotion from you? If so, reflect on why this might be so.
- What common themes do you identify as you read the definitions? Write these out on a sheet of paper.
- Appraise each definition for its applicability to practice. What might be the possible implications for assessment and care of clients using each of the definitions of spirituality?

As previously stated, there is no one universal definition of spirituality. One of the major reasons behind this is that each person's conception of what spirituality means to him or her is unique. That reality is repeated frequently in the nursing literature and is an important point to remember when working with clients. It is the client's view of his or her own personal spirituality that is important if nurses are committed to client-centered care (widely touted in the nursing literature as the "paramount approach" to care). Unruh (2007) says, "A person-centered approach is key to ensuring that the patient's spirituality is understood from his or her perspective" (pp. 78–79). Kevern (2012) agrees with this perspective: "Only the patient can decide what is to count as a 'spiritual value' for them, and the existential weight that must be accorded to it" (p. 982).

As may be gleaned from Reflection 1.2, there *are* themes that are common to a variety of descriptions of spirituality. If a number of clients were asked what spirituality means to them, then there should be common themes in *their* responses. Some of those common themes, as described in the nursing literature, are addressed next.

THEMES IN DESCRIPTIONS OF SPIRITUALITY

Identifying themes in how spirituality is described not only enables a more in-depth understanding of the concept of spirituality, but also provides "signposts" for clinical focus. In a review of how the concept of spirituality is considered in the health sciences literature between 1991 and 2000, Chiu and colleagues (2004) found the following themes: existential reality (experiences, meaning and purpose, and hope); transcendence (i.e., beyond current reality, exceeding the physical); connectedness (to self, others, nature, and a higher being); and power/force/energy (life giving, allowing integration and healing, and driving force). Drawing on the reviews of several authors on the concept of spirituality, Paley (2008) identified the following array of themes related to spirituality:

> . . . religious faith . . . relationship between self, others and God; belief in a "higher power" or "transcendence"; an expression of integrative energy; "connectedness" or "ultimate reality"; reverence, awe, and other "numinous emotions"; a search for meaning and purpose; hope; the person's highest values; close relationships; various complementary therapies; art, poetry, music; the contemplation and enjoyment of nature; personal well-being; political ideals; work or physical activity; personal gain (for reviews, see Ross, 1994, Dyson et al., 1997, Coyle, 2002, Bash, 2004, Miner-Williams, 2006, Ross, 2006). (p. 179)

Ellor (2011), who conducted a review of the definitions of spirituality and religion in the *Journal of Religion, Spirituality and Aging* from its inception in 1984, was more succinct in concluding that spirituality is often linked to being human, to meaning, to wholeness, to a divine being, and to creation. McSherry and Cash (2004) conducted a literature review of definitions of spirituality in the nursing literature from 1985 through 2002 and identified a "spiritual taxonomy" (p. 152) to further clarify the concept of spirituality. The descriptors found in this taxonomy included the following (p. 155):

- Theistic—belief in God, a Supreme Being, deity

- Religious—affiliation with a religion and undertaking religious practices, customs, and rituals

- Language—using certain language to describe spirituality such as "inner strength" or "inner peace"

- Cultural, political, and social ideologies—subscribing to an ideology that influences and governs attitudes and behaviors

- Phenomenological—learning about life from living and learning in negative and positive experiences and situations

- Existential—"a semantic philosophy of life and being, finding meaning, purpose and fulfillment in all life's events" (p. 155)

- Quality of life—implicit in definitions in that spirituality contributes to quality of life

- Mystical—"a relationship between the transcendent, interpersonal, transpersonal, life after death" (p. 155)

Surbone, Konishi, and Baider (2011) identified central aspects of spirituality that they appraised as relevant for health care: meaning and purpose (in life and in life events); values, beliefs, and standards (related to beauty, worth, and truth); transcendence (someone or something beyond the self); connecting (to self, others, God or a higher power, the environment); and becoming (the unfolding of life that is reflected and experienced by the person). Similar themes can be found in other reviews of definitions of spirituality, for example, in Zinnbauer, Pargament, and Scott (1999), Martsoff and Mickley (1998), and Sessanna and colleagues (2007).

From the aforementioned review, it is obvious that there are recurring themes associated with the word "spirituality" and the accompanying descriptors.

Reflection 1.3

Review the themes described in the literature and also those identified in Reflection 1.2. Write these on a sheet of paper and reflect on the following questions:

- Are there additional themes that you would add; and why?
- If you were to rank each theme in order of its importance in terms of your own personal beliefs, values, and life experiences, then which would be ranked as the most important? And which would be the least important?
- In considering each theme, how might it guide you in terms of discussing spirituality with clients and in terms of providing spiritual care to clients?

METAPHORS OF SPIRITUALITY

Definitions and descriptions of spirituality are important, but another way to expand understanding of spirituality is through the use of metaphors. There are three metaphors that are particularly helpful in further expanding the concept of spirituality: wind, mountain range/journey, and soccer ball.

WIND

Hoshiko (1994) developed a practical model to facilitate spiritual assessment and spiritual care based on "worldview." Hoshiko likened spirituality to wind. A person cannot see wind, but can certainly see the impact of wind: tree branches sway, hair blows in a million directions, balance is hard to maintain while walking, and many more. Wind can be particularly strong one day and the next day it may recede to a gentle breeze; or even be nonexistent. When the weather is particularly hot, wind is welcomed as it provides comfort and relief. Wind spreads new life as it disperses seeds over wide distances. There are patterns to wind, such as seasonal patterns. For example, in some places it can be very windy in the spring. Wind can also blow in a particular direction, but this aspect is constantly changing. Wind can create energy by windmills strategically placed to capture it. And when paired with other phenomena such as thunderstorms or heavy snow, wind can create havoc; and at times, that havoc can have long-term impact.

In comparing the characteristics of wind to spirituality, there are many similarities. One cannot see spirituality, but the effects of spirituality on a person's life can be readily visible, for example, a person's search for meaning in illness, or his or her sense of peace during adverse life events. A person's sense of his or her spirituality may be strong at different points in time, for example, at the time of the birth of a child, during hard times, or while hiking in the mountains. At other times, he or she may not be aware of his or her spirituality and may not feel that it is important or relevant at that particular time. Like the wind on a hot day, spirituality can provide comfort and peace, in life generally and also in specific experiences such as illness. Spirituality can generate new life: new insights and new beginnings in a person's life and relationships. It can also be different during the various seasons of life as spiritual development occurs over one's life span. Spirituality can provide direction and energy in a person's life in terms of a general life direction, and it can also be a strong force in a particular direction during a life experience. Moreover, when spirituality is coupled with a phenomenon such as illness or loss, disequilibrium in one's spirituality may occur to create havoc for a period of time or even permanently (spiritual distress, spiritual pain, etc.; Hoshiko, 1994).

Mountain Range/Journey

To describe spirituality, McSherry (2006) uses the analogy of a mountain range, with life seen as a journey or pilgrimage. The steep slopes of the mountain may be hard to navigate and tax the emotional and physical resources of the person, sometimes to the extreme. Yet, along the journey, there may be periods when the path is quite easy. And at pivotal points in the journey, such as when one takes a turn in the steep path and can see towering mountains and green plains, one is particularly moved to experience awe, wonder, and joy.

McSherry (2006) compares the steep slopes of a mountain to times of hardship and conflict in a persons' life, such as times of illness, loss, or other adversity. One's spirituality may come to the forefront at such times, for example, when the person asks, "Why is this happening to me?" Such a question may signify a crisis of meaning. Spiritual resources may be accessed at this time to try to deal with the stress, such as prayer or meditation. New insights can also be gained that can be quite powerful and life-changing, such as when a person almost dies of a heart attack. During recovery, the person may reevaluate his or her life's goals and purpose, instigating changes that are conducive not only to physical health but also to social, emotional, and spiritual health. Often, nurses are at the juncture of such periods and will be privy, and influential, to the spiritual impact of such events. The scenic routes on the journey can be described as periods when life is smooth and calm, and everything is falling into its place—a great job, good relationships, and enough money for one's needs and pleasures. At such times, the person experiences spirituality as joy, contentment, and peace. In referring to the journey of life, McSherry states, "It is during this journey that a person's spirituality is shaped and developed" (p. 51). Although McSherry likens life to a journey in this analogy, some people comment on just their spiritual experience as a journey when they describe the events that are contributing to their "spiritual journey."

Soccer Ball

McSherry and Draper (1998) give the analogy of a football (soccer ball in North America) to illustrate the integrating and unifying force of spirituality. A standard soccer ball consists of 32 synthetic leather patches, usually black and white; high-quality balls are stitched together with thread strong enough to withstand the play of the game.

The football represents the whole person as defined by Rogers (1980). Each leather patch represents a different dimension and facet of our nature and being. The black patches may represent the physical, psychological or social domains of our life. . . . The white patches symbolize our ideologies, creeds, beliefs and values. They can even represent factors or forces which determine our disposition and attitude to life in general. The leather patches are all tightly stitched together by a strong thread, symbolically representing the unifying force of spirituality. The majority of patches are diametrically and symmetrically equal in size and shape, all sharing the same structural value. The life force of an individual is represented by the air which gives the ball its shape and form. The air touches all patches of the ball in an even and equal manner. . . . Yet each patch is specific having characteristics unique to itself (Labun, 1988) . . . should the thread become worn or should a patch be punctured then the entire function and nature of the ball is impaired. (p. 689)

In McSherry and Draper's (1998) analogy, the dark patches on the ball can perhaps be readily seen; the lighter patches not so much. The "thread" of spirituality can become weak or worn, or a "patch" can become punctured (e.g., if illness or stress of some other crisis occurs). If this occurs, then the entire function of the "ball" (i.e., the person's spiritual being) can be compromised.

Reflection 1.4

Think about your own concept of spirituality as well as the information given about spirituality in this chapter. What metaphor might you use to explain the concept of spirituality to another person? How does your metaphor describe the nature and characteristics of spirituality?

SPIRITUALITY AND WORLDVIEW

The concept of worldview can be helpful in understanding spirituality as it is a more tangible concept that can help translate the theoretical concepts of spirituality to something more practical that is useful for nursing practice. Worldview is pertinent to every religion or spiritual perspective; it shapes the person's perceptions of his or her physical, emotional, social, and spiritual being (Kumar, 2004).

Sire (2004) proposes that all people have a worldview that he describes as "a set of presuppositions (or assumptions) which we hold (consciously or subconsciously) about the basic makeup of our world" (p. 17). Discovering one's worldview is seen by Sire as being an important step toward "self-awareness, self-knowledge and self-understanding" (p. 17). Sire proposes:

A well-rounded worldview includes basic answers to each of the following questions. (1) What is prime reality—the really real? . . . (2) Who is man? . . . (3) What happens to man at death? . . . (4) What is the basis of morality? . . . (5) What is the meaning of human history? (p. 18)

Such questions are intricately connected to spirituality.

Worldview is helpful in identifying and quantifying spirituality as a person's spiritual perspective can be evident to some degree in his or her particular worldview. For example, if a person is committed to a Christian worldview, then that spiritual perspective will be evident in all aspects of his or her life: How he or she sees himself or herself as a person; how he or she takes his or her relationships with self, others, and God; how he or she sees his or her responsibility to the environment; what he or she thinks about the purpose of life; and similar considerations. Hoshiko (1994) sees worldview as a visible indicator of spirituality in the meanings of the six relationships identified in her definition (Table 1.1). These meanings are dynamic, interrelated, and constantly changing. In fact, Hoshiko's use of the word "worldview" is seen by her to be more comprehensive, less emotionally charged, and a more communicable term than the word "spirituality." Hoshiko describes worldview as that which

> . . . gives coherence, direction, and meaning to life. It is what makes sense out of life. A worldview is one's perspective on the world and on oneself in the midst of that world. A worldview answers such questions as: What is life all about? Who am I? Where have I come from? What community am I a part of? What am I doing here? What should I be doing? And where am I going? These questions reflect the six relationships . . . [described in Hoshiko's definition of spirituality]. Thus a person's worldview can be defined as the meaning or significance that a person attaches to these six relationships. (p. 6)

Hoshiko's model of spirituality as worldview is a practical one in that it provides a focus for the nurse in assessing the impact of illness or some other adverse event in the person's life with respect to these six relationships. It also provides direction for spiritual care. Smith (2008), drawing on the work of nursing in the area of spirituality, also developed a spiritual framework based on worldview for use by occupational therapists in their practice.

Reflection 1.5

Reflect on the six relationships that Hoshiko (1994) proposes to be intricately connected to one's spirituality:

1. To God or whomever or whatever is considered ultimate reality (a transcendent reality)

(continued)

> ### Reflection 1.5 (continued)
>
> **2.** To self (includes self-esteem and self-image)
> **3.** To others (includes other people such as family, friends, as well as the community and society)
> **4.** To the environment (how resources are created and used, pattern of consumption, and productivity)
> **5.** To the past (beliefs about the past, origins, and their influence on the present)
> **6.** To the future (means hope or hopelessness, purpose or lack of purpose, and beliefs about death and afterlife; pp. 5–6)
>
> - Do you consider all of these relationships to be relevant to spirituality? If not, which ones are relevant for you?
> - How is your own spirituality seen in each of the relationships that you see as relevant to your own personal understanding of spirituality, that is, what meaning or significance do you attach to each?
> - How might you determine or assess the meaning of these relationships to clients? What questions might you ask?

SPIRITUAL WELL-BEING

Spiritual well-being is intricately related to the concept of spirituality, and this relationship is emphasized in the nursing literature, in practice, and in research. Perhaps one reason for this emphasis is that spiritual well-being is seen to be an approximate indicator of spiritual health, and it is considered to be the behavioral expression of spiritual health (Carson & Stoll, 2008).

There are various definitions and descriptions of spiritual well-being. A widely quoted definition in the literature is that provided by the National Interfaith Coalition on Aging (NICA, 1975): Spiritual well-being is "the affirmation of life in a relationship with God, self, community and environment that nurtures and celebrates wholeness" (p. 1). The quality of a person's relationship with these four domains is indicative of a person's spiritual health (Fisher & Brumley, 2008). Ellison (1983), whose Spiritual Well-Being Scale (SWBS) is perhaps the most widely used in research pertaining to spirituality, suggests that the definition of spiritual well-being provided by the NICA involves both a religious component and a social-psychological component. Ellison's SWBS includes both a measurement of religious well-being and existential well-being. Another description of spiritual well-being is provided by Hungelmann, Kenkel-Rossi, Klassen, and Stollenwerk (1985), who developed the JAREL SWBS:

Spiritual well-being [is] a sense of harmonious interconnectedness between self, others/nature, and Ultimate Other which exists throughout and beyond time and space. It is achieved through a dynamic and integrative growth process which leads to a realization of the ultimate purpose and meaning of life. (p. 152)

Previously discussed themes with respect to the concept of spirituality can be seen in these descriptions of spiritual well-being.

SPIRITUALITY AND CULTURE

In any discussion with clients about spirituality, culture should be considered as the "backdrop" within which that conversation takes place. It should also be present within the context of nursing care. This is not only the case for culture in its broadest sense but also in terms of the various subcultures that exist in society. A person can belong to a certain culture, but simultaneously be a part of various subcultures within that culture; or even part of another distinctive culture. For example, a 17-year-old person may belong to the African American culture but within that culture the person may concurrently be part of a number of subcultures such as a youth subculture, or a particular religious subculture.

Based on her earlier work, Leininger (1988) provided a classic definition of culture: "Culture refers to the learned, shared, and transmitted values, beliefs, norms and life practices of a particular group that guides thinking, decisions, and actions in patterned ways" (p. 156). Spirituality can be influenced by culture (Reinert & Koenig, 2013). For example, if the dominant culture is secular, then people within that culture may not normally see themselves as spiritual (McSherry, Cash, & Ross, 2004). Spiritual (and religious) values, beliefs, norms, and practices can be culturally shaped, which is true not just in terms of the broader culture, but also in terms of multiple subcultures. Thus, the meaning ascribed to spirituality depends on the cultural context.

It is often the case that a person's spiritual or religious belief system originates from a cultural or ethnic heritage. For example, the province in which I live has a long cultural heritage involving the sea, as well as a Christian worldview. Its people are known to be fatalistic, perhaps because the sea was a significant factor regarding life and death in the history of the province; and also because God's will was seen to be present in life events. When faced with various life events, people may say something like: "Well, it was meant to be"; or "Everything happens for a reason." Such beliefs about life and its events will then be naturally carried over into how illness and loss is perceived.

In an analysis of cultural and religious beliefs and practices related to the concept of spirituality in health sciences research, Chiu and colleagues (2004) found similar themes regarding the concept of spirituality in both culturally focused studies and nonculturally focused studies. However, some concepts related to spirituality were culturally specific. For example, in the Native American culture, there is the pursuit of harmony with nature and the prominence of supernatural forces; whereas in the Hispanic culture, there is the centrality of religious faith.

It is important to note that not all people from a particular cultural heritage will share the same views. Some people may develop spiritual beliefs and practices that will be in direct opposition to cultural norms. Life experiences also interact with culture, as for example, when a person travels to a new cultural setting and develops new spiritual beliefs/values that are influenced by the norms in that new culture. As such, it is helpful for a nurse to know the spiritual beliefs and values of a dominant culture. However, because spirituality is a highly individualized concept, the nurse must also carefully assess whether a person shares the beliefs and values of the dominant culture. If the person does not share the dominant beliefs/values, then it can be helpful to know what experiences the person has had to shape his or her particular spiritual perspective.

Reflection 1.6

Reflect on your own dominant culture as well as various subcultures with which you are affiliated within that broader culture. What aspects of these cultural groups are connected to spirituality? How have those cultural factors shaped your own spirituality?

THE EXPRESSION AND NURTURING OF SPIRITUALITY

Many people share the view that the concept of spirituality is related *only* to religion—including nurses. It is important to remember that for some people, their spirituality is so intricately connected to religion that the two concepts are inseparable. However, if one accepts the premise that spirituality is a universal characteristic of all people, then it will be expressed in multiple ways, including nonreligious expression, as not all people are connected to a religion. Most people will have multiple ways of expressing and nurturing their spirituality, an important point to remember in terms of implications for nursing practice.

THE ARTS

The arts can be described as all of the creative ways that people respond to their surroundings, using a variety of media such as words, music, film, paint, clay, yarn, and so on (Bailey, 1997). The arts can meet an individual's basic spiritual needs, such as the need for meaning and purpose, or the need for hope. For example, many artists comment on how their particular art medium provides meaning and purpose in their lives, and additional meaning is derived from sharing their art with others. The arts can also regenerate the spirit. The arts can connect the person to the source of life itself, and create joy and delight within the person, for example, the satisfaction experienced in capturing nature on canvas as the Creator made it.

The arts are considered as a means of facilitating healing of the whole person, as witnessed by their prominence in various treatment modalities (Bailey, 1997; Lane, 2005). In fact, Lane (2005) states, "Nurses are discovering ways they can care for the whole person through creative interventions because art and meditation automatically put patients into the place where healing flows . . . . Creativity and spirituality allow nurses to transform healing and change nursing care" (p. 125). Nurses will likely encounter in their clinical practice the use of the arts to facilitate healing, and, indeed, may initiate this use of the arts.

Reflection 1.7

Reflect on Coles's *The Voyage of Life* paintings, which can be found on the following website (www.explorethomascole.org/tour/items/73/series). These paintings illustrate stages of life as a journey on a river during which the landscape is constantly changing. Reflect on where you are on your journey of life with respect to spirituality. Which of these paintings would best represent where you are (Becker, 2009)?

NATURE/ENVIRONMENT

Many people connect their spirituality with nature—some do this in a profound manner. Engaging with nature directly, such as a walk in the woods, or watching a sunset, can create within the person a profound sense of something or someone beyond the self and a sense of awe and mystery. Rejuvenation of spirit can also occur. There can also be an indirect engagement with nature, for example, examining a painting that someone has completed, or watching a television program on some aspect of nature, which can create a spiritual experience for the person. Passion for the environment can also provide meaning and purpose in a person's life.

MEANINGFUL WORK

Work can be seen as a career engaged in to provide a living, such as a business or some kind of helping profession. Work can also be unpaid, such as caring for a child at home or volunteering in the community. Meaningful work can contribute to a person's spirituality as well as be a source of spirituality (Hasselkus, 2002). Sometimes, a person can feel a "calling" to a particular work, such as was the case for Mother Teresa. It must be understood that engaging in whatever the person considers to be work can provide meaning and purpose for the person, nurturing his or her spirituality and expressing it through the work completed. Work can also provide a sense of connection for the person, not only to the work itself, but also to the people encountered in that work.

MYSTICAL EXPERIENCES

Mystical experiences can be described as experiences that are inspirational for a person, make the person happy, create a feeling of well-being, and provide some sense of meaning for that person. Examples include a meditational state, a physically induced ecstasy, and esoteric religious experiences (Taylor, 2012). Other examples include pilgrimages to sacred sites; visions; an experience of a Supreme Being, which is felt as a powerful presence in the person's life; or feelings that are hard to put into words that a person experiences while engaging in a religious or spiritual practice. Many clients will describe such mystical experiences in relation to their illness. For example, one person who experienced a deep depression for which she was hospitalized described "hands" that raised her up from her bed and enabled her to engage in self-care activities. "Near-death" experiences can also be counted as mystical experiences. Sometimes, mystical experiences can be life-changing for a person, creating new behaviors and new ways of being.

Reflection 1.8

Reflect on the place of religion, the arts, nature/the environment, work, or mystical experiences in the nurturing and expression of your own spirituality:

- Which of these are the most important ways that you nurture and express your spirituality?
- How would you describe how each of these ways actually contributes to your sense of spiritual well-being?
- When you have faced adversity in your life (an illness, a loss, stress, etc.), what changes have occurred in how your spirituality was nurtured or expressed? For example, while experiencing illness, did work provide a sense of purpose and hope for you in the midst of the illness?
- How have you seen spirituality expressed and nurtured in your family, your friends, and clients with whom you have worked? What has been the impact on the person?

  It can be helpful to use a house as a visualization of the different ways that spirituality is expressed and nurtured.

In Figure 1.2, we see that spirituality is the overarching concept (the roof) under which all of the other expressions of spirituality (the rooms) are subsumed. For example, those who see their religion and spirituality as one and the same might have both religion and spirituality at the roof of their house. Depending on the importance of each expression of spirituality to the person, the rooms representing those expressions could be drawn in different sizes. For example, a man who is dealing with Parkinson's disease (PD) comments about the place of spirituality/religion in his life and in terms of the illness. For most of the conversation, he spoke about his strong connection with nature, which he experienced not only in terms of being out in nature (going for walks in wooded areas, snowshoeing, etc.), but also in terms of bringing nature into his home in the form of a greenhouse. He also painted nature scenes and carved figures out of wood. That person's "room" for the expression of his spirituality through nature would indeed be large. This example also shows that a person can express and nurture his or her spirituality through a primary mode, but other modes of expression can also be present and operative. Not only was nature a prime example of the expression of spirituality for this individual, but also artistic endeavors were of overlapping importance to him. He also spoke about his relationship with God as important to his spirituality.

The expressions of spirituality described are foundational expressions of spirituality. When illness or some other significant life stressor occurs in a person's life, his or

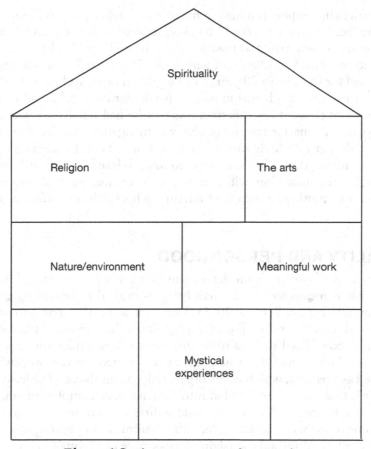

Figure 1.2 The expressions of spirituality.

her spirituality may be expressed in "distressing" terms—in spiritual pain, spiritual anger, spiritual guilt, and so on. Moreover, because people are integrated beings, psychosocial and physical signs and symptoms may be present, such as anxiety, depression, or somatic or actual illness. This is in keeping with the assertion that what is happening in one dimension of a person may impact all of the other dimensions of personhood.

Cox (2003) discusses a couple of case studies that illustrate some of the expressions of spirituality, including a discussion of how these different expressions can be useful in caring for clients. The first case Cox explores is that of a 37-year-old client who was hospitalized for a major depressive disorder/acute psychotic reaction and attempted suicide. It was found that this person adhered to common aboriginal traditions, such as respecting the land and all natural forms of life in the environment, such as plant and animal life. He had verbalized to staff that he was on a spiritual quest, and was having spiritually enriching visions. He had sold some of the art work that he had created. He had also regularly engaged in hunting expeditions on the land. The nurse noticed that when he talked about his spiritual beliefs, his mood improved and he became more peaceful and coherent. Among other interventions, the nurse encouraged him to continue to express his spirituality, supported him in his spiritual beliefs, and facilitated access to a location at the facility where he could be close to nature. Subsequently, the client expressed feeling more powerful and positive about himself and his life.

The second case that Cox (2003) presents is of a 58-year-old aboriginal man who had been hospitalized for more than 20 years in a long-term care psychiatric facility. Because of poor dental care, his speech was impaired, particularly when he had emotional outbursts. One issue of concern for this man was that he had refused to sleep in a bed for more than 8 years. A behavior treatment plan was instigated with the client to deal with this issue, but this met with little success. A nurse noticed that he frequently sang a religious song, and during those times, he seemed more relaxed. When such music was introduced into the treatment plan, within a short time the man started to sleep in his bed. Providing access to music as a means of nurturing his spirit was effective in the treatment plan.

SPIRITUALITY AND PERSONHOOD

The primary focus of nursing is on the human being as a person; therefore, an understanding of what it means to be a human being is critical to providing good nursing care (Hammoud, White, & Fetters, 2005). There are some differences in how "person" is conceptualized within nursing. For example, within the reciprocal interaction worldview, a person is considered to be a multidimensional being (biological, psychological, social, spiritual) who is viewed as a whole. In the simultaneous action worldview, the person is described as a pattern, which is self-organized, changeable, and orderly. The person is seen as a unit that cannot be divided into dimensions (Alimohammadi, Taleghani, Mohammadi, & Akbarian, 2013). There are also differences in how various religions define the concept of person. For example, Alimohammadi and colleagues (2013), using philosophical inquiry, identified the Islamic perspective of a human being:

> In the Islamic view, the human being is a unit of reality, a unique nature and a unitary being created of two aspects: the material aspect [body] and the immaterial aspect [soul] . . . . The soul (Ruh) is incorporated within the body so that they seem to be a single unit. (p. 123)

In Islamic thought, a human being is also seen as having cognitive, emotional, social, and spiritual dimensions.

A common general assertion in the nursing literature is that spirituality is part of being human. This means that all people are spiritual beings, whether they are aware of it or not (Hay & Hunt, 2002; Hay & Nye, 1998; Newberg, D'Aquili, & Rause, 2002; Smart, 1996). Burkhardt and Nagai-Jacobson (2002) capture the idea well: "By virtue of being human, all persons, at all ages, in all cultures, whether or not they are religious are biopsychosocialspiritual beings" (p. 8). Burkhardt and Nagai-Jacobson also state, "Rather than separate parts, the body-mind-spirit being is in essence an intertwined and interpenetrating unity" (p. 5). Long (1997) points out the close connection between spirituality and personhood by maintaining that being spiritual is being fully human and that being fully human is being spiritual. Yet, it is important to remember that not all people would see personhood in this way. Even though the description of the human being in Islamic thought described in the previous paragraph would appear to be overtly similar to that described by Burkhardt and Nagai-Jacobson, Alimohammadi and colleagues (2013) state, "In the Islamic view, the human is not formed by two separate elements of body and mind, or the three elements of bio–psycho–social, but is a single reality in two material and immaterial constructs" (p. 126). Pesut and colleagues (2009) make the point that, as nurses "we must be careful to preserve a space in the professional domain for diverse understandings such as those espoused by the people who reject, or suspend judgment, of the existence of a spiritual reality" (p. 340). Pesut and colleagues also state in this regard: "If the human spirit is characterized by choice and will, then an essential human freedom is the ability to choose whether to believe in a metaphysical spiritual world or a purely naturalistic one" (p. 340). It is important to remember that this statement applies not only to clients, but also to health care professionals.

The goal of nursing is to provide holistic care and to provide this care for all, regardless of whether a nurse is able to converse with clients about spirituality or not. If people are spiritual simply because they are human, then those limited by cognitive ability, those with dementia, and those who are in a comatose state are still spiritual beings. McSherry and Cash (2004) make this point in their criticism of many contemporary definitions of spirituality in the literature, stating that such definitions "are restrictive, implying that a functional intellect, and the ability to reason, are prerequisite for developing spirituality, thereby potentially excluding individuals with severe language difficulties or degenerative disorders of the brain, such as dementia" (p. 152). This is an important point to remember. People can be described not as physical beings who have a spirit, but as spiritual beings who have psychosocial and physical dimensions.

Haase, Britt, Coward, Leidy, and Penn (1992) provide a distinction between "spirituality" and "spiritual perspective," which can be helpful for practical reasons. Spirituality is seen as "a basic and inherent quality of all humans" (p. 142). Spiritual perspective, as described by Reed in Haase et al. (1992), "varies between individuals [and is] a highly individualized awareness of one's spirituality and its qualities" (p. 143). Haase and colleagues go on to state that spiritual perspective is "an integrating and creative energy based on belief in, and a feeling of interconnectedness with, a power greater than self" (p. 143).

Therefore, nurses must respond to clients as spiritual beings irrespective of the clients' physical or emotional states. However, nurses *can* converse with those who will be aware of the attributes of their own spirituality.

Reflection 1.9

Do *you* see people as spiritual beings or as having a spiritual dimension?

- If so, do you respond to clients in a way that honors your view of personhood? If not, what keeps you from doing this?
- If not, what is your view of personhood? How does this view impact your work with clients?

Reflection 1.10

Think of one person who you would deem to be a "spiritual person." What qualities, attitudes, beliefs, and other characteristics does this person possess that would lead you to believe that he or she is a spiritual person (Lemmer, 2010)?

SPIRITUAL DEVELOPMENT

No discussion of spirituality would be complete without some reference to spiritual development. Nurses work with people across the life span. Therefore, it is necessary to appreciate developmental tasks and issues at all stages of growth and development. In nursing textbooks, much attention has been given to physical, mental, and social growth and development; but spiritual development has received far less coverage. However, if nurses are to be involved in holistic care, where the spirituality is included, then it is incumbent upon them to know something about spiritual development as well. Being able to assess at what stage a client may be in terms of his or her spiritual development can be valuable to his or her care.

Some developmental specialists include and discuss spiritual development in their developmental models, such as Maslow (1971) who described "being values" or peak experiences that can be deemed to be spiritual, involving transcendence. When it comes to spiritual development, perhaps the most widely quoted person is James Fowler, who developed seven age-related stages of faith development (Fowler, 1981). Taylor (2002) points out that although the word "faith" can refer to various religious faiths, Fowler's view of the term was to see it as "a universal human phenomenon that leads persons to need and find meaning, an understanding of themselves in relation to their world" (p. 22). Barnum (2011) adds that Fowler also saw faith as resting in "beliefs concerning ultimate meaningful values in a person's life" (p. 18). As such, Fowler's stages can apply both to those who identify with a particular religion and to those who do not. Taylor (2002) summarizes Fowler's stages quite well (pp. 22–24) but refers to Fowler's original work for a more in-depth discussion of the seven stages. A summary of Taylor's discussion of Fowler's stages is presented in Table 1.2.

The idea of spiritual development as a process is consistent with all of the other types of development of a person. Unlike physical development, which declines with age, spiritual development can continue to expand until the point of death, as new spiritual insights, beliefs, and values are attained. In fact, there is reference in the literature and in later chapters to spiritual development in end-of-life contexts. As a process, spiritual development may occur when a person becomes aware of what is meaningful in his or her life, or what or who provides purpose in his or her life. It can also occur as spirituality is expressed by the person in various ways. Some people may develop a sense of the transcendent, albeit not all people will connect this to a Supreme Being. Carson and Stoll (2008) describe the process of developing spirituality because of a relationship with a Supreme Being as being a vertical process, whereas spiritual development that does not include a relationship with a Supreme Being is described by Carson as a horizontal process.

Table 1.2 **Fowler's Stages of Faith Development**

1. *Undifferentiated faith* (infancy–3 years). The child's task at this stage is to acquire "the fundamental spiritual qualities of trust and mutuality as well as courage, hope, and love" (Taylor, 2002, p. 22). Parental responses to a child can undermine or enhance these qualities.

2. *Intuitive-projective faith* (3–7 years). "Children relate intuitively to the ultimate conditions of existence through stories and images, the fusion of fact and feelings. What is make-believe or magically concocted is what reality is" (Taylor, 2002, p. 22). Stories, actions, examples, and moods influence and shape the child's view of reality. For example, Santa Claus may be seen as real and, depending on the stories told to the child, God may be seen as an old man in the sky.

3. *Mythic-literal faith* (school-aged up to 12 years but can extend to adulthood). In this stage, fantasy is sorted out from fact. Stories help children find meaning and give organization to experience. Beliefs and practices of the community are learned, which help the child make sense of the community and the world of which he or she is part. However, stories, beliefs, and practices are taken literally rather than with abstract meanings. For example, a child will learn stories from a particular faith tradition and accept them at face value, which provides him or her with a means of making sense of the community and the world around him or her.

4. *Synthetic-conventional faith* (child/adolescent but can extend to adulthood). In this stage, the experience of the world goes beyond that experienced in the family unit. This stage must provide a helpful understanding of this extended environment. The synthesis of values and information provides the basis of identity. Conforming to the beliefs of others around them is common because these beliefs have not yet been reflected on or studied objectively. For example, teens may observe the rituals and traditions of a particular faith and accept parents' beliefs.

5. *Individuative-reflective faith* (young adults but can extend to later adulthood). In this stage, self-identity and worldview are developed, which are unique to the person. Independent commitments, lifestyle, beliefs, and attitudes are formed. The "demythologizing of symbols into conceptual meanings" (Taylor, 2002, p. 23) occurs as the literal changes into the meaning underlying it. For example, someone who has been taught not to touch the "holy water" in the parent's home sees this not as a religious edict but as a means of respect for what is sacred.

6. *Conjunctive faith* (adults past midlife). "Adults find new appreciation for their past, value their inner voices, and become aware of deep-seated myths, prejudices and images that are indwelling because of their social background. An individual with conjunctive faith 'strives to unify opposites in mind and experience' and allows 'vulnerability to the strange truths of those who are other' (p. 198*). For example, instead of trying to dissuade or avoid others with differing spiritual beliefs, a person in this stage would embrace persons of other faith traditions, recognizing that in their faith may be new understanding" (p. 23).

(continued)

Table 1.2 **Fowler's Stages of Faith Development (*continued*)**
7. *Universalizing stage of faith* (infrequently reached by many people). "Those in this stage of faith have a 'sense of an ultimate environment [that] is inclusive of all being. They have become incarnators and actualizers of the spirit of an inclusive and fulfilled human community' (p. 200*). These persons work to unshackle social, political, economic, or ideological burdens in society. They fully love life, yet simultaneously hold it loosely" (Taylor, 2002, p. 23). Examples of people whom Fowler identified as achieving this stage include Dr. Martin Luther King, Mahatma Gandhi, and Mother Teresa.

*Taylor quoting Fowler (1981).

This chapter has examined the concept of spirituality. Although spirituality is a complex concept, there are identifiable aspects that can be described and considered, which can make the concept more comprehensible. A fundamental understanding and appreciation of spirituality is essential to incorporating spirituality into nursing practice.

The Bottom Line

- Spirituality is inherent in what it means to be human. All people are spiritual beings.

- Understanding one's own spirituality is critical to addressing spirituality with clients.

- Nurses need to be aware of the variety of definitions and descriptions of spirituality; but the client's concept of spirituality is the pivotal point from which the nurse proceeds.

- Spirituality and religion are intricately connected but each has its distinguishing characteristics. However, for some people, spirituality and religion are one and the same.

- Spirituality can be expressed and nurtured in a variety of ways.

- All definitions and descriptions of spirituality have their roots in the author's underlying philosophy.

- Culture is an important contextual factor in a person's spiritual positioning. Culture is also contextual in the spiritual assessment and care of clients.

- Approximate measures of spiritual health can be obtained from clients.

- Spiritual development needs to be considered when working with clients.

Taking It Further

1. Create a poster using a variety of materials such as magazines, string, markers, and glitter. Endeavor to have the poster express your spiritual perspective during a particularly difficult time in your life (e.g., when you experienced illness,

loss of some kind, an inordinate amount of stress). Reflect on the use of art as a methodology to express your feelings, beliefs, and questions during this particular time.

2. Read more about Fowler's stages of faith development in Fowler (1981). Which stage would you say applies to your life at this point in time? What factors or experiences have contributed to your spiritual growth? Are there ways that you can contribute further to your spiritual growth? Critique Fowler's stages of spiritual development with respect to their potential use in clinical practice.

3. Develop a timeline of your own spiritual development, noting significant factors, events, and people that may have contributed to this development (Meyer, 2003). This exercise can be completed in a group such that the group can discuss the exercise, including identifying common themes in the spiritual growth of its members.

4. Read discussions of spirituality from a variety of perspectives—for example, the Christian theological perspective, the existential perspective, and the biological perspective (Narayanasamy, 1999). Reflect on each of these perspectives (and perhaps discuss them with colleagues) using the following questions:

    a. Which perspective, if any, correlates with your personal and subjective perspective of spirituality?

    b. What are the implications for client care for health care professionals operating from each of these different philosophies?

5. For a period of time (e.g., 6 months), keep a personal journal that documents your spiritual growth, issues that you encounter related to your spirituality, and experiences that have occurred with respect to your spirituality (Meyer, 2003). Reread your journal at the end of the time period that you kept it. What insights about spirituality do you gain from your journaling?

6. Review a number of definitions and descriptions of spirituality in the nursing literature (endeavor to collect approximately 25 distinctive definitions). On a scale of 1 to 10, with 1 being "not spiritual" and 10 being "very spiritual," rate yourself on how spiritual you are in terms of the way spirituality is described in these definitions (van Leeuwen, Tiesinga, Middel, Post, & Jochemsen, 2008).

7. Dawson (1997) states that " . . . science does not have the copyright on truth . . . " (p. 289). Discuss in a group the following: What "truths" are found in science? What "truths" are found in spirituality? How is Dawson's statement relevant for the "truth" found in spirituality? What are the implications for nursing practice?

8. Conduct a debate to argue both sides of the question: Is there an interest in spirituality and spiritual issues in society today?

9. Conduct a comprehensive review of the nursing literature for definitions of spirituality from 1970 to the present:

    a. What observations do you have about the evolution of the definitions over time?

    b. What common themes do you see in the definitions in the 1970s, 1980s, 1990s, and from 2000 onward?

   c. Which of the definitions comes closest to your own personal definition of spirituality?

   d. Which definition(s) might be most useful for use in your practice setting?

10. Conduct a survey of the research on the biological basis of spirituality. What conclusions can you draw from your analysis of the research?

11. Review the spiritual framework developed by Smith (2008) for use by occupational therapists. What is your appraisal of the potential of this framework for your practice setting?

12. Formulate a number of research questions pertaining to spirituality. Conduct a review of the nursing literature to see if these questions have been addressed and what the findings were.

13. Research the concept of "person" or "human being" in various nursing theories. Document the various conceptualizations, reflecting on the implications of the concept of personhood for nursing practice from each of these theoretical frameworks.

14. Howden (1992), quoted in Meyer (2003), identifies four attributes of spirituality: meaning and purpose in life (sees life as meaningful); inner resources (possesses inner peace and balance); interconnectedness (is connected to life, a higher power, other people, has a desire to be of service); and transcendence (achieves new perspectives within oneself). Rate yourself on a scale of 1 to 10, with 1 being "not present/manifested in my life" and 10 being "very present/manifested in my life." Discuss these attributes and your personal scores in a small group setting. Focus on your own self-assessment as well as the spiritual attributes of your peers and of clients whom you may have encountered in practice (Meyer, 2003).

15. Review the work of such existentialists/theologians as Sartre, Kierkegaard, Heidegger, and Jung. How does each of their worldviews connect to the concepts relevant to spirituality?

REFERENCES

Alimohammadi, N., Taleghani, F., Mohammadi, E., & Akbarian, R. (2013). The nursing metaparadigm of human being in Islamic thought. *Nursing Inquiry, 21*(2), 1–9. doi:10.1111/nin.12040

Bailey, S. S. (1997). The arts in spiritual care. *Seminars in Oncology Nursing, 13*(4), 242–247. doi:10.1016/S0749-2081(97)80018-6

Barnum, B. S. (2011). *Spirituality in nursing: The challenges of complexity* (3rd ed.). New York, NY: Springer Publishing Company.

Becker, A. L. (2009). Ethical considerations of teaching spirituality in the academy. *Nursing Ethics, 16*(6), 697–706. doi:10.1177/0969733009342639

Buck, H. G. (2006). Spirituality: Concept analysis and model development. *Holistic Nursing Practice, 20*(6), 288–292.

Burkhardt, M. A. (1989). Spirituality: An analysis of the concept. *Holistic Nursing Practice, 3*(3), 69–77.

Burkhardt, M. A., & Nagai-Jacobson, M. G. (2002). *Spirituality: Living our connectedness.* Albany, NY: Delmar.

Carson, V. B. (Ed.). (1989). *Spiritual dimensions of nursing practice.* Philadelphia, PA: W. B. Saunders.

Carson, V. B., & Stoll, R. (2008). Spirituality. In V. B. Carson & H. G. Koenig (Eds.), *Spiritual dimensions of nursing practice* (Rev. ed., pp. 3–32). West Conshohocken, PA: Templeton Foundation.

Chiu, L., Emblen, J. D., van Hofwegen, L., Sawatzky, R., & Meyerhoff, H. (2004). An integrative review of the concept of spirituality in the health sciences. *Western Journal of Nursing Research, 26*(4), 405–428. doi:10.1177/0193945904263411

Clarke, J. (2009). A critical view of how nursing has defined spirituality. *Journal of Clinical Nursing, 18*(12), 1666–1673. doi:10.1111/j.1365-2702.2008.02707.x

Cohen, M. Z., Holley, L. M., Wengel, S. P., & Katzman, M. (2012). A platform for nursing research on spirituality and religiosity: Definitions and measures. *Western Journal of Nursing Research, 34*(6), 795–817. doi:10.1177/0193945912444321

Cox, T. (2003). Theory and exemplars of advanced practice spiritual intervention. *Complementary Therapies in Nursing and Midwifery, 9*(1), 30–34. doi:10.1016/S1353-6117(02)00103-8

Coyle, J. (2002). Spirituality and health: Towards a framework for exploring the relationship between spirituality and health. *Journal of Advanced Nursing, 37*(6), 589–597. doi:10.1046/j.1365-2648.2002.02133.x

Dawson, P. J. (1997). A reply to Goddard's "spirituality as integrative energy." *Journal of Advanced Nursing, 25*(2), 282–289. doi:10.1046/j.1365-2648.1997.1997025282.x

Deal, B., & Grassley, J. S. (2012). The lived experience of giving spiritual care: A phenomenological study of nephrology nurses working in acute and chronic hemodialysis settings. *Nephrology Nursing Journal, 39*(6), 471–496.

Delaney, C. (2005). The Spirituality Scale: Development and psychometric testing of a holistic instrument to assess the human spiritual dimension. *Journal of Holistic Nursing, 23*(2), 145–167. doi:10.1177/0898010105276180

Ellison, C. W. (1983). Spiritual well-being: Conceptualization and measurement. *Journal of Psychology & Theology, 11*(4), 330–338.

Ellor, J. W. (2011). Reflections on the words "religion," "spiritual well-being," and "spirituality." *Journal of Religion, Spirituality & Aging, 23*(4), 275–278. doi:10.1080/15528030.2011.603074

Fisher, J., & Brumley, D. C. (2008). Nurses' and carers' spiritual well-being in the workplace. *Australian Journal of Advanced Nursing, 25*(4), 49–57.

Fowler, J. (1981). *Stages of faith development: The psychology of human development and the quest for meaning.* San Francisco, CA: Harper & Row.

Fowler, M., & Peterson, B. S. (1997). Spiritual themes in clinical pastoral education. *Journal of Supervision and Training in Ministry, 18*, 46–54.

Gallison, B. S., Xu, Y., Yurgens, C. Y., & Boyle, S. M. (2013). Acute care nurses' spiritual care practices. *Journal of Holistic Nursing, 31*(2), 95–103. doi:10.1177/0898010112464121

Goddard, N. C. (1995). "Spirituality as integrative energy": A philosophical analysis as requisite precursor to holistic nursing practice. *Journal of Advanced Nursing, 22*(4), 808–815. doi:10.1046/j.1365-2648.1995.22040808.x

Haase, J. E., Britt, T., Coward, D. D., Leidy, N. K., & Penn, P. E. (1992). Simultaneous concept analysis of spiritual perspective, hope, acceptance and self-transcendence. *Journal of Nursing Scholarship, 24*(2), 141–147.

Hammoud, M. M., White, C. B., & Fetters, M. D. (2005). Opening cultural doors: Providing culturally sensitive health care to Arab American and American Muslim patients. *American Journal of Obstetrics and Gynecology, 193*(4), 1307–1311.

Hasselkus, B. R. (2002). Occupation as a source of spirituality. In B. R. Hasselkus (Ed.), *The meaning of everyday occupation* (pp. 101–112). Thorofare, NJ: Slack.

Hay, D., & Hunt, K. (2002). *Understanding the spirituality of people who don't go to church: The final report of the adult spirituality project.* Nottingham, England: University of Nottingham.

Hay, D., & Nye, R. (1998). *The spirit of the child.* London, England: HarperCollins.

Hoshiko, B. R. (Spring, 1994). *Worldview: A practical model of spirituality.* Lecture given at Kent State University, Kent, Ohio.

Hungelmann, J., Kenkel-Rossi, E., Klassen, L., & Stollenwerk, R. (1985). Spiritual well-being in older adults: Harmonious interconnectedness. *Journal of Religion & Health, 24*(2), 147–153. doi:10.1007/BF01532258

Kevern, P. (2012). Who can give "spiritual care?" The management of spiritually sensitive interactions between nurses and patients. *Journal of Nursing Management, 20,* 981–989. doi:10.1111/j.1365-2834.2102.01428.x

Kreitzer, M. J. (2012). Spirituality and well-being: Focusing on what matters. *Western Journal of Nursing Research, 34*(6), 707–710. doi:10.1177/0193945912448315

Kumar, K. (2004). Spiritual care: What's worldview got to do with it? *Journal of Christian Nursing, 21*(1), 24–28. doi:10.1097/01.CNJ.0000262275.10582.66

Lane, M. R. (2005). Creativity and spirituality in nursing: Implementing art in healing. *Holistic Nursing Practice, 19*(3), 122–125. doi:10.1097/00004650-200505000-00008

Leininger, M. M. (1988). Leininger's theory of nursing: Cultural care diversity and universality. *Nursing Science Quarterly, 1*(4), 152–160. doi:10.1177/089431848800100408

Lemmer, C. M. (2010). Reflections on teaching "Spirituality in the Healthcare Environment." *Journal of Holistic Nursing, 28*(2), 145–149. doi:10.1177/0898010109350770

Lincoln, V. (2000). Ecospirituality: A pattern that connects. *Journal of Holistic Nursing, 18*(3), 227–244. doi:10.1177/089801010001800305

Linhares, C. H. (2012). The lived experience of midwives with spirituality in childbirth: Mana from heaven. *Journal of Midwifery & Women's Health, 57*(2), 165–171. doi:10.1111/j.1542-2011.2011.00133.x

Long, A. (1997). Nursing: A spiritual perspective. *Nursing Ethics, 4*(6), 496–510.

MacDonald, D. A. (2011). Studying spirituality scientifically: Reflections, considerations, recommendations. *Journal of Management, Spirituality & Religion, 8*(3), 195–210. doi:10.1080/14766086.2011.599145

Markani, A. K., Yaghmaei, F., & Fard, M. K. (2013). Spirituality as experienced by Muslim oncology nurses in Iran. *British Journal of Nursing, 22*(4), S22–S28. doi:10.12968/bjon.2013.22.Sup2.S22

Maslow, A. H. (1971). *The farther reaches of human nature* (2nd ed). New York, NY: Viking.

McBrien, B. (2006). A concept analysis of spirituality. *British Journal of Nursing, 15*(1), 42–45.

McSherry, W. (2006). *Making sense of spirituality in nursing and health care practice: An interactive approach* (2nd ed.). London, England: Jessica Kingsley.

McSherry, W., & Cash, K. (2004). The language of spirituality: An emerging taxonomy. *International Journal of Nursing Studies, 41*(2), 151–161. doi:10.1016/S0020-7489(03)00114-7

McSherry, W., Cash, K., & Ross, L. (2004). Meaning of spirituality: Implications for nursing practice. *Journal of Clinical Practice, 13*(8), 934–941. doi:10.1111/j.1365-2702.2004.01006.x

McSherry, W., & Draper, P. (1998). The debates emerging from the literature surrounding the concept of spirituality as applied to nursing. *Journal of Advanced Nursing, 27*(4), 683–691. doi:10.1046/j.1365-2648.1998.00585.x

McSherry, W., & Jamieson, S. (2013). The qualitative findings from an online survey investigating nurses' perceptions of spirituality and spiritual care. *Journal of Clinical Nursing, 22*(21–22), 3170–3182. doi:10.1111/jocn.12411

Meyer, C. L. (2003). How effectively are nurse educators preparing students to provide spiritual care? *Nurse Educator, 28*(4), 185–190.

Mok, E., Wong, F., & Wong, D. (2010). The meaning of spirituality and spiritual care among the Hong Kong Chinese terminally ill. *Journal of Advanced Nursing, 66*(2), 360–370. doi:10.1111/j.1365-2648.2009.05193.x

Murray, R. B., & Zentner, J. B. (1989). *Nursing: Concepts for health promotion.* London, England: Prentice-Hall.

Narayanasamy, A. (1999). A review of spirituality as applied to nursing. *International Journal of Nursing Studies, 36*(2), 117–125. doi:10.1016/S0020-7489(99)00007-3

National Interfaith Coalition on Aging (NICA). (1975). *Spiritual well-being: A definition.* Athens, GA: NICA.

Newberg, A., D'Aquili, E., & Rause, V. (2002). *Why God won't go away: Brain science and the biology of belief.* New York, NY: Ballantine.

O'Connor, C. I. (2001). Characteristics of spirituality, assessment, and prayer in holistic nursing. *Holistic Nursing Care, 36*(1), 33–45.

Ozbasaran, F., Ergul, S., Temel, A. B., Aslan, G. G., & Coban, A. (2011). Turkish nurses' perceptions of spirituality and spiritual care. *Journal of Clinical Nursing, 20*(21–22), 3102–3110. doi:10.1111/j.1365-2702.2011.03778.x

Paley, J. (2008). Spirituality and secularization: Nursing and the sociology of religion. *Journal of Clinical Nursing, 17*(2), 175–186. doi:10.1111/j.1365-2702.2006.01917.x

Pesut, B. (2002). The development of nursing students' spirituality and spiritual care-giving. *Nurse Education Today, 22*(2), 128–135. doi:10.1054/nedt.2001.0664

Pesut, B., Fowler, M., Reimer-Kirkham, S., Taylor, E. J, & Sawatzky, R. (2009). Particularizing spirituality in points of tension: Enriching the discourse. *Nursing Inquiry, 16*(4), 337–346. doi:10.1111/j.1440-1800.2009.00462.x

Reinert, K. G., & Koenig, H. G. (2013). Re-examining definitions of spirituality in nursing research. *Journal of Advanced Nursing, 69*(12), 2622–2634. doi:10.1111/jan.12152

Rew, L. (1989). Intuition: Nursing knowledge and the spiritual dimension of persons. *Holistic Nursing Practice, 3*(3), 56–68. doi:10.1097/00004650-198905000-00010

Rockwood Lane, M. (2005). Creativity and spirituality in nursing: Implementing art in healing. *Holistic Nursing Practice, 19*(3), 122–125.

Salmon, B., Bruick-Sorge, C., Beckman, S. J., & Boxley-Harges, S. (2010). The evolution of student nurses' concepts of spirituality. *Holistic Nursing Practice, 24*(2), 73–78. doi:10.1097/HNP.0b013e3181d39aba

Seeber, J., Park, M. O., & Kimble, M. A. (2001). Pathogenic-salugenic faith and integrative wellness. *Journal of Religious Gerontology, 13*(2), 69–81. doi:10.1300/J078v13n02_07

Sessanna, L., Finnell, D., & Jezewski, M. A. (2007). Spirituality in nursing and health-related literature: A concept analysis. *Journal of Holistic Nursing, 25*(4), 252–262. doi:10.1177/0898010107303890

Shirahama, K., & Inoue, E. M. (2001). Spirituality in nursing from a Japanese perspective. *Holistic Nursing Practice, 15*(3), 63–72.

Sire, J. W. (2004). *The universe next door* (4th ed.). Downers Grove, IL: Intervarsity.

Smart, N. (1996). *The religious experience of mankind* (5th ed.). Englewood Cliffs, NJ: Prentice-Hall.

Smith, A. R. (2006). Using the synergy model to provide spiritual care in critical care settings. *Critical Care Nurse, 26*(4), 41–47.

Smith, S. (2008). Toward a flexible framework for understanding spirituality. *Occupational Therapy in Health Care, 22*(1), 39–54. doi:10.1080/J003v22n01_04

Stoll, R. (1989). The essence of spirituality. In V. Carson (Ed.), *Spiritual dimensions of nursing practice* (pp. 4–23). Philadelphia, PA: W. B. Saunders.

Surbone, A., Konishi, T., & Baider, L. (2011). Spiritual issues in supportive cancer care. In I. Olver (Ed.), *The MASCC textbook of cancer supportive care* (pp. 419–425). New York, NY: Springer Publishing Company.

Tanyi, R. A. (2002). Toward clarification of the meaning of spirituality. *Journal of Advanced Nursing, 39*(5), 500–509. doi:10.1046/j.1365-2648.2002.02315.x

Taylor, E. J. (2002). *Spiritual care: Nursing theory, research, and practice.* Upper Saddle River, NJ: Prentice-Hall.

Taylor, E. J. (Ed.). (2012). *Religion: A clinical guide for nurses.* New York, NY: Springer Publishing Company.

Taylor, E. J. (2013). New Zealand hospice nurses' self-rated comfort in conducting spiritual assessment. *International Journal of Palliative Nursing, 19*(4), 178–185. doi:10.12968/ijpn.2013.19.4.178

Taylor, E. J., & Brander, P. (2013). Hospice patients and family carer perspectives on nurse spiritual assessment. *Journal of Hospice & Palliative Nursing, 15*(6), 347–354. doi:10.1097/NJH.0b013e3182979695

Tiew, L. H., Creedy, D. K., & Chan, M. F. (2013). Student nurses' perspectives of spirituality and spiritual care. *Nurse Education Today, 33*(6), 574–579. doi:10.1016/j.nedt.2012.06.007

Tiew, L. H., Kwee, J. H., Creedy, D. K., & Chan, M. F. (2013). Hospice nurses' perspectives of spirituality. *Journal of Clinical Nursing, 22*(19–20), 2923–2933. doi:10.1111/jocn.12358

Tinley, S. T., & Kinney, A. Y. (2007). Three philosophical approaches to the study of spirituality. *Advances in Nursing Science, 30*(1), 71–80.

Unruh, A. M. (2007). Spirituality, religion, and pain. *Canadian Journal of Nursing Research, 39*(2), 66–86.

van Leeuwen, R., Tiesinga, L. J., Middel, B., Post, D., & Jochemsen, H. (2008). The effectiveness of an education programme for nursing students on developing competence in the provision of spiritual care. *Journal of Clinical Nursing, 17*(20), 2768–2781. doi:10.1111/j.1365-2702.2008 .02366.x

Wasner, M., Longaker, C., Fegg, M. J., & Borasio, G. D. (2005). Effects of spiritual care training for palliative care professionals. *Palliative Medicine, 19*(2), 99–104. doi:10.1191/0269216305pm995oa

Zinnbauer, B. J., Pargament, K. I., & Scott, A. B. (1999). The emerging meanings of religiousness and spirituality: Problems and prospects. *Journal of Personality, 67*(6), 889–919. doi:10.1111/1467 -6494.00077

2

Religion, Spirituality, and Health

W hat do you think of when you hear the word "religion?" Some may think of a particular Christian denomination or of one of the major world religions such as Islam or Buddhism. Others may think of a place of worship such as a church, mosque, or synagogue. For others, the word may be associated with persons who are thought of as religious, such as Mother Teresa, priests, or other religious leaders. Still others may think of various religious rituals such as a baptism, wedding, or funeral. Some may think of the tensions or conflicts that often occur between religious groups, some resulting in wars. Not only could the word "religion" evoke one or more of the images described, but it can also engender strong emotional reactions, particularly if there has been some conflict or trauma associated with religion in a person's background.

Reflection 2.1

Reflect on the word "religion" in terms of its personal meaning to you. What images or thoughts come to your mind? What is your personal definition of "religion?" Are you aware of any emotions evoked in you as a result of this word? If so, then what is the origin of these emotions?

Chapter 1 explored the concept of spirituality, which is considered to be a broader concept than religion. In fact, religion is usually seen to be subsumed under the concept of spirituality. However, a point made in Chapter 1 is that for some people, their spirituality is so intricately connected to religion that they are considered as one and the same. For example, I had a conversation with a nurse who works in an intensive care unit and when she was asked what spirituality meant to her, she replied, "My spirituality and my religion are one." As a demographic, Muslims generally consider spirituality and religion to be one. For example, Markani, Yaghmaei, and Fard (2013) state, "In the Islamic contexts there is no spirituality without religious thoughts and practices; religion provides the spiritual path for salvation and a way of life (Karimollahi, Abedi, & Yousefi, 2007)" (p. S23). Yet, the common assumption that spirituality and religion are the same, an assumption held by many health care professionals, is not necessarily accurate for all people. As stressed in Chapter 1, even if people do not indicate an overt connection to religion, they may still have a desire to believe in something beyond themselves and they have spiritual beliefs (Kevern, 2012; Timmins & McSherry, 2012). However, it is important and appropriate to look more closely at the concept of religion because of its importance in many peoples' lives in some form, and because it can also impact their health and well-being.

THE CONCEPT OF RELIGION

The word "religion" has its roots in the Latin *religare*, which means "to bind together" (Wasner, Longaker, Fegg, & Borasio, 2005, p. 100). This bond can be between people themselves, and/or between people and a higher power. It is appropriate to examine some definitions and descriptions of religion in the literature as summarized in Table 2.1.

Reflection 2.2

Reflect on each of the descriptions or definitions of religion in Table 2.1. Which comes closest to your own understanding of religion that you constructed in Reflection 2.1?

- What common themes do you see in the definitions?
- Appraise each definition for its applicability to nursing practice. What might be the possible implications for assessment and care of clients?

Some people may declare themselves to be affiliated with or committed to one of the major world religions such as Christianity, Hinduism, or Islam. Others may refer to other species of spirituality such as aboriginal spirituality, Wicca, Celtic spirituality, or New Age spirituality (Pearson, 2002) and they may consider one of those worldviews as their "religion." Others may refer to particular causes such as environmentalism, humanism, or feminism as their "religion." As with spirituality, it is important in a clinical setting to determine how each client describes his or her religion. In comparing the definitions and descriptions of spirituality with those of religion, it should be apparent that religion can be more easily observed than spirituality. This may be due to observable religious rituals and practices.

The terminology associated with religion can mean different things to different people. For example, when asked, "What religion are you?" some people may identify that they are Roman Catholic, Baptist, or Muslim. In this sense, they are identifying with a

Table 2.1 Definitions/Descriptions of Religion

[Religion is] 1. Belief in and reverence for a supernatural power or powers regarded as creator and governor of the universe. 2. A system grounded in such belief and worship.... 3. A set of beliefs, values, and practices based on the teachings of a spiritual leader. 4. A cause, a principle, or an activity pursued with zeal or conscientious devotion (Green & Harkness, 1997, p. 1158).

...religion offers a participant a specific worldview and answers to questions about ultimate meaning. Religion can also offer guidance about how to live harmoniously with self, others, nature, and god(s). This direction is presented through a religion's belief system (e.g., its myths, doctrines, stories, dogma) and is acknowledged when one participates in rituals or other religious practices and observances (Taylor, 2002, p.10).

Religion means the organized beliefs, rituals, and practices with which a person identifies and wishes to be associated. It generally involves worshipping a deity or Supreme Being and gathering with those of like faith or similar beliefs (Mauk & Schmidt, 2004, p. 3).

"A religion organizes the collective spiritual experiences of a group of people into a system of beliefs and practices" (Wasner et al., 2005, p. 100).

"Religion refers to an organized system of beliefs regarding the cause, purpose, and nature of the universe that is shared by a group of people and to the practices, including worship and ritual, related to that system" (Burkhardt & Nagai-Jacobson, 2002, p. 13).

"*Religion* involves public and private practices and rituals, beliefs, and a creed with dos and don'ts. It is community-oriented and responsibility-oriented" (Koenig, 2008, p. 33).

"[Religion is]...an organization that binds people together in many ways. Part of the binding comes from its shared beliefs, part from communal membership, and part from shared rituals. Among its parts, for many members, will be that component we call spirituality" (Barnum, 2011, p. 3).

"system," a term used to describe many religions. However, they may be only loosely affiliated with such a system as opposed to being committed to the beliefs, values, and practices associated with that system. Sometimes such identification with a religion is based solely on heritage or culture without any comprehension, understanding, or overt acceptance of the belief system. If asked, "Are you a religious person?" then one might answer, "No, I never attend church," or, "Yes, I attend church quite regularly." Such a response is indicative of that person equating the word "religious" with an institution. Another response such as "I don't consider myself religious, but I do have a personal relationship with God" is demonstrating a differentiation of religion from faith. The point here is that it is important to be aware that words can have a variety of meanings—including ones that are in variance to literal definitions and/or the understanding of the listener. In practice settings, therefore it is imperative to ascertain the intended meanings attached to certain words by clients, and not to assume that clients have the same meanings as that possessed by the nurse.

COMPARISON OF RELIGION AND SPIRITUALITY

A perusal of the health care literature will reveal that there have been many attempts to analyze spirituality and religion, each in relation to the other. Examination of a few examples will bring about an understanding of the connection between these two concepts.

Hillet and colleagues (2000) define spirituality and then add a definition of religion. They provide a summary of the definitional criteria for religion and spirituality. For example, the criterion for both spirituality and religion includes

> the feelings, thoughts, experiences, and behaviors that arise from a search for the sacred. The term "search" refers to attempts to identify, articulate, maintain or transform. The term "sacred" refers to a divine being, divine object, Ultimate Reality, or Ultimate Truth as perceived by the individual. (p. 66)

One criterion for religion that Hillet and colleagues add, which is in addition to the aforesaid criterion, is "A search for non-sacred goals (such as identity, belongingness, meaning, health, or wellness) in a context that has as its primary goal the facilitation of [the above criterion for spirituality and religion]" (p. 66). A second criterion for religion that Hillet and colleagues add, which is also additional to the aforesaid criterion, includes "The means and methods (e.g., rituals or prescribed behaviors) of the search that receive validation and support from within an identifiable group of people" (p. 66).

Rankin and DeLashmutt (2006) describe the relationship between religion and spirituality: "spirituality is more basic than and precedes religious expression (religiosity) because it is an inherent human quality. Religion and religious needs are tradition and practice specific, whereas the existential need of spirituality exists regardless of religious practice or affiliation" (p. 283).

Pesut, Fowler, Taylor, Reimer-Kirkham, and Sawatzky (2008) acknowledge complexity in the relationship between spirituality and religion. They note in the nursing literature that spirituality is portrayed as separate from religion but related to it. Spirituality is also portrayed as an umbrella under which religion can be subsumed. This demonstrates the importance of being sensitive to the manner in which the connection between spirituality and religion is described when reading the nursing literature.

Moberg (2008) notes that spirituality and religion can be distinguished, but they also can be addressed together. Moberg describes "religiosity," a term often discussed in the literature on religion and health, as "membership and participation in the organizational structures, beliefs, rituals, and other activities related to a religious faith like Judaism, Hinduism, Islam, or Christianity" (p. 101). He describes spirituality as having "a more existential and experiential focus upon an individual's internalized faith, values, and beliefs, along with their consequences in daily behavior" (p. 101). In this sense, both terms enjoy significant overlap and both can be part of a person's everyday life, as well as in his or her response to illness and other adversities. Religiosity is further described by Ellor (2011) as a characteristic of an individual or as the importance of religion in an individual's life. Larson, Swyers, and McCullough (1998) also discuss religiosity as connected to religion in terms of religious systems, beliefs, practices, and rituals, but they also include the feelings, attitudes, and responses that a person has toward a higher power as being relevant to this term.

The concepts of spirituality and religion are significantly interconnected, but there can be distinctions made between the two that are important to consider in nursing practice. It is also important to remember that a person's spirituality and/or religion cannot be separated from other dimensions of his or her personhood due to the holistic nature of persons. Any examination of one to the exclusion of the other is merely for the purposes of focused analysis.

RELIGION IN THE WORLD, THE UNITED STATES, AND CANADA

Religion is important to many people. Considering the place of religious adherence from a worldwide perspective, there is evidence that it is growing (Fowler, 2009b; Ross, 2008). It is beyond the scope of this chapter to provide a detailed analysis of geographic variations of religious affiliation. However, it is interesting to touch upon a few statistics to springboard further independent exploration (a good resource is www.worldreligionda tabase.org).

More than 85% of the world's population identify adherence to some religious affiliation. The religion with the largest number of adherents is Christianity (33%) followed by Islam (22.5%) and Hinduism (13.6%; Turner, 2010). It is important to remember when looking at such statistics that *adherence* to a particular religion is not synonymous with overt *commitment* to its doctrines, beliefs, and practices, that is, an internalization of the religion. For example, in North America, many people may say that they are "Christian" when asked what their religion is, but Christian beliefs and practices may play no part in their everyday lives. In fact, many professing Christians may not even know much about the basic or essential tenets of Christianity. However, I have noted in my own practice, and it has been substantiated in the health care literature, that when faced with illness or some other significant life event, many people will return or engage in enhanced attention to some of the beliefs and practices of the religion with which they affiliate. Thus, in nursing practice, when clients may present themselves in the context of such a significant life event, it is important to conduct a more in-depth assessment. The nurse practitioner should explore beyond the mere identification of religious affiliation, but further consider how the person's religion may or may not impact his or her health or how he or she perceives and experiences illness. Knowing the place, scope, and importance of religion in a client's life is essential to providing effective religious care.

Recently, North America has become very pluralistic with respect to a multiplicity of religions—a function of enhanced immigration to North America from other countries. There is more variation in both clients' and nurses' religious orientations than in the past, and there is the possibility of enhanced polarization in terms of each other's religious perspective. In the mid-2000s in the United States, Christianity was the dominant religion, with 85% claiming adherence (Encyclopedia Britannica Online, 2010). The Canadian percentage is lower: 67%. The percentage of Muslims in the United States and Canada is low, 2% to 3%, with a recognition that this religion is growing (Hasmain,

Connell, Menon, & Tranmer, 2011; Lawrence & Rozmus, 2001). Approximately 24% of the Canadian population claim to not be affiliated with any religion (Statistics Canada, 2011), which constitutes a higher percentage than the 8% in the United States who claim to be "nonreligious" (Turner, 2010). Within Canada, there has been a trend toward a greater number of the population indicating "no religion" on census surveys (Reimer-Kirkham, 2009). However, Reimer-Kirkham notes that other than for church attendance, other measures of religiosity in Canada are stable. This observation suggests that people may be engaging in religious practices outside of organized religion. In addition to the growth of non-Christian religions in Canada, Reimer-Kirkham also notes an increased affiliation with evangelical and charismatic Christian churches due to the influx of immigrants with these religious traditions.

RELIGIOUS DEVELOPMENT

Fowler's stages of faith development, discussed in Chapter 1 (see section on Spiritual Development), can be applied to religious development as well as spiritual development. Peck's spiritual development stages are similar to Fowler's in terms of their connection to age groups, but Peck's stages are more closely related to religion, and, in particular, to the Judeo-Christian tradition (Peck, 1987, 2003). Carson (1989) describes religious development as related to a person's acceptance of a particular religion and its beliefs, values, rituals, and so forth. In this sense, religious development can occur at any age.

Reflection 2.3

- Review Fowler's stages of spiritual development in Chapter 1 (see section on Spiritual Development). If you identify with a particular religion, then apply these stages to your own religious growth and development.
- Reflect on your own spiritual development in terms of what factors contributed to your religious growth, and whether this growth was a gradual process or a sudden occurrence. If you identify with a Judeo-Christian faith perspective, then you may also want to consult Peck's stages of spiritual development as part of your reflection (Peck, 1987, 2003).

RELIGION AND CULTURE

As in the case of spirituality, religion can also be connected to culture. For example, a person can become affiliated with a particular religion simply because of the dominant culture around him or her. As Fowler (2009b) states, "religion and culture interpenetrate so that culture may shape the symbols of religious tradition . . . some cultures are suffused with religious influence where adherence may not be widespread" (p. 394). Fowler goes on to state, "some religious traditions may so co-mingle with culture that the actual religious content may, in an accommodationist syncretism, become a variant form of nationalism (Reimer-Kirkham, 2009)" (p. 395). Culture can influence the development of religious beliefs, values, and practices.

An example of culture shaping religious symbols can be found in the culture of the province of Newfoundland and Labrador, Canada. Newfoundland has a rich history of fishing as the main source of employment for its population, particularly in coastal regions. Most people in the province also adhere to the Christian faith. A local wood carver recently completed a nativity scene depicting the birth of Jesus Christ: Joseph (Jesus's father) was carved in the likeness of a local fisherman; Mary (Jesus's mother) as a locally dressed woman; the "stable" where Jesus was born was carved as a typical Newfoundland fishing shed; and the "wise men," who from the biblical account came to visit Jesus and who brought gifts of gold, frankincense, and myrrh, were carved presenting "fish" to the family. The entire religious tradition of the nativity scene was infused with local cultural overtones.

Culturally appropriate care is an integral part of religious nursing care. Clients who are connected to various religions can be seen as belonging to subcultures within the dominant culture, and knowledge of such subcultures is important for nurses (Miller, 1995). For example, gender issues may be important and distinctive in various religious contexts and such issues will necessarily have to be considered in nursing care.

RELIGION AND BELIEFS/PRACTICES

All religions have distinctive beliefs and practices—many of which relate to health, illness, and health care. It is beyond the scope of this chapter to identify such beliefs for all the major world religions as well as how these are interconnected to health and illness. Some religious practices are common to all religions. For example, prayer is commonly practiced by all religions whether they are theistic or nontheistic (Fowler, 2009a). However, to whom the person prays, and other logistics of how prayer is carried out, may vary widely from religion to religion (and indeed, may vary significantly within a given religion).

Religious practices related to health, illness, and health care may vary widely among different religions. Some examples include the lighting of candles as part of a prayer practice; blessing the throat to prevent illness; circumcision, which demonstrates a covenantal relationship between God and man (DeFazio Quinn, 2006); various practices associated with birth and death; dietary restrictions; and so on. Fowler (2009a) maintains that when a person is committed to a particular religion, religious practices that are rooted in the person's inner life are foundational to how that person understands and lives his or her life in terms of the meaning, beliefs, and values that stem from that commitment.

An important point with respect to a particular religion and the beliefs and practices that accompany that religion is that there may be significant variation among people associated with that religion in terms of what they believe and practice and how such are expressed in their lives. One cannot assume that a person who is committed to the Christian faith will hold the same beliefs as all others committed to this faith, engage in the same practices, or carry out these practices in the same manner. Within any religion there will invariably be distinctive subgroups. For example, in Christianity, there are such traditions as Orthodox, Protestant, and Roman Catholic—each again with multiple subgroups and further divisions. In Judaism, there are groups that are Orthodox, Conservative, Reform, and so on. While each subgroup of a religion will generally identify with the basic tenets of its religion, how that religion is "lived out," and the application of the beliefs and practices that accompany it may be quite distinctive for each subgroup (Fowler, 2009b). As previously emphasized, assessment of individual clients and any relevant religious context is crucial.

Religious beliefs and practices have been used in health promotion, and in particular, in terms of health education. For example, in the eastern Mediterranean, a series of eight booklets on the Islamic position with respect to various health issues (e.g., smoking and healthy lifestyle) have been produced. One of the eight booklets, the one on AIDS, was jointly developed by Muslim and Christian leaders (Khayat, 1998).

Reflection 2.4

- What religious beliefs, values, and practices do you hold, if any? Which of these would correspond to the common beliefs, values, and practices of the religion with which you are connected? Which, if any, might be at variance to the common beliefs, values, and practices?
- What purpose(s) do your religious beliefs, values, and practices serve in your life?

RELIGION/SPIRITUALITY IN HEALTH AND ILLNESS

Much has been written about the relationship between spirituality/religion and health/illness. Studies exploring the connection between the two are prolific and growing, including the nature of this connection (Koenig, 2008). Entire journals have been devoted to the topic. For example, the *Journal of Religion and Health*, the *Journal of Religion and Spirituality in Social Work*, and the *Journal of Religion, Spirituality and Aging*, and multiple other journals on spirituality/religion specifically include information on health/illness in their articles. Discussions/studies on the topic include a variety of aspects related to spirituality/religion and health/illness and health/nursing care. Examples include the examination of the values and beliefs of particular religious groups with the corresponding implications for nursing practice (Charles & Daroszewski, 2012; Glick, 2012; Lawrence & Rozmus, 2001); what sacred writings such as the Bible and the Quran say about clients' health rights with respect to care from health care professionals (Hatami, Hatami, & Hatami, 2013); how spirituality/religion impacts clients' experiences, including coping, with various illnesses or health experiences (e.g., perioperative care by DeFazio Quinn, 2006; HIV infection by Walulu, 2011, and breast cancer by Schreiber, 2011). Some of the discussion and studies pertaining to specific health problems/illnesses are covered in the later chapters of this book; at this point, only a brief overview of the role of spirituality/religion in health and illness is sufficient.

RELIGION/SPIRITUALITY AND HEALTH

Religiosity is a social determinant of health (Maselko, Hughes, & Cheney, 2011). It is also related to other social determinants of health. Some of these determinants include the following:

- *Poverty*—The research on poverty and health shows the faith of the poor as being instrumental in their dealing with all the ramifications of poverty, finding meaning and purpose, developing hope and empowerment, and transcending their circumstances (Delashmutt, 2007).

- *Social support*—Having social support from others in one's faith community and from God or a higher power is known to contribute to health and well-being, and to promote spiritual growth, which contributes to overall personal growth (Koenig, 1997; Taylor, 2012).

- *Culture*—The connection between culture and religion has been described earlier in this chapter.

- *Personal health practices* (related to physical and mental health)—These can be impacted by religious beliefs and values (Koenig, 1997), and religion/spirituality has been shown to be intricately connected to coping skills, in particular coping with illness, loss, and other adversities (Koenig, 2008).

- *Child development*—Spirituality is part of overall child development.

Religion is also related to a number of components and concepts of health promotion, which is defined by the WHO as "the process of enabling people to increase control over, and to improve, their health. It moves beyond a focus on individual behavior towards a wide range of social and environmental interventions" (WHO, 2016). For example, health promotion may involve increasing a person's resilience, which is the ability to not only deal with adversity but also grow in the face of it. Studies have shown that clients identify spirituality as one way to enhance their resilience. Spirituality/religious practices are also connected to a number of positive health indicators such as experiencing peace, joy, a sense of wellness, optimism, and hope (Narayanasamy, 2004; Shoqirat & Cameron, 2013; Taylor, 2012). Religious beliefs and practices have also been linked to avoidance of smoking and alcohol abuse, dietary practices that support health, social support, and enhanced mental well-being, all of which are known to contribute to good health (Astedt-Kurki, 1995; Koenig, 1997; Taylor, 2012). Religious involvement is seen as a protective factor with adolescents, as those who are religiously committed are less likely to smoke, abuse alcohol or other drugs, engage in less risky behaviors, and have a better attitude toward life (Cotton, Larkin, Hoopes, Cromer, & Rosenthal, 2005; Rew & Wong, 2006). Studies also show spirituality/religion to be associated with increased quality of life, effective coping skills, and better mental health (decreased anxiety and depression, greater hope and optimism, lower rates of suicide, greater marital satisfaction, and less substance abuse) (Koenig, 2008; Mueller, Plevak, & Rummans, 2001; Post, Puchalski, & Larson, 2000; Townsend, Kladder, & Ayele, 2002; van Leeuwen, 2008).

It is interesting to note that in 1985, the executive board of the WHO adopted a resolution to modify the preamble of the WHO constitution to contain a definition of health that included spiritual as well as physical, mental, and social well-being. The WHO also included spirituality as a component of quality of life (Khayat, 1998). Furthermore, in May 1984, the 37th World Health Assembly adopted a resolution that made the spiritual dimension a part of the health strategies of the WHO member states (WHO, 1985). Well-being has been described as "a state of being in balance and alignment in body, mind and spirit. It is a state in which people describe themselves as feeling healthy, content, purposeful, peaceful, energized, in harmony, happy, prosperous, and safe" (Kreitzer, 2012, p. 707). In Chapter 1, spirituality was presented as being an integrating force in terms of the physical, emotional, and social dimensions of a person. Religiosity is a dimension of well-being (Astedt-Kurki, 1995). Spiritual well-being and religious well-being are commonly referred to in the health care literature as "measurable constructs."

Koenig (2008) and Taylor (2012) identify religious beliefs as assisting people to cope with or make sense of life in general, and of dealing with changes and stressful events that occur in their lives. Religious practices such as prayer or reading sacred writings can provide hope and consolation in the face of illness or other adversity. The support of a religious community can be very helpful. An example that comes to mind is that of a Christian family that immigrated to Canada from a war-torn country. In conversation with this family, they readily identified their religious faith, their religious practices, and their faith community as all helpful in not only dealing with past trauma, but also in enabling them to adjust to life in Canada.

Drawing from a variety of sources, Coyle (2002) concludes that spirituality can

> provide us with a mental attitude, which promotes health either through our actions (behaviour) or our way of being (calm and balanced); or, if things don't go well, spirituality appears to help us to accept adversity and cope with change. Studies suggest that this type of spirituality fosters a positive calm, peaceful, harmonious state of mind, a belief in oneself through connectedness with the divine that has given one's life meaning, purpose, and hope. From an intrapersonal perspective, it may well provide us with a resource or reserve, which we can draw on in times of need. (p. 596)

Coyle also identifies connection to God or a higher power as providing meaning and purpose for religiously committed people. However, one must be careful in ascribing only "positive emotional states" to a description of spirituality, as suffering, a basic human experience, may then be seen as a pathological state (Pesut, 2008).

What aspects of religion are most closely associated with positive health? There has been significant research on the practice of prayer as a coping mechanism (e.g., McCaffrey, Eisenberg, Legedza, Davis, & Phillips, 2004). Attendance at religious services or gatherings is also strongly connected to positive health outcomes and support during illness (e.g., Koenig, McCullough, & Larson, 2001). Taylor (2011) identifies religiosity and intrinsic personal spirituality as being the most adaptive healthful aspects for clients. Personal devotion and a relationship with God or a higher power have also been identified as salient factors that promote health (Hackney & Sanders, 2003; Krause, 2006; Polzer & Miles, 2007; Siegel & Schrimshaw, 2002). Harris, Allen, Dunn, and Parmelee (2013) suggest that the ongoing presence of spirituality/religion in a person's life is key: "It might be that the daily, lived experience of engaging in the coping practice (guided by one's religion/spirituality) is what imparts emotional benefit" (p. 778). As Koenig (1997) states:

> Research has shown that persons who use religion as a means to an end do not experience the psychological benefits of religious practice (Alvarado, Templer, Bresler, & Thomas-Dobson, 1985; Batson & Ventis, 1982). Rather it is those who involve themselves in religion as an end in itself (i.e., persons with intrinsic faith) who are more likely to experience mental health, greater life satisfaction, and less worry and anxiety. (p. 126)

From these brief comments about the role of spirituality/religion in health, one can see that these concepts need to be considered by nurses as factors that contribute to the resilience and the health of people. Asking "What makes people healthy?" is just as important a question as "What makes people unhealthy?"

RELIGION/SPIRITUALITY AND STRESS/ILLNESS

There is a growing body of evidence that spirituality and religion impact not only health and well-being, but they are also operant in times of illness and other health concerns (Loeb, Penrod, Falkenstern, Gueldner, & Poon, 2003; Tyler & Raynor, 2006). Spiritual/religious beliefs and/or supports are drawn upon by people to help them cope and make sense of illness and loss (de Jager Meezenbroek et al., 2012; Narayanasamy, 2002; Surbone, Konishi, & Baider, 2001). Religion has been seen to contribute to the creation of a sense of control during illness (Mueller et al., 2001) as well as contributing to the development of meaning in and of the illness (Thuné-Boyle, Stygall, Keshtgar, & Newman, 2006). Koenig (2008) notes that, when compared to nonreligious people, religious people experience faster recovery from illness, fewer heart attacks, are more likely to recover from heart surgery, experience less disability and slower cognitive decline as they grow older, and generally live longer (especially if they are involved in a religious community). Koenig goes on to identify some mediating factors with respect to the impact of religion during illness: immune, endocrine, genetic, cardiovascular, central nervous system influences, and supernatural mechanisms. With respect to mental illness, religion has been known to enable coping with stress, anxiety, and despair; and a religious faith is a protective factor in the occurrence of depression (Koenig, 1997). Koenig (1997) also notes that, for clients who are experiencing anxiety or depression and who identify with a religion, incorporation of religion into their treatment plan was more effective than if only nonreligious approaches had been used. It is uncertain whether the specific findings from the research that Koenig examined on religion and illness can be more generally applied to the broader concept of spirituality, pointing to the need for further research.

For both acute and chronic illness, it is the case that the nature of illness itself is known to stimulate questions related to life, mortality, suffering, and death. These questions may include:

- Why is this happening to me?

- Where is God in the midst of all of this?

- What does all of this (illness) mean for my life?

- Why is God allowing this suffering?

These, and many others like them, are questions intricately related to spirituality and religion (Molzahn & Shields, 2008). Furthermore, in the midst of illness, suffering, loss, and grief, many people examine beliefs, including religious and spiritual beliefs that they may have had since childhood (Mauk & Schmidt, 2004). There will be a closer examination of religion and spirituality as they relate to specific client contexts in later chapters, but here it is appropriate to offer just a few general comments about the connection between spirituality/religion and illness.

Ano and Vasconcelles (2005) conducted a meta-analysis of 46 empirical studies on religious coping and psychological adjustment to stress. They concluded from their analysis that spiritual/religious resources were connected to significant positive health outcomes. Overall, the body of literature on religion as an aid to coping with stress is impressive in terms of positive outcomes (e.g., Folkman, 2008; Harris et al., 2013; Koenig, 2008; Pargament, 1997).

From a literature review of the findings examining the impact of spirituality/religion on pain, Unruh (2007) concluded that spirituality/religion is part of daily life for many living with pain. Spirituality/religion can impact a client's beliefs about pain, his or her preferences for pain management strategies, and is an important resource in his or her coping with pain. Unruh noted that a wide variety of spiritual/religious practices are often incorporated into pain management, such as meditation, spiritual/religious music, prayer, and sacred readings. Spirituality has also been linked to acceptance of chronic pain (Risdon, Eccleston, Crombez, & McCracken, 2003).

Religious belief is also connected to healing. Mystical experiences that are associated with many religions can activate a healing energy in people. For example, experiences such as prayer, music, and the "laying on of hands" can be accompanied by feelings of joy and well-being, which can contribute to the healing response. Divine intervention that leads to healing is also accepted by many religious believers, although interpretations of how this occurs vary with religious tradition (Taylor, 2012). One does not have to be affiliated with the health care system for very long in order to encounter instances in which medical science cannot explain a positive change in the health status of a client after prayer had been offered up on behalf of that client.

Reflection 2.5

- Reflect on your own health. What spiritual/religious beliefs, values, and practices contribute to your health and well-being? How/why do they do so?
- Reflect on the impact of religion on health, both positively and negatively. If you are connected to a religious framework, what has been the impact of your religious beliefs and practices upon your health in times of illness or during some other significant life event? What spiritual/religious beliefs, values, and practices enabled you to cope or even grow in the midst of your adversity? What effects of religion have you witnessed on the health of family, friends, and clients?

RELIGION/SPIRITUALITY AS A SOURCE OF STRUGGLE

It is important to note that religion and spirituality *can* be a source of struggle for those facing illness and loss. For example, Pargament and Ano (2006) identify several such struggles associated with spirituality/religion during illness:

- The questioning of previously held spiritual/religious assumptions
- The questioning of one's relationship with God or a higher power

- Strain in relationships within one's faith community
- Doubting spiritual/religious beliefs and values previously held

For example, a person who is committed to the Christian faith and who is experiencing an illness (either his or her own, or in a loved one) can believe that God has abandoned him or her or perhaps that the illness is caused by some sin in his or her life (Pulchalski, 2001). He or she may feel that his or her prayers "don't go beyond the ceiling of the room" and may not be able to concentrate on reading the Bible as he or she had previously. Such struggles can cause spiritual distress, which can be just as crippling—or even more crippling—as the illness itself. Nurses need to be alert to signs of spiritual or religious struggle in clients' lives in order to open up conversations about such struggle and take appropriate measures to resolve or alleviate it.

RELIGION/SPIRITUALITY AND SUFFERING

Suffering is common when people experience physical and emotional pain. It is also important to note that spiritual pain and distress is a type of suffering in and of itself. Raholm, Lindholm, and Eriksson (2002) explored the essence of suffering, noting that suffering can be a path to spirituality, while at the same time, spirituality can make suffering bearable, meaningful, and understandable. Raholm and colleagues developed a model to illustrate the connection between spirituality and suffering for appraisal and discussion by clinicians, nurse educators, and researchers. McSherry and Jamieson (2013) also found that spirituality was connected to suffering and that nurses perceived part of their role as supporting those who suffer.

Religion in particular has been noted to assist people to interpret suffering in meaningful ways (Koenig, 2008). For example, I spoke with a client who was dealing with severe fibromyalgia. She was very active in the local Fibromyalgia Association and told me that she believed that God had allowed her suffering so that she, in turn, could offer more relevant help to others struggling with the condition. As Pesut, Fowler, Reimer-Kirkham, Taylor, and Sawatzky (2009) state, "Spiritual health and suffering are no longer antithetical states but can co-exist with the potential for the personal interpretation of suffering to contribute positively to the spiritual journey" (p. 341).

Reflection 2.6

- Have you ever experienced struggle related to your spiritual/religious beliefs during illness or some other significant life event? What was the nature of that struggle? What was (or what might have been) useful in helping you deal with the struggle?
- What have you witnessed about the impact of spirituality/religion on suffering, either in your own life or another's life in terms of spirituality/religion being a resource during suffering or in the development of meaning in and of the suffering?

RELIGION AND NEGATIVE IMPACT ON HEALTH/WELL-BEING

No discussion of religion and health would be complete without reference to the potential negative impact that religion can have on health. We will look more closely at the "neurotic" uses of religion (Koenig, 1997) in Chapter 8. In that chapter, we look at how mental illness can sometimes create bizarre religious beliefs. Suffice to say that the nurse must be aware of uses of religion that do not contribute positively to a person's health. For example, an individual may cite statements from religious writings out of context to support a particular position on health and illness. Or, a person may believe that God will take care of him or her and conclude that there is no need for medical treatment.

How does a nurse decide whether the particular beliefs and practices of a given religion are "healthy" or "unhealthy?" Although one must proceed with caution in answering this question, there are some general guidelines to follow in terms of deciding whether a particular religious perspective is "healthy" or "sick." For example, Pesut, Fowler, Taylor, Reimer-Kirkham, and Sawatzky (2008) indicate:

> A healthy spirituality or religion will transcend itself in compassion; recognize the inevitability of suffering; seek to redress that suffering at the individual and societal level; make room for difference while searching for commonality; and refuse to reduce discourse to an idolatrous search for personal, political or economic gain. (p. 2809)

Furthermore, if the religious practices and beliefs of the client result in feelings of false guilt, anxiety, or some other emotion that is psychologically distressing for the client, then Pesut and colleagues (2008) would deem the particular religion (or the client's interpretation of it) is "unhealthy." The point about the *client's interpretation of the religion* is an important one. The guidelines given by Rao and Katze (1979), quoted in Schnorr (1983) and Graves (1983), are still relevant today in terms of discerning a "healthy" from a "sick" religion: whether the religion acts as a vice; whether the religion deviates from a client's premorbid religious belief system (i.e., deemed to be normative for people in that belief system); whether the client's religion differs significantly from others in the same religion; whether the religion overwhelms the client with guilt that is not based in reality; whether false humility is manifested by the client or he or she denies personal abilities and resources; and whether the religion urges the client to deny feelings, especially negative feelings. Shelly and John (1983), again, a classic work on mental health and spirituality, add to the guidelines provided by Rao and Katze, in their description of what constitutes a healthy versus an unhealthy spiritual life (pp. 61–71; seen on a continuum). As can be seen, there is somewhat of a bias toward the Christian religion in some of the items on the continuum. On the unhealthy end of the continuum of spiritual life, the following can be present:

- Beliefs that separate/fragment the person and that create separation from others by withdrawal

- Beliefs that cause a person to be absorbed into a group identity, with no personal identity present, that cause the person to manipulate others, and that see God as a "magical being"

- Preoccupation with wrongdoing and an inability to forgive or to be forgiven—or, an absence of a sense of wrongdoing and lack of values and standards of what is right and wrong

- Total freedom without sanctions, or lack of freedom with no responsibility for one's actions

- Legalism

- A feeling of being driven with no enjoyment of life

- Repressed feelings and thoughts

- Poor self-esteem or grandiosity

- Unhealthy view of suffering, for example, that it is a form of punishment stemming from the person's "not being good enough"

On the healthy side of the continuum of spiritual life, the following are characteristics:

- Beliefs that contribute to a sense of wholeness; that strengthen one's view of self as a person of worth and value as well as the ability to accept oneself; that see God as good and controlling the universe, but giving people free choice and responsibility; and that build bridges, not barriers between people and foster interdependence with others; supportive, mutual relationships are normative

- Acknowledgment of wrongdoing and an ability to be forgiven as well as to forgive and to reconcile with others

- Living with the freedom of a full range of emotional expressions, tolerating ambiguity, appreciating humor, and expressing spiritual feelings and thoughts honestly

- A healthy view of suffering, that is, that suffering is part of the human condition (Drawing on resources such as God's strength to deal with suffering is also characteristic, resulting in growth in suffering.)

Reflection 2.7

Review the indicators of a "sick" and "healthy" religion, as well as a "healthy" and "unhealthy" spiritual life.

- Appraise each indicator in terms of its applicability to your life. For example, you may not identify with a particular world religion so items dealing with religion may not be as relevant for you. However, in some instances, you may be able to modify the indicator to apply to yourself.

(continued)

> *Reflection 2.7* **(continued)**
>
> - Put each indicator on a Likert scale, with 1 being the "unhealthy" end of the scale, and 10 being the "healthy" end of the scale.
> - Rate your own religion/spiritual life on the scale. Which indicators fall on the "healthy" end of the scale, and which fall on the "unhealthy" end of the scale?
> - What insights have you gained from this exercise?

Taylor (2012) also writes about the negative impact of religion on health. Citing the works of several authors, she gives several examples of how religiosity can have a deleterious impact on health. It can cause "confusion, despair, isolation, helplessness, meaninglessness, detachment or resentment . . . unhelpful guilt or shame . . . passivity . . . a sense of abandonment . . . " (p. 11). These are states that are known to be associated with poor health and religiosity may be a catalyst for such negative results in multiple ways (Taylor, 2012):

- Attributing health events to demonic forces

- Abdicating any personal responsibility for a health outcome but instead believing that God will magically solve the problem

- Engaging in beliefs and practices that are significantly at variance with the normative beliefs and practices of the person's particular religion

- Being connected to a religion that, in and of itself, isolates the person from others and engages in practices known to be harmful to the person's well-being, such as can be found in some cults

Taylor concludes that when someone who is religious has beliefs that do not comfort or assure him or her, that result in him or her feeling guilt or shame, that create passivity within him or her or make him or her feel abandoned, then such religious beliefs are harmful to the person. Koenig (2008) also comments upon the negative impact of religion in situations where religions engender fear, and when persons use religion to avoid issues and to resist making changes. If a nurse is unfamiliar with a particular religion in terms of its beliefs, tenets, values, and practices, it would be wise to consult with a religious leader of that particular religion in order to obtain information about the religion so that the nurse can determine whether the client's interpretation is appropriate and/or healthy.

RELIGION AND ETHICAL/LEGAL ISSUES

There are a number of factors related to religion and the law within the context of health/nursing care. These factors overlap with multiple ethical issues and dilemmas. This topic is not extensively explored within this work, but two excellent books that cover the area in a comprehensive manner are recommended: *Religion: A Clinical Guide for Nurses* (Taylor, 2012) and *Religion, Religious Ethics, and Nursing* (Fowler, Reimer-Kirkham, Sawatzky, & Taylor, 2011). A few comments are offered here to whet appetites.

Taylor (2012) identifies several aspects of religion and the law in terms of nursing practice (within the context of U.S. health care). Some of those aspects covered by Taylor include the following:

- The legality of nurse behaviors related to religious beliefs and values

- Laws that protect the rights of nurses who are religious persons

- How religious nurses can avoid conflict with the law and yet remain true to their religious beliefs

This work cannot authoritatively canvass the relevant law operant with respect to health care issues but it is important for nurses to know such laws in the respective countries in which they practice. Taylor discusses such law in the United States, and concludes that there *are* provisions within ethical codes of nursing to protect religious nurses. However, such protections are limited. For example, Tayler points out that proselytization, or the attempt to convert the client to the nurse's own religion, is not appropriate from a legal as well as ethical perspective; nor is the withdrawal of safe and compassionate care. In her book she outlines practice guidelines and obligations for religious nurses.

Another context in which law and ethics may be pertinent is when certain religious groups hold views that conflict with health care practices. Perhaps the most widely known group in this regard is the Jehovah's Witnesses, who refuse blood transfusions based on their interpretation of certain Biblical texts. Another group, the Scientologists, believes in faith healing (Taylor, 2012) and may generally refuse modern medical interventions such as drug therapy. An important point to remember in caring for such clients is that persons who are committed to such groups may experience spiritual distress when faced with a medical choice that violates their religious beliefs. Often, the client's spiritual leader or a pastoral care professional/chaplain can be helpful in such situations. For example, Jehovah's Witnesses representatives can give information about alternate medical care, which is acceptable to their faith perspective and thereby assist the health care team to manage the situation. Sometimes, in the case of children, temporary custody can be awarded to the state in order for medical treatment to occur over the religious objections of parents or guardians. In the case of adults, however, clients' decisions generally prevail if they are considered to be of sound mind. If a client dies because of refusal to accept a potentially life-saving treatment or procedure, this loss can be particularly distressing for a nurse who does not share the same religious perspective. In this case, the nurse can proceed in a manner consistent with any ethical dilemma, for example, consulting with other members of the health care team (Taylor, 2012).

Sometimes, a client's religious beliefs and practices may cause him or her to prefer, or even insist upon, being cared for by a nurse with similar beliefs and practices. For example, nurses have advised that many female Mormon clients ask to have a nurse assigned to them from their own faith because of their particular religious beliefs about undergarments. It is less stressful for such clients if the nurse caring for them understands their perspective. Although such preference may not always be logistically possible, if clients do make such requests, and if there is a nurse from the same religion as the clients, then it does make sense for that nurse, if possible, to care for the clients. Another example would be the case of a Christian client with spiritual/religious concerns who would prefer to be cared for by a Christian nurse who he or she may perceive to be capable of greater understanding of his or her particular situation and concerns.

Reflection 2.8

- Are you aware of your ethical decision making being grounded in a spiritual/religious belief system? If not, in what is it grounded?
- Reflect on any clinical situation where the client's decisions about care were based on religious beliefs. How was the situation dealt with? What feelings did you experience in this situation and how did you deal with these feelings?

RELIGION IN NURSING PRACTICE

Fowler (2009a) maintains that the religious dimension of human experience has been largely neglected in nursing. This is an assertion supported by other authors. Taylor (2012) identifies a number of reasons why religion should be considered in nursing care (pp. 3–8), many pertaining to what has already been discussed in this chapter:

- Many clients are religious.

- Religiosity is associated with health outcomes.

- Regular religious fellowship benefits health by offering support that buffers the effects of stress and isolation.

- Participation in worship and prayer benefits health through the physiological effects of positive emotions.

- Faith benefits health by leading to thoughts of hope, optimism, and positive expectation.

- Mystical experiences benefit health by activating a healing bioenergy, or life force, or altered states of consciousness.

- Divine intervention allows healing.

Nurses need to assess how clients perceive religion to be operating in their lives, and they should also be sensitive to both positive and negative overtones from clients. Spiritual/religious assessment is discussed in Chapter 5. There will be particular nursing interventions that may be pertinent to specific world religions. Referencing Taylor (2012) for information in this regard will be informative.

Unruh (2007), Taylor (2002), and Koenig (1997) identify more general practice guidelines for nurses in dealing with the religious aspects of care:

- The nurse needs to inquire about the religious background, beliefs, values, and practices of clients, including how they perceive these aspects may impact their health. A person-centered approach is imperative in such an inquiry.

- The nurse needs to be supportive and respectful of clients' religious beliefs, values, and practices, even if they are at odds with what the nurse subjectively believes. This is part of the nurse's ethical practice. It also implies that the nurse needs to be open to discussion about religion with the client.

- The nurse should affirm the religious beliefs and practices that clients identify as being sources of strength and hope for them, providing that such beliefs or practices are not known to be harmful to clients.

- For clients who are committed to a particular religion, the nurse needs to encourage them to actively participate in their faith community as a way of gaining social and spiritual support. When clients are unable to participate with their community due to illness or hospitalization, the nurse can refer them to pastoral care professionals/chaplains, if clients so desire. Members of the faith community can also be encouraged to visit clients, assist them with religious practices, and provide other supports. Faith communities can be invaluable resources to the physical, emotional, and spiritual care of clients and their families.

- The nurse can integrate religious beliefs and practices into treatment/nursing care strategies if clients so choose. Of utmost importance is that input from clients and their families is crucial in this regard so that what is integrated is compatible with the clients' faith perspectives.

- Pastoral care professionals/chaplains need to be seen as integral members of the health care team. Nurses need to develop collegial relationships with these professionals so as to adequately meet the religious needs of clients.

- The nurse needs to be aware of any personal subjective biases with respect to religion in general, and any specific biases toward a particular religion. These biases may adversely affect the assessment and care of clients.

- If the situation warrants it, the nurse needs to assist clients in thinking about potentially harmful religious beliefs, values, and practices. Consultation with religious leaders, pastoral care professionals/chaplains is advisable in such a situation.

Reflection 2.9

Reflect on the aforementioned guidelines for nurses in dealing with the religious aspects of care. On a scale of 1 to 10, with 1 being "not at all effective" and 10 being "very effective," how many of these guidelines do you incorporate into your current nursing practice? How might you improve in this area?

RELIGIOSITY IN THE NURSE'S LIFE

The role of religiosity in the nurse's life is important to consider. After all, nurses are people, and, as such, are spiritual beings who may choose to express and nurture their spirituality through a particular religion. As Taylor (2012) states, "we all bring who we are to the bedside" (p. 88). You may be concerned that because religion has not played a significant role in your own life, you will not be able to attend to the religious expression of spirituality in a satisfactory manner. If you have had negative experiences with religion, then you may fear that such experiences may impede your ability to engage with clients who are religious. Or, you may describe yourself as being "religious" and fear that you may inadvertently "push" your religious views on clients. These are all natural and normative concerns.

Cusveller (1995) presents an interesting discussion with respect to the presence and function of religious commitment in the nurse. He questions the claim by some that nursing care is "morally and religiously neutral" (p. 973). He maintains that nurses bring their own particularities to nursing, and rather than perceiving them as "private matters," he suggests that accounting for them is perhaps the better alternative. Operating from this premise, Cusveller believes that it is possible and justifiable for certain nursing decisions to reflect religious convictions. He gives an example of a client with terminal cancer who wished to stay alive to celebrate the upcoming Christmas, which presented as an important time for that client. The physician had decided to discontinue treatment, which could have resulted in the client's imminent death. A religiously committed nurse saw it within her professional duty to advocate for continuation of care to try to keep the client alive until after the celebration of Christmas. In this instance, the options for care were affected not only by a client-centered stance, but also affected by the nurse's religious commitment.

In addition to religious commitment impacting various options in nursing care, Cusveller (1995) maintains that religious commitment may give some nurses a sense of what care or for whom care is important. For example, on the basis of their religious commitment, the nurses in Mother Teresa's order, the Missionaries of Charity, have decided to focus on care for the poorest of the poor. Cusveller goes on to identify that religious commitment may also influence a nurse's perception of situations, a nurse's motivation, a nurse's sensitivity to spiritual needs, and a nurse's ethical position(s) on various health care matters. Of course, it is never appropriate to proselytize or to attempt to "convert" the client to the nurse's subjective religious views and beliefs as it would be in direct violation of codes of ethics that direct the nurse to respect clients' religious perspectives. Cusveller concludes:

> Just as scholars cannot rid themselves of their particular points of view, but have to discuss them in order to develop the best theories, so nurses have to bring their particular points of view to nursing and to discuss them in order to provide the best possible care. Moral, philosophical and religious convictions are not just bias, although they may be, but they can also have a positive function. (p. 977)

Reflection 2.10

What do you think of Cusveller's ideas? Are you aware of your own or some other nurses' religious convictions impacting on nursing care in some manner; or how nursing itself is viewed? What have been the impacts of such convictions, both positive and negative?

Like Cusveller, Pesut (2008) identifies as problematic the assumption that nurses should lay aside their developed spiritual worldviews as potential biases in caring for clients. Pesut states, "We need to move from the naive view that [the nurse's] personal beliefs have little or no place in spiritual care to a more sophisticated understanding of how those beliefs should be negotiated within a profession that has a public trust with patients in positions of vulnerability" (p. 172). Markani and colleagues (2013) also support the view that there is room for the personal convictions of nurses in terms of providing care and they propose that the ability of nurses to care holistically is connected in part to their spiritual development. Taylor (2012) should be referenced for a more in-depth discussion of integrating personal religiosity with professional nursing practice.

A final point with respect to religion and nursing practice is the importance of knowing how to converse with clients about their religious beliefs and practices. This is discussed later in this work. The information in this chapter not only provides knowledge about the religious aspects of care, but it also provides a foundation from which to explore religious aspects of care with clients.

The Bottom Line

- You should know the basic tenets and practices of major world religions, especially those that may be specifically relevant to health/illness.

- You should be aware of your own religious positioning and biases.

- You should know and comply with ethical practice that includes respecting clients' religious beliefs, values, and practices.

- Supporting clients' religious beliefs and values and facilitating their religious practices is part of good religious nursing care.

- Referral of clients to pastoral care professionals/chaplains/other team members may be warranted.

- You should be open to discussion of religion with clients as such is foundational to good religious nursing care.

- Assessment of the religious perspectives of clients is necessary to ensure appropriate nursing care.

- Because culture and religion are intricately connected, culturally appropriate care is relevant to good religious nursing care.

- Proselytization is never appropriate or ethical in a nursing care context.

- Client-centered care is critical.

Taking It Further

1. Research each of the major world religions (Christianity, Judaism, Islam, Buddhism, Hinduism), noting the basic beliefs, values, and practices of each. Imagine, in sequence, that you are a member of each of these religions. What benefits and issues might you experience in terms of your own health and health practices? How might you envision this religion helping you if you were experiencing illness or some other adverse life event? How can this reflection serve to enhance your clinical practice with various religious groups? (If this reflection is done as a group activity, each group member can choose one religion, research it, and report findings back to the group. The entire group should discuss the benefits and issues pertaining to each religion in terms of health and illness, and how the learning attained from this exercise can benefit clinical practice.)

2. Review the major world religions to determine how each would describe spirituality and the spiritual dimension of personhood. What are the implications for nursing practice for clients who may be committed to each of these religions?

3. Have a conversation with a client this week who has identified with a particular religion. Ask him or her how his or her religious beliefs and practices impact on his or her health, including how it helps him or her cope with his or her illness or health problem. Compare the client's responses with findings identified in this chapter and in any other readings that deal with the area of religion and health.

4. Choose a spiritual leader who is important to you in terms of the values/teachings of this person in guiding your life (e.g., Jesus Christ, the Dalai Lama, Mohammed, Confucius):

   a. Identify aspects of this person's philosophy that are congruent with those of the nursing profession.

   b. Identify qualities/values associated with spirituality that this particular leader may advocate. Which parallel those found in professional nursing?

   c. Envision yourself as possessing the qualities/values in (b). How might these enhance your nursing practice? How can they assist you to cope and even flourish in today's health care system (Hermann, 2003)?

5. Review the major world religions (e.g., Christianity, Judaism, Islam, Buddhism, Hinduism). Postulate what you would include in a nursing education program pertaining to each of these religions to increase awareness in nursing students/nurses about the religious/cultural aspects of care for clients from each of these groups. (This exercise can be completed as a group, with each group member

researching a particular religion, and then collectively discussing aspects to include in an education program.)

6. If you identify with a particular religion, reflect on how you might handle your own faith perspective when encountering clients in various nursing contexts. Do you have particular beliefs, values, or convictions that could pose challenges for you? How might your beliefs, values, or convictions be supportive to you in your role as a nurse? What beliefs, values, and convictions of clients would prove to be challenging for you? And how might you handle these challenges? (This exercise can be completed in a group of people with mixed religions or of the same religion.)

7. What religious experiences have you had that might impact your work with clients, both positively and negatively? For those experiences that have engendered a negative impact for you, how can you deal with them in order to better care for clients who are religious?

8. VanLeeuwen, Tiesinga, Jochemsen, and Post (2009) describe the regulative side of nursing practice as the personal beliefs, motives, objectives, and expectations of the nurse. What beliefs, motives, objectives, and expectations do you have that are connected to religion or spirituality in general? How do these interact with the religious/spiritual care of clients?

9. It has been argued in this chapter that nursing has largely neglected the religious/spiritual dimension of care. Do you agree? If so, then why do you think this is so? How might the study of the religious domain of care be incorporated into nursing in an ethical and responsible manner?

10. If you were to incorporate the religious aspect of care into the nursing practice setting in which you currently operate, what principles would you suggest for nurses to follow? What aspects of nursing care would be affected (e.g., dietary implications, decisions about medical/nursing care, cultural aspects)?

11. If you identify with a particular religion, or have strong religious beliefs, reflect on the following questions:

    a. How did your faith influence your choice of nursing as a career?

    b. How has your faith helped you in your nursing career so far?

    c. Has your faith hindered you in any way in your nursing career to date? If so, in what way(s)?

    d. How have clients/colleagues reacted to your religious beliefs/values?

    e. Has your faith ever caused conflict in terms of nursing professional codes of ethics? If so, what was the nature of this conflict, and how did you resolve it (Timmins & Narayanasamy, 2011)?

12. How does viewing religion as a social determinant of health legitimize its place in health/nursing care? How does such a view of religion impact its place as a focus on population health? How might this determinant of health impact the

health of a population as a whole and for any subgroups within the population (Maselko et al., 2011)?

13. Reflect on various world religions, or on particular subgroups within a religion. Are there any toward which you are biased, either positively or negatively? What factors contribute to your bias (e.g., their beliefs, media reports, personal experience)? How might your bias potentially impact your nursing care of clients from that religion/group? How might it potentially impact your work with colleagues who are from that religion/group?

14. What are the religious/spiritual aspects of the dominant culture and subcultures of which you consider yourself to be a part? Which of these would you desire and/or expect a nurse to consider if you were a client? What would you want them to do (Giger & Davidhziar, 1990)?

15. Discuss with a group of colleagues how religious/spiritual beliefs and values facilitate or constrain the development of a therapeutic relationship with clients (Olson et al., 2003).

16. Review a number of studies reported in the literature on religion/spirituality and health/illness. Record the following about each study: weaknesses and strengths of the various measures of religion/spirituality; quality of study design; study outcomes; and the study's limitations. Report your findings to a group of peers and discuss the implications for nursing practice as well as any directions for further research.

17. Interview pastoral care professionals/chaplains about the following:

    a. Their role in terms of the religious/spiritual care of clients as well as of staff in the institution/agency

    b. Their experiences as part of the health care team and what they feel they contribute to the team

    c. Their educational preparation for their role

    d. Their perspectives on the role of nurses in religious/spiritual care and in the referral process

    e. Their experiences in working with nurses in terms of religious/spiritual care, including what factors contribute to an effective working relationship

    (Alternatively, you can convene a panel of pastoral care professionals/chaplains to address these topics with a nursing class or a group of practicing nurses.)

18. Research the major world religions (e.g., Christianity, Judaism, Islam, Buddhism, Hinduism) to determine how ethical decision making is impacted by the beliefs and values of that particular religion. Identify specific examples to illustrate. (This exercise can be completed in a group with each group member researching one religion and reporting back to the group for information and collective discussion.)

19. Convene a panel of nurses to discuss how they deal with situations where clients may have very different religious/spiritual values from their own. Ask them

to describe specific clinical examples, and also to discuss helpful guidelines that they endeavor to follow to deal appropriately with such situations.

20. Reimer-Kirkham and colleagues (2011) outline several recommendations for health care providers and health care organizations from their study on the negotiation of religious and spiritual pluralism in health care: creating and maintaining designated ecumenical spaces as well as creative informal sacred spaces in health care institutions; intentionality on the part of health care providers to "nurture relational spaces for enhanced healing" (p. 210); attending to spiritual practices at the organizational level; supporting pluralistic religious and spiritual expressions by providing diverse services with broad mandates; employing specialists in religion; ensuring that representatives of specific religious/ spiritual traditions are present in an institution. Discuss the following questions with respect to the above recommendations:

    a. In the health care institution/agency in which you practice nursing, how many of these recommendations are currently being implemented? How many are being deliberately or inadvertently ignored?

    b. If any recommendations are not being currently implemented in your health care institution/agency, what role can nurses and other health care professionals play to ensure that they are duly implemented?

    c. Would you add other recommendations based on your own experience or readings?

21. Cockell and McSherry (2012) indicate that nurse managers need to be proactive in supporting and educating nurses to understand spirituality and the influence of religion on clients. This would include the impact on their spiritual needs, and how clients' beliefs may influence nursing care. Which specific strategies can you identify for each of these responsibilities? What resources are available to ensure that these responsibilities are adequately carried out?

22. If the spiritual/religious dimension of care were to be adequately addressed in the geographic region in which you practice, what would need to change in terms of the delivery of health care in your region? What particular groups, agencies, or interested bodies could possibly work together to ensure adequate spiritual/ religious care? For what health issues could religious leaders be of assistance to health care professionals; and how might this be accomplished (Khayat, 1998)?

23. Research the concept of "person" in various nursing theories/models and in various religions. How congruent is nursing's view of personhood with each religion's view? Are there aspects of personhood in various religions that could inform nursing practice in a positive way? What are the implications for nursing for each view of personhood in each of the religions?

24. Interview a person, or several people, who are involved in a local religious community. Ask them the following questions:

    a. How does involvement in your religious community influence your own sense of health and well-being and/or the health and well-being of the community?

b. What aspects of the experience in a religious community are particularly important for you with respect to your health and well-being?

c. If you were ill and unable to be physically present in your religious community, how might they still be of help to you? How might you still be able to be involved in the activities of the community?

Share your findings with a group of peers and discuss the impact of involvement in a religious community on health and well-being.

25. Consider the following options in order to raise awareness of the research on religion/spirituality in the institution or agency in which you practice:

a. Organize a discussion group on the topic, or have someone who does research in the area provide a presentation on the subject.

b. Organize a workshop or conference on the topic.

c. Develop a special interest group focusing on the topic.

d. Engage researchers to conduct research in your institution/agency on the topic, perhaps with you as part of the research team.

e. Obtain further education and training on conducting research on the topic (e.g., at the Center for Spirituality, Theology and Health at Duke University Medical Center; Aten & Schenck, 2007).

REFERENCES

Ano, G. G., & Vasconcelles, E. B. (2005). Religious coping and psychological adjustment to stress: A meta-analysis. *Journal of Clinical Psychology, 61*(4), 461–480. doi:10.1002/jclp.20049

Astedt-Kurki, P. (1995). Religiosity as a dimension of well-being. *Clinical Nursing Research, 4*(4), 387–396. doi:10.1177/105477389500400405

Aten, J. D., & Schenck, J. E. (2007). Reflections on religion and health research: An interview with Dr. Harold G. Koenig. *Journal of Religion & Health, 46*(2), 183–190.

Barnum, B. S. (2011). *Spirituality in nursing: The challenges of complexity* (3rd ed.). New York, NY: Springer Publishing Company.

Burkhardt, M., & Nagai-Jacobson, M. (2005). Spirituality and health. In B. Dossey, L. Keegan, & C. Guzzetta (Eds.), *Holistic nursing: A handbook for practice* (4th ed., pp. 168–172). Sudbury, MA: Jones & Bartlett.

Carson, V. B. (Ed.). (1989). *Spiritual dimensions of nursing practice*. Philadelphia, PA: W. B. Saunders.

Charles, C. E., & Daroszewski, E. (2012). Culturally competent nursing care of the Muslim patient. *Issues in Mental Health Nursing, 33*(1), 61–63. doi:10.3109/01612840.2011.596613

Cockell, N., & McSherry, W. (2012). Spiritual care in nursing: An overview of published international research. *Journal of Nursing Management, 20*(8), 958–969. doi:10.1111/j.1365-2834.2012.01450.x

Cotton, S., Larkin, E., Hoopes, A., Cromer, B. A., & Rosenthal, S. L. (2005). The impact of adolescent spirituality on depressive symptoms and health risk behaviors. *Journal of Adolescent Health, 36*(6), 529–535. doi:10.1016/j.jadohealth.2004.07.017

Coyle, J. (2002). Spirituality and health: Towards a framework for exploring the relationship between spirituality and health. *Journal of Advanced Nursing, 37*(6), 589–597. doi:10.1046/j.1365-2648 .2002.02133.x

Cusveller, B. (1995). A view from somewhere: The presence and function of religious commitment in nursing practice. *Journal of Advanced Nursing, 22*(5), 973–978. doi:10.1111/j.1365-2648.1995 .tb02650.x de Jager Meezenbroek, E., Garssen, B., van den Berg, M., van Dierendonck, D., Visser, A., & Schaufeli, W. B. (2012). Measuring spirituality as a universal human experience: A review of spirituality questionnaires. *Journal of Religion & Health, 51*(2), 336–354. doi:10.1007/s10943-010 -9376-1

DeFazio Quinn, D. M. (2006). How religion, language and ethnicity impact perioperative nursing care. *Nursing Clinics of North America, 41*(2), 231–248. doi:10.1016/j.cnur.2006.01.002

Delashmutt, M. B. (2007). Students' experience of nursing presence with poor mothers. *Journal of Obstetric, Gynecologic & Neonatal Nursing, 36*(2), 183–189. doi:10.1111/j.1552-6909.2007.00135.x

Ellor, J. W. (2011). Reflections on the words "religion," "spiritual well-being," and "spirituality." *Journal of Religion, Spirituality & Aging, 23*(4), 275–278. doi:10.1080/15528030.2011.603074

Encyclopedia Britannica Online. (2010). Religion: Year in review 2010: Worldwide adherents of all religions. Retrieved from https://www.britannica.com/topic/religion-Year-In-Review-2010/World wide-Adherents-of-All-Religions

Folkman, S. (2008). The case for positive emotions in the stress process. *Anxiety, Stress, & Coping, 21*(1), 3–14. doi:10.1080/10615800701740457

Fowler, M. (2009a). Preface to thematic section: Religions, spirituality, ethics and nursing. *Nursing Ethics, 16*(4), 391–392. doi:10.1177/0969733009104603

Fowler, M. (2009b). Religion, bioethics and nursing practice. *Nursing Ethics, 16*(4), 393–405. doi:10.1177/0969733009104604

Fowler, M., Reimer-Kirkham, S., Sawatzky, R., & Taylor, E. J. (Eds.). (2011). *Religion, religious ethics and nursing.* New York, NY: Springer Publishing Company.

Giger, J. N., & Davidhziar, R. (1990). Contextual care: Religious considerations for culturally appropriate nursing care. *Advancing Clinical Care, 5*(4), 48–51.

Glick, L. H. (2012). Nurturing nursing students' sensitivity to spiritual care in a Jewish Israeli nursing program. *Holistic Nursing Practice, 26*(2), 74–78. doi:10.1097/HNP.0b013e31824621e6

Graves, C. G. (1983). Counterpoint: Cause or cure? *Perspectives in Psychiatric Care, 21*(1), 27. doi:10.1111/j.1744-6163.1983.fb00169.x

Green, S., & Harkness, J. (Eds.). (1997). *ITP Nelson Canadian Dictionary of the English Language: An encyclopedic reference.* Scarborough, ON, Canada: Thomson.

Hackney, C. H., & Sanders, G. S. (2003). Religiosity and mental health: A meta-analysis of recent studies. *Journal for the Scientific Study of Religion, 42*(1), 43–55. doi:10.1111/1468-5906.t01-1-00160

Harris, G. M., Allen, R. S., Dunn, L., & Parmelee, P. (2013). "Trouble won't last always": Religious coping and meaning in the stress process. *Qualitative Health Research, 23*(6), 773–781. doi:10 .1177/1049732313482590

Hasmain, M., Connell, K. J., Menon, U., & Tranmer, P. A. (2011). Patient-centered care for Muslim women: Provider and patient perspectives. *Journal of Women's Health, 20*(1), 73–83. doi:10.1089/ jwh.2010.2197

Hatami, H., Hatami, M., & Hatami, N. (2013). The religious and social principles of patients' rights in the Holy Books (Avesta, Torah, Bible, and Quran) and in traditional medicine. *Journal of Religion & Health, 52*(1), 223–234.

Hermann, M. L. S. (2003). Keeping the magic alive in nursing care: Advice from the Dalai Lama. *Nurse Educator, 28*(6), 245–246.

Hill, P. C., Pargament, K. I., Hood, R. W., McCullough, M. E., Swyers, J. P., Larson, D. B., & Zinnbauer, B. J. (2000). Conceptualizing religion and spirituality: Points of commonality, points of departure. *Journal for the Theory of Social Behaviour, 30*(1), 51–77. doi:10.1111/1468-5914.00119

Larson, D. B., Swyers, J. P., & McCullough, M. E. (Eds.). (1998). *Scientific research on spirituality and health: A report on the scientific progress in spirituality conferences.* Rockville, MD: National Institute of Healthcare Research.

Karimollahi, M., Abedi, H. A., & Yousefi, A. (2007). Spiritual needs as experienced by Muslim patients in Iran: A qualitative study. *Research Journal of Medical Science, 1*(3), 183–190.

Kevern, P. (2012). Who can give "spiritual care?" The management of spiritually sensitive interactions between nurses and patients. *Journal of Nursing Management, 20*(8), 981–989. doi:10.1111/ j.1365-2834.2012.01428.x

Khayat, M. H. (1998). Spirituality in the definition of health: The WHO's point of view. Retrieved from http://www.tinyurl.com/9edlyk7

Koenig, H. G. (1997). *Is religion good for your health? The effects of religion on physical and mental health.* London, England: Routledge.

Koenig, H. G. (2008). Religion, spirituality and health: Understanding the mechanisms. In V. B. Carson & H. G. Koenig (Eds.), *Spiritual dimensions of nursing practice* (pp. 33–61). West Conshohocken, PA: Templeton Foundation Press.

Koenig, H. G., McCullough, M. E., & Larson, D. B. (2001). *Handbook of religion and health.* New York, NY: Oxford University Press.

Krause, N. (2006). Gratitude toward God, stress, and health in late life. *Research on Aging, 28*(2), 163–183. doi:10.1177/0164027505284048

Kreitzer, M. J. (2012). Spirituality and well-being: Focusing on what matters. *Western Journal of Nursing Research, 34*(6), 707–710. doi:10.1177/0193945912448315

Lawrence, P., & Rozmus, C. (2001). Culturally sensitive care of the Muslim patient. *Journal of Transcultural Nursing, 12*(3), 228–233. doi:10.1177/104365960101200307

Loeb, S. J., Penrod, J., Falkenstern, S., Gueldner, S. H., & Poon, L. W. (2003). Supporting older adults living with multiple chronic conditions. *Western Journal of Nursing Research, 25*(1), 8–29. doi:10.1177/019394590223883

Markani, A. K., Yaghmaei, F., & Fard, M. K. (2013). Spirituality as experienced by Muslim oncology nurses in Iran. *British Journal of Nursing, 22*(4), S22–S28. doi:10.12968/bjon.2013.22.Sup2.S22

Maselko, J., Hughes, C., & Cheney, R. (2011). Religious social capital: Its measurement and utility in the study of the social determinants of health. *Social Science & Medicine, 73*(5), 759–767. doi:10.1016/j.socscimed.2011.06.019

Mauk, K. L., & Schmidt, N. K. (Ed.). (2004). *Spiritual care in nursing practice.* Philadelphia, PA: Lippincott Williams & Wilkins.

McCaffrey, A. M., Eisenberg, D. M., Legedza, A. T. R., Davis, R. B., & Phillips, R. S. (2004). Prayer for health concerns: Results of a national survey on prevalence and patterns of use. *Archives of Internal Medicine, 164*(8), 858–862. doi:10.1001/archinte.164.8.858

McSherry, W., & Jamieson, S. (2013). The qualitative findings from an online survey investigating nurses' perceptions of spirituality and spiritual care. *Journal of Clinical Nursing, 22*(21–22), 3170–3182. doi:10.1111/jocn.12411

Miller, M. A. (1995). Culture, spirituality and women's health. *Journal of Obstetric, Gynecologic, & Neonatal Nursing, 24*(3), 257–263. doi:10.1111/j.1552-6909.1995.tb02471.x

Moberg, D. O. (2008). Spirituality and aging: Research and implications. *Journal of Religion, Spirituality & Aging, 20*(1–2), 95–134. doi:10.1080/15528030801922038

Molzahn, A. E., & Shields, L. (2008). Why is it so hard to talk about spirituality? *Canadian Nurse, 104*(1), 25–29.

Mueller, P. S., Plevak, D. J., & Rummans, T. A. (2001). Religious involvement, spirituality, and medicine: Implications for clinical practice. *Mayo Clinic Proceedings, 76*(12), 1225–1235. doi:10.4065/76.12.1225

Narayanasamy, A. (2002). Spiritual coping mechanisms in chronically ill patients. *British Journal of Nursing, 11*(22), 1461–1470. doi:10.12968/bjon.2002.11.22.10957

Narayanasamy, A. (2004). The puzzle of spirituality for nursing: A guide to practical assessment. *British Journal of Nursing, 13*(19), 1140–1144. doi:10.12968/bjon.2004.13.19.16322

Olson, J. K., Paul, P., Douglass, L., Clark, M. B., Simington, J., & Goddard, N. (2003). Addressing the spiritual dimension in Canadian undergraduate nursing education. *Canadian Journal of Nursing Research, 35*(3), 94–107.

Pargament, K. (1997). *The psychology of religion and coping: Theory, research, practice.* New York, NY: Guilford Press.

Pargament, K. I., & Ano, G. G. (2006). Spiritual resources and struggles in coping with medical illness. *Southern Medical Journal, 99*(10), 1161–1162. doi:10.1097/01.smj.0000242847.40214.b6

Pearson, J. (Ed.). (2002). *Beliefs beyond boundaries: Wicca, Celtic spirituality and the new age.* Bath, England: Ashgate/Open University Press.

Peck, S. (1987). *The different drum: Community making and peace.* New York, NY: Touchstone

Peck, M. S. (2003). *The road less travelled, timeless edition: A new psychology of love, traditional values and spiritual growth.* New York, NY: Touchstone.

Pesut, B. (2008). Spirituality and spiritual care in nursing fundamentals textbooks. *Journal of Nursing Education, 47*(4), 167–173. doi:10.3928/01484834-20080401-05

Pesut, B., Fowler, M., Reimer-Kirkham, S., Taylor, E. J., & Sawatzky, R. (2009). Particularizing spirituality in points of tension: Enriching the discourse. *Nursing Inquiry, 16*(4), 337–346. doi:10.1111/j.1440-1800.2009.00462.x

Pesut, B., Fowler, M., Taylor, E. J., Reimer-Kirkham, S., & Sawatzky, R. (2008). Conceptualizing spirituality and religion in healthcare. *Journal of Clinical Nursing, 17*(21), 2803–2810. doi:10.1111/j.1365-2702.2008.02344.x

Post, S. G., Puchalski, C. M., & Larson, D. B. (2000). Physicians and patient spirituality: Professional boundaries, competency, and ethics. *Annals of Internal Medicine, 132*(7), 578–583. doi:10.7326/0003-4819-132-7-200004040-00010

Raholm, M., Lindholm, L., & Eriksson, K. (2002). Grasping the essence of the spiritual dimension reflected through the horizon of suffering: An interpretive research synthesis. *The Australian Journal of Holistic Nursing, 9*(1), 4–73.

Rankin, E. A., & DeLashmutt, M. B. (2006). Finding spirituality and nursing presence: The student's challenge. *Journal of Holistic Nursing, 24*(4), 282–288. doi:10.1177/0898010106294423

Reimer-Kirkham, S. (2009). Lived religion: Implications for nursing ethics. *Nursing Ethics, 16*(4), 406–417. doi:10.1177/0969733009104605

Reimer-Kirkham, S., Sharma, S., Pesut, B., Sawatzky, R., Meyerhoff, H., & Cochrane, M. (2011). Sacred spaces in public places: Religious and spiritual plurality in health care. *Nursing Inquiry, 19*(3), 202–212. doi:10.1111/j.1440-1800.2011.00571.x

Rew, L., & Wong, J. Y. (2006). A systematic review of associations among religiosity/spirituality and adolescent health attitudes and behaviors. *Journal of Adolescent Health, 38*(4), 433–442. doi:10.1016/j.jadohealth.2005.02.004

Risdon, A., Eccleston, C., Crombez, G., & McCracken, L. (2003). How can we learn to live with pain? A Q-methodological analysis of the diverse understandings of acceptance of chronic pain. *Social Science & Medicine, 56*(2), 375–386. doi:10.1016/S0277-9536(02)00043-6

Ross, L. (2008). Commentary on Paley, J. (2008) spirituality and secularization: Nursing and the sociology of religion. *Journal of Clinical Nursing, 17*(2), 175–186. *Journal of Clinical Nursing, 17*(20), 2795–2798. doi:10.1111/j.1365-2702.2008.02401.x

Schnorr, M. A. (1983). Point: Religion. *Perspectives in Psychiatric Care, 21*(1), 26. doi:10.1111/j.1744-6163.1983.fb00168.x

Schreiber, J. A. (2011). Image of God: Effect on coping and psychospiritual outcomes in early breast cancer survivors. *Oncology Nursing Forum, 38*(3), 293–301. doi:10.1188/11.ONF.293-301

Shoqirat, N., & Cameron, S. (2013). A qualitative study of hospital patients' understanding of health promotion. *Journal of Clinical Nursing, 22*(19–20), 2714–2722. doi:10.1111/jocn.12212

Siegel, K., & Schrimshaw, E. (2002). The perceived benefits of religious and spiritual coping among older adults living with HIV/AIDS. *Journal for the Scientific Study of Religion, 41*(1), 91–102. doi:10.1111/1468-5906.00103

Statistics Canada. (2011). 2011 National household survey: Data tables. Retrieved from http://www12.statcan.gc.ca/nhs-enm/2011/dp-pd/dt-td/Rp-eng.cfm?LANG=E&APATH=3&DETAIL=0&DIM=0&FL=A&FREE=0&GC=0&GID=0&GK=0&GRP=0&PID=105470&PRID=0&PTYPE=105277&S=0&SHOWALL=0&SUB=0&Temporal=2013&THEME=95&VID=0&VNAMEE=&VNAMEF=

Surbone, A., Konishi, T., & Baider, L. (2011). Spiritual issues in supportive cancer care. In I. Olver (Ed.), *The MASCC textbook of cancer supportive care* (pp. 419–425). New York, NY: Springer Publishing Company.

Taylor, E. J. (2002). *Spiritual care: Nursing theory, research, and practice.* Upper Saddle River, NJ: Prentice-Hall.

Taylor, E. J. (2011). Religion and patient care. In M. Fowler, S. Reimer-Kirkham, R. Sawatzky, & E. J. Taylor (Eds.), *Religion, religious ethics and nursing* (pp. 313–338). New York, NY: Springer Publishing Company.

Taylor, E. J. (Ed.). (2012). *Religion: A clinical guide for nurses.* New York, NY: Springer Publishing Company.

Thuné-Boyle, I. C., Stygall, J. A., Keshtgar, M. R., & Newman, S. P. (2006). Do religious/spiritual coping strategies affect illness adjustment in patients with cancer? A systematic review of the literature. *Social Science & Medicine, 63*(1), 151–164. doi:10.1016/j.socscimed.2005.11.055

Timmins, F., & McSherry, W. (2012). Spirituality: The Holy Grail of contemporary nursing practice. *Journal of Nursing Management, 20*(8), 951–957. doi:10.1111/jonm.12038

Timmins, S., & Narayanasamy, A. (2011). How do religious people navigate a secular organisation? Religious nursing students in the British National Health Service. *Journal of Contemporary Religion, 26*(3), 451–465. doi:10.1080/13537903.2011.616040

Townsend, M., Kladder, V., & Ayele, H. (2002). Systematic review of clinical trials examining the effects of religion on health. *Southern Medical Journal, 95*(12), 1429–1434.

Turner, D. J. (2010). Religion: Year in Review 2010. Worldwide adherents of all religions. *Encyclopaedia Britannica.* Retrieved from http://www.britannica.com/topic/religion-Year-In-Review-2010/Worldwide-Adherents-of-All-Religions

Tyler, I. D., & Raynor, J. E. (2006). Spirituality in the natural sciences and nursing: An interdisciplinary perspective. *The ABNF Journal, 17*(2), 63–66.

Unruh, A. M. (2007). Spirituality, religion, and pain. *Canadian Journal of Nursing Research, 39*(2), 66–86.

vanLeeuwen, R. R. (2008). *Towards nursing competencies in spiritual care* (Doctoral dissertation, University of Groningen). Retrieved from http://www.rug.nl/research/portal/publications/towards-nursing-competencies-in-spiritual-care(4e556c37-6639-4b36-9065-f37a63dbeb87).html

vanLeeuwen, R., Tiesinga, L. J., Jochemsen, H., & Post, D. (2009). Learning effects of thematic peer-review: A qualitative analysis of reflective journals on spiritual care. *Nurse Education Today, 29*(4), 413–422. doi:10.1016/j.nedt.2008.10.003

Walulu, R. N. (2011). Role of spirituality in HIV-infected mothers. *Issues in Maternal Health Nursing, 32*(6), 382–384. doi:10.3109/01612840.2011.568160

Wasner, M., Longaker, C., Fegg, M. J., & Borasio, G. D. (2005). Effects of spiritual care training for palliative care professionals. *Palliative Medicine, 19*(2), 99–104. doi:10.1191/0269216305pm995oa

World Health Organization. (1985). *Handbook of resolutions and decisions of the World Health Assembly and the Executive Board* (Vol. 2, pp. 1973–1984). Retrieved from http://apps.who.int/iris/handle/10665/79012

World Health Organization. (2016). *Definition of health promotion.* Retrieved from http://www.who.int/topics/health_promotion/en

3

Rationale and Challenges for Spirituality in Nursing

Having examined the concepts of spirituality and religion, as well as how these two concepts are connected to illness, health, and well-being, it is appropriate to explore how they are relevant to health care professionals and, in particular, nurses. A foundational rationale for the inclusion of spirituality into nursing practice is important. The identification and articulation of such a rationale enables nurses to explain why spirituality is important to clients and families, colleagues, and others both within and outside of the health care system. It also enables nurses to more articulately advocate for incorporating spirituality into nursing practice. Challenges to incorporating spirituality into nursing practice are also important to consider and are discussed later in this chapter (see section on Challenges to Incorporating Spiritual Care Into Nursing Practice, Education, and Research).

The following is an outline of some of the rationales for integrating spirituality into health care and nursing. Each rationale could have a distinct chapter devoted to it. Some of the rationales are explored in more detail in other chapters of this book. However, the intent here in this chapter is to provide an overview of the rationales as well as to provide references for further exploration.

RATIONALE FOR SPIRITUALITY IN HEALTH CARE AND NURSING

SIGNIFICANT INTEREST IN THE TOPIC ON HEALTH CARE AND NURSING

The proliferation of articles, books, dissertations, and theses on the topic of spirituality in health care has been profound in recent years, and continues to grow, especially since the 1970s. Not only is this growth evident in the Western world, but also in countries in Asia, such as China and Iran. Spirituality and spiritual/religious care has also been a focus in many recent nursing and health-related conferences. Some conferences, such as the 4th European Conference on Religion, Spirituality and Health in Malta, the 5th

Conference on Compassion, Spirituality and Health in Australia, and conferences of the National Institutes of Health in the United Kingdom focus totally on the topic of spirituality. Multiple health institutes and centers are devoted to the topic of spirituality in health care. For example, there are the Institute for Spirituality and Health (www .ish-tmc.org) and the Center for Spirituality, Theology and Health (www.spiritualityand health.duke.edu) in the United States; and in Canada, there is the Institute of Spirituality and Aging (www.uwaterloo.ca/grebel/academics/continuing/institute-spirituality-and -aging). There are multiple websites that are devoted to spirituality, such as (www.sacred space.org.uk). As Timmins and McSherry (2012) state, "interest in spirituality within the context of nursing and health care has 'mushroomed' internationally" (p. 951). All of this interest in spirituality, religion, and health is evident not only in the nursing context, but also in other health-related professions, such as medicine, social work, occupational therapy, and rehabilitative therapy.

Within nursing education, electives on the spiritual dimension of nursing care have been developed, and spirituality is often a thread in the nursing curriculum. Nursing textbooks have been written on the topic, and many textbooks contain chapters specifically dealing with the topic of spirituality/religion. Special interest groups have been established. Some groups have focused on generic spirituality, whereas other groups consider spirituality from a particular worldview. Examples of the latter type are Nurses Christian Fellowship (an international organization) and the Spirituality, Religion, and Health Interest Group (at the Hospital of the University of Pennsylvania). At least one nursing journal focuses solely on the aspects of spiritual/religious care in nursing (the *Journal of Christian Nursing*) and many other nursing journals are also regularly published on the topic. Sometimes, all issues of a volume are devoted to the topic, for example, the *Journal of Clinical Nursing*, Volume 15 (2006). Critiques of spirituality in nursing are also appearing: for example, Clarke (2009) and Pesut, Fowler, Reimer-Kirkham, Taylor, and Sawatzky (2009). There is also growth in the area of parish nursing as a recognized subspecialty in nursing (Ruder, 2013).

SOCIETAL INTEREST IN SPIRITUALITY

In Western society, there has been a well-documented intensification of interest in spirituality (Davie, 1994; Hufford, Fritts, & Rhodes, 2010; Pesut, 2003). In particular, there has been growth in nonreligious spirituality (Sharma, Reimer-Kirkham, & Fowler, 2012). Pesut (2009a) states that society is "increasingly enchanted with the idea of the sacred" (p. 17). She acknowledges the diversity in views pertaining to spirituality, arguing that this is a rationale for not having a "unified ontology" of spirituality in nursing. Becker (2009) sees such an interest, in North American society at least, as a search for meaning and purpose (a concept connected closely to spirituality). Becker states: "Interest in spirituality is not a fleeting trend . . . . It is becoming increasingly difficult for the academy to ignore these trends, especially among students and faculty members in higher education who value spirituality because it informs their lives" (p. 705). Becker goes on to say: "The freedom to engage (or not) in spiritual beliefs and practices must be honored but not at the expense of silence in the guise of privacy . . . meaningful interdisciplinary dialogue about the issues is warranted to respond respectfully to this contemporary call" (p. 705).

The evidence for interest in spirituality in society can be seen readily. Multiple books on the subject are available at local bookstores. Workshops are often devoted to some aspects of spirituality (e.g., mindfulness workshops). There are many movies and television shows that focus on some spiritually related themes. Even book clubs focusing on spiritual matter are not uncommon. Public interest in alternative and complementary therapies has grown, and spirituality is often integral to such therapies (Barnum, 1996; Canadian Nurses Association [CNA], 2008). In fact, the CNA has specifically identified alternative and complementary therapies as a trend and opportunity for the coming decade. Finally, myriad products have been brought into the market with an emphasis on spirit/soul as part of the marketing approach for these products.

Nursing has long responded to the needs of the broader society within which it is situated, so it is not surprising that in a spirituality-focused society, spirituality has made its inroads into the nursing profession. As Pesut (2009b) states, "The burgeoning interest in spirituality within health care reflects a societal interest" (p. 17). The diversity of understandings of spirituality in society certainly poses challenges for nurses (Reimer-Kirkham, Pesut, Sawatzky, Cochrane, & Redmond, 2012).

Reflection 3.1

Reflect on the references to spirituality in society in general; for example: books you have seen in local bookstores; popular magazine articles or advertisements related to some aspects of spirituality; local advertisements in your community for workshops and courses related to spirituality (e.g., mindfulness workshops); websites of popular fitness or health clubs in your community advertising programs beneficial for body, mind, and spirit; websites of local churches regarding programs that are directed at a person's spiritual life; the presence of aspects of spirituality in broadcast media and in social media. What concepts of spirituality are inherent in each of these examples? Are they a generic, universal spirituality or a spirituality focused on religious beliefs and values?

THE NATURE OF BEING HUMAN

As discussed in Chapter 1 (see section on Spirituality and Personhood), spirituality is an integral part of being human (Burkhardt & Nagai-Jacobson, 2002; McSherry & Jamieson, 2013). In fact, some would say that it is the essence of being human. The idea of spirituality as a universal phenomenon means that all people have spiritual needs whether they overtly embrace a religious framework or not. They include the need for meaning and purpose in life or in life events, and the need for love and relatedness (Smith, 2009). Therefore, regardless of the age, gender, cognitive, physical or psychological ability of the client, or the specific health issue at play, it is noted that spirituality is relevant to all.

IMPORTANCE TO CULTURE

The connection between spirituality/religion and culture was also discussed in Chapter 1 (see section on Spirituality and Culture). Spirituality is a well-recognized concept in all known cultures (Olson et al., 2003), although it manifests and presents itself in multiple varied forms and practices. In some instances, spirituality and religion can be the central feature of a cultural identity (Karairmak, 2004; Ozbasaran, Ergul, Temel, Aslan, & Coban, 2011; Tisdell, 2006). Such is the case, for example, in some aboriginal cultures, the Haitian culture, and the African American culture.

Culturally sensitive care is one of the hallmarks of good nursing care, particularly important in today's increasingly culturally diverse society (CNA, 2008). Such sensitivity extends to the spiritual and religious beliefs, tenets, and practices within each culture. It should also be pointed out here that various religious or spiritual groups can be considered to be subcultures within the broader culture; therefore, awareness and appreciation of these groups is also important so that nurses can be sensitive to clients within such subcultures.

IMPORTANCE IN HEALTH/ILLNESS

The significance of spirituality and religion to health and illness was discussed in Chapter 2 (see section on Religion/Spirituality in Health and Illness). There is strong empirical evidence of a significant link between the two (Baldacchino, 2011; Biro, 2012; Callister, Bond, Matsumura, & Mangum 2004; Maj, 2010; Moberg, 2008; Reimer-Kirkham et al., 2011; Ruder, 2013). In fact, Ribaudo and Takahashi (2008) noted a steady increase in research studies on spirituality and health since the 1980s (14.9 studies per year in the 1980s; 209.5 studies per year in the early 2000s). Discussions on issues related to spirituality and research abound; for example, the discussions by Reinert and Koenig (2013) and MacDonald (2011). Authors who have conducted research reviews generally conclude that there is ample evidence to promote the inclusion of spirituality into health and illness care. For example, Sessanna, Finnell, and Jezewski (2007) maintain that psychosocial, biochemical, and neuroscientific research supports the role of spirituality and religion in health, healing, and well-being. Cockell and McSherry (2012), after reviewing research papers on spiritual care in nursing from 2006 to 2010, conclude: "While there is much still to learn, [about spiritual care] enough is known to provide a solid evidence base . . . . A rapidly growing body of research indicates that [spiritual care] is too important to be ignored, for the sake of both practitioners and patients" (p. 966). Narayanasamy (2011), who has published prolifically in the area of spirituality in nursing education and practice, maintains that there is sufficient empirical information to warrant the inclusion of spirituality into nursing care. Many research studies are referenced in this book to support such claims.

If spirituality and religion are positively linked to health, resilience, and healthy lifestyles; if spirituality and religion are positively connected to adaptation to chronic and acute illness, making sense of illness and other adversity; and if spirituality is related to quality of life, including the end of life, then it is definitely the case that spirituality is a powerful resource for nurses in working with clients. In fact, certain clinical contexts are known to be particularly connected to spirituality and spiritual needs, such as life-threatening illness, palliative care, and mental health (Highfield, Taylor, & Amenta, 2000; WHO, 2016). The suffering inherent in those contexts of health and illness often stimulates spiritual exploration (Becker, 2009).

The concepts of health and illness are core to the focus of nursing practice. Each is connected to spirituality. With respect to the concept of health, it is interesting to note that prior to Hippocrates, health was broadly seen as a divine gift (Bonting, 2005), a view that still persists in some people to this day. There are a myriad of descriptions and definitions of "health" by various organizations and authors, many referring implicitly to spirituality, but other health definitions are much more explicit with respect to spirituality. A definition that implies spirituality is one given in Stanhope, Lancaster, Jessup-Falcioni, and Viverais-Dresler (2011): "Community health nursing practice supports the World Health Organization (WHO) definition, which views health positively as a resource for everyday living that is holistic and includes physical, social, and personal capabilities (World Health Organization [WHO], 2006)" (p. 9). Describing health as a resource for living that is holistic would include all of the resources that a person uses to effect health, including spiritual resources. In an example of a more explicit definition, O'Brien (2011) refers to being truly healthy as not primarily related to physical health as much as being "solidly grounded spiritually" (p. 9). O'Brien and many others also refer to "holistic health" as encompassing not only the health of the body and mind, but also the health of the spirit.

As discussed in Chapter 2 (see section on Religion/Spirituality and Stress/Illness), illness is known to stimulate spirituality/religious searching or questioning of the "deeper questions of life." In fact, a critical illness can be the client's first awareness of an encounter with the spiritual self. Clients also use a wide range of religious and spiritual beliefs to cope with illness and promote healing (Brady, Peterman, Fitchett, Mo, & Cella, 1999; McCord et al., 2004; Molzahn & Sheilds, 2008; Reimer-Kirkham et al., 2011). Swinton (2005) sums up the relationship between spirituality and religion well when he states:

> Spirituality sits at the heart of . . . [illness] experiences. A person's spirituality, whether religious or non-religious, provides belief structures and ways of coping through which people begin to rebuild and make sense of their lives in times of trauma and distress. It offers ways in which people can explain and cope with illness experiences and in so doing discover and maintain a sense of hope, inner harmony and peacefulness in the midst of the existential challenges illness inevitably brings. [These experiences] are crucial to the complex dynamics of a person's movement towards health and fullness of life even in the face of the most traumatic illness. (p. viii)

If health and illness are the "business" of nursing, and if spirituality is inherent in both the concepts, then spirituality is necessarily the "business" of nursing.

SPIRITUALITY AS A FACTOR IN RESILIENCE

Spirituality is one of the protective factors that serve to foster resilience (Battey, 2012; Bonanno, 2004). Resilience is described by Bonanno (2004) as "the ability of adults [and children] in otherwise normal circumstances who are exposed to an isolated and potentially highly disruptive event [such as a health crisis] to maintain relatively stable, healthy levels of psychological and physical functioning" (p. 20). Based on earlier work (Bonanno, Papa, & O'Neill, 2001), Bonanno (2004) goes on to indicate that, although resilient individuals may experience a temporary disruption in normal functioning, they can also have "the capacity for generative experiences and positive emotions" (p. 21). As Mattison (2006) maintains, spirituality is an internal experience that can transform an external situation that sometimes cannot be altered in any other way. The life and writings of Viktor Frankl illustrate this point well. Frankl was a Jewish psychiatrist who was interned in several concentration camps during World War II. He maintained that people can find meaning regardless of their external situation, an observation he made regarding survivors of the Holocaust. Frankl went on to develop logotherapy, a therapy focusing heavily on the process and nature of meaning making (Frankl, 1985).

Fostering resilience in clients and families is one of the goals of nursing; therefore, the connection between spirituality and resilience cannot be ignored. There is also an interrelationship between resilience and holistic health, discussed later in this chapter (see section on Nature, Values, and Goals of Nursing): "Holistic health affects the patient's resiliency or the ability to recover quickly or move on to a peaceful death" (Battey, 2012, p. 1016).

Reflection 3.2

- Would you consider yourself to be a resilient person? If so, does spirituality or the religious expression of spirituality contribute to your resilience? If "yes," how does it do this?
- Reflect on a time when you felt desperate, hopeless, or troubled and yet felt that you were able to maintain some sense of "well-being" in spite of the situation, perhaps even generating growth as a result of the situation. What role, if any, did spirituality play in working through this situation? How did this occur and what were the specific outcomes?
- Reflect on ways that nurses can use spirituality/religion to foster resilience in clients. What do you need to do in your own practice to consider this factor in promoting resilience in clients/families?

ECONOMIC FACTORS

Economic factors related to health care are always first and foremost in the popular and professional media today. It seems as if "cuts" in health-related programs and services occur on a regular basis, and everyone waits anxiously for news about health care with every national and provincial/state budget announcement. The economic concerns and struggles that characterize the current health care system fuel the search for less costly alternatives. Spiritual therapies are one such alternative (Cohen, Holley, Wengel, & Katzman, 2012; Olson et al., 2003). Unruh (2007) also supports this economic interest in spirituality in health care when she identifies the growing aging population in society, with its increasing demand on the health care system as a reason for an enhanced focus on spirituality as a factor that promotes health and resilience.

Another impact of economic factors with respect to spiritual care in health care is related to the place of such care in clinical practice. As Swinton and McSherry (2006) maintain, the current "political, economic and financial constraints placed on many health care systems inevitably deprioritizes the spiritual and despiritualizes those who work within it" (p. 801).

CLIENTS' PERSPECTIVES

According to the research, and further borne out by anecdotal comments by health care professionals and clients alike, many clients want health care professionals to talk about spiritual/religious concerns that the clients may have—as well as to support their spirituality/religiosity (Battey, 2012; Daaleman, Cobb, & Frey, 2001; Molzahn & Sheilds, 2008; Taylor, 2002). Many nurses encounter clients who are religious or are influenced by religion (Taylor, 2012). Moreover, for many clients, religion is important in maintaining health in the midst of illness or adversity (Pesut, Fowler, Taylor, Reimer-Kirkham, & Sawatzky, 2008; Ross, 2006). Nurses also report regularly encountering (as frequently as on a daily basis) clients with spiritual needs (McSherry & Jamieson, 2011).

If the religious and spiritual needs of clients and their families are not met, then they can experience spiritual distress, which may lead to negative client outcomes (Hexem, Mollen, Carroll, Lanctot, & Feudtner, 2011; Taylor, 2003). For example, it is suggested that in some instances, spiritual distress and anguish can actually exacerbate the clients' perceptions of pain, anxiety, restlessness, and other symptoms that are present during the dying process (Wasner, Longaker, Fegg, & Borasio, 2005). Conversely, when spiritual and religious needs are met, clients are more satisfied (Lind, Sendelback, & Steen, 2011). Evidence of positive client outcomes provides one of the most important rationales for spirituality/religion to be incorporated into client care. There is ample evidence to indicate that the quality of care improves when spirituality/religion is considered in that care (Pesut, 2009c). Not only does this relate to client outcomes, but also to the improvement of client-centered care (Hoover, 2002), which occurs as nurses strive to assess spirituality from the client's perspective and tailor spiritual care to each client's situation. It is clear, then, from the client's perspective, that the client's spirituality/religion is important to be considered and addressed.

Reflection 3.3

- Reflect on clinical situations where clients have given "cues" that they might like to discuss spiritual or religious issue with you, either with respect to themselves or to loved ones. For example, joking about "the man upstairs" (referring to God), or asking "Why" questions, such as "Why is this happening to me (him, her)?" or "What did I (he, she) do to deserve this" or "Why do I (he, she) have to suffer so?"
  a. What feelings or thoughts are evoked in you in such situations?
  b. How do you respond in such situations? Are you comfortable in proceeding to conversation that will focus on some aspect of spirituality, or do you largely

(continued)

Reflection 3.3 (continued)

> ignore such cues? If the latter, why is this so? And how might you respond differently so as to meet the clients' spiritual needs?
>
> • What outcomes have you noted in clients whose spiritual/religious needs are met, either by themselves or by the intervention of health care professionals?

HISTORICAL ROOTS OF NURSING

The historical roots of nursing provide a foundation for the inclusion of spirituality/ religion into nursing practice. Tracing the history of nursing is an interesting exercise. For example, Taylor (2002) describes the history of nursing from the time of Jesus Christ. In her review of the history of nursing, it is seen that the origins of nursing, and also the development of nursing as a profession, grew out of a worldview that saw people as spiritual beings. The writings of early nurse leaders such as Florence Nightingale abound with references to the need of care for the whole person. The spiritual and religious roots of nursing are discussed in more detail in Chapter 6.

NATURE, VALUES, AND GOALS OF NURSING

The very nature of nursing supports the inclusion of spirituality into nursing practice. As Highfield and colleagues (2000) state:

> Nursing centers on strengthening patient resources and relationships, facilitating growth and wholeness, and empowering the person and family. In this respect, nursing is a profession that, by its very nature, lends itself to spiritual caregiving—the facilitating of satisfying intrapersonal, interpersonal and transpersonal relatedness. (p. 62)

As can be observed from this quote, nursing is relational in nature, as is spiritual care (Stern & James, 2006). The client is known to the nurse through the nurse–client relationship, and this relationship is at the heart of spiritual care. Critical to the nature of nursing is nurses being available and present to clients. Availability and presence are also crucial in the provision of spiritual care (Hoglund, 2013).

Nursing is also focused on peoples' experiences as well as their responses to such experiences across their life spans (American Nurses Association [ANA], 2011). These experiences include life events, such as illness, dying, grief, and maintaining or facilitating health. As discussed earlier, spirituality is an intrinsic part of being human, which makes it inevitable that for many peoples' experiences, spirituality will necessarily play a part in such experiences. Two student nurses summed up the connection between nursing and spirituality well in a study by Callister and colleagues (2004): "Nursing is a career drenched in spirituality" (p. 165); and "Nursing is more than just caregiving; it is nourishing the human spirit" (p. 165).

Values of nursing are connected to spirituality. Curlin and colleagues (2001) observe that nursing values underlie the professional mandate to promote peoples' health. Horton, Tschudin, and Forget (2007) maintain that nursing values are expressed in behaviors normally exhibited by nurses in their practice. For example, the nursing values of compassion, loving kindness, integrity, autonomy, altruism, social justice, patience, recognition of the sacred, and preserving human dignity are also seen as spiritual values (Cameron, 2003; Fahrenwald et al., 2005; International Council of Nurses [ICN], 2012; Meehan, 2012).

Nursing focus on holistic care is central to its nature and many definitions of nursing include holistic care as a defining feature of nursing (O'Brien, 2011). In fact, Tyler and Raynor (2006) describe holistic care as "the crux of nursing practice in the 21st century" (p. 65). Holistic nursing is seen as a combination of the science of nursing with the art of nursing (Ross & McSherry, 2010; Timmins & McSherry, 2012). As holistic care is so central to the nature of nursing, it is also critical to the practice of nursing (Battey, 2012; Carr, 2010; Jackson, 2011; Lemmer, 2010; Miner-Williams, 2006; Ruder, 2013). Holistic nursing recognizes the unity and balance of the mind, body, spirit, and social dimensions of a person, as well as the interdependence of these dimensions (Narayanasamy & Owens, 2001; Swinton, 2001). In fact, the nursing profession has had a rich history in providing holistic care and has provided a leadership role in promoting consideration of the client's spirituality as part of holistic care (Burkhardt & Nagai-Jacobson, 2002, 2005). Nursing associations such as the American Holistic Nurses Association (AHNA) and the CNA challenge nurses to have a holistic view of persons and include the spiritual dimension as part of this view (American Holistic Nurses Association, 2009; CNA, 2008). Holistic nursing practice is also central to most nursing theories—for example, Leininger's theory of cultural diversity and Watson's human caring theory (Becker, 2009).

Lundberg and Kerdonfag (2010) connect the goal of nursing to a holistic perspective when they identify this goal as " . . . to help people gain harmony in body, mind, and spirit and find meaning in their existence and experiences . . . . Nurses are responsible for creating the most conducive physical, social and spiritual conditions for their patients' recovery" (p. 1122). Others, for example O'Brien (2011), also connect holistic care to the goal of nursing. Therefore, if nurses ignore spiritual needs, holistic care is actually impaired (Baldacchino, 2011) and the goal of nursing is not achieved. As Plato so aptly put it (Jowett, 1871):

[A]s you ought not to attempt to cure the eyes without the head, or the head without the body, so neither ought you to attempt to cure the body without the soul . . . for the part can never be well unless the whole is well. (p. 11)

Reflection 3.4

Reflect on the quotes given in the discussion of the nature, values, and goals of nursing (see section on Nature, Values, and Goals of Nursing). Do you concur with the perspectives of the persons authoring the quotes? Why or why not? How do your views of the nature, values, and goals of nursing direct your nursing practice?

NURSING CODES OF ETHICS

Codes of ethics in nursing guide nursing actions and also provide "a framework for the standards of conduct" (ICN, 2012, p. 6). They are to be used by nurses along with professional standards, laws, and regulations that guide nursing practice (CNA, 2008). Specifically, codes of ethics "assist nurses in practicing ethically and working through ethical challenges that arise in practice with individuals, families, communities and public health systems" (CNA, 2008, p. 1). Furthermore, codes of ethics provide

> guidance for ethical relationships, responsibilities, behaviors and decision-making . . . a means of self-evaluation and self-reflection for ethical nursing practice . . . [and] an ethical basis from which nurses can advocate for quality work environments that support the delivery of safe, compassionate, competent and ethical care. (CNA, 2008, p. 2)

Nursing codes of ethics refer to spirituality as "an obligation of care" (Pesut, 2009b, p. 16). The ICN *Code of Ethics* (ICN, 2012) states: "Inherent in nursing is a respect for human rights, including cultural rights, the right to life and choice, to dignity and to be treated with respect. Nursing care is respectful of and unrestricted by considerations of age, colour, and creed" (p. 2). The word "creed" is defined by Green and Harkness (1997) as: "**1.** A formal statement of religious belief; a confession of faith. **2.** A system of beliefs, principles, or opinions" (p. 325). The ICN *Code of Ethics* goes on to say: "In providing care, the nurse promotes an environment in which the human rights, values, customs, and spiritual beliefs of the individual, family and community are respected" (p. 3). Nurses and nurse managers are to be "sensitive to the values, customs, and beliefs of people" (ICN, 2012, p. 7). Inherent in these statements is the assumption that the clients' spiritual and religious beliefs are to be ascertained by the nurse. Otherwise, how can there be intentional sensitivity and respect of such beliefs? An important point that Pesut (2008) makes is that the nursing literature goes beyond the "respecting" and "supporting" of clients' spirituality/religion (as phrased in codes of ethics) to actual intervention in this dimension of care.

The ICN *Code of Ethics* also focuses on the spirituality of the nurse when it states that nurses and nurse managers are to "monitor and promote the personal health of nursing staff" (ICN, 2012, p. 8). Personal health is defined by the ICN *Code of Ethics* as: "Mental, physical, social and spiritual wellbeing of the nurse" (p. 11). With respect to a nurse's own health, the ICN *Code of Ethics* also directs nursing associations to "promote healthy lifestyles for nursing professionals [and to] lobby for healthy workplaces and services for nurses" (p. 8). Presumably, such directives refer to the fostering of spiritual well-being as well as physical, social, and emotional well-being.

Both the CNA (2008) *Code of Ethics* in Canada and the ANA (2011) *Code of Ethics* in the United States have information similar to the ICN *Code of Ethics* with respect to the spiritual and religious care of clients and with respect to the spirituality of the nurse. Examining these codes will provide specific details.

From the discussion so far, it can be concluded that it is not surprising that ignoring the spiritual dimension in nursing practice would be unethical (Post, Puchalski, & Larson, 2000; Wright, 1998). In fact, referring to the inclusion of religion/spirituality into nursing practice, Sampson (1982) terms it "the neglected ethic"—neglected not due to a deliberate act, but because of a lack of information on this aspect of nursing care.

NURSING AND RELATED THEORISTS

Because nursing needs to be evidence based and grounded in theory, it is appropriate to observe whether nurse theorists incorporate spirituality into their nursing theories, models, and frameworks. Many contemporary nurse theorists advocate for holistic nursing care, which includes spiritual care. For example, Chung, Wong, and Chan (2007) conducted a review of nurse theorists and concluded that "nursing scholars agree that humans are bio-psycho-social-spiritual beings. Some scholars consider spirituality as the core (e.g., Nightingale, Watson) but others treat it as an isolated dimension without any integration (e.g., Henderson's)" (p. 160).

With respect to examining the place of spirituality in nurse theorists' work, there have been several reviews conducted. Oldnall (1996) reviewed 26 nurse theorists examining the inclusion of spirituality into their theories. Twelve theorists were deemed not to include spirituality in theories, whereas some others referred to it implicitly without explanation of terminology used (with the exception of Watson's theory). Only two theorists, Watson and Neuman, were identified as acknowledging spirituality in a significant way within the development of their theories. Martsolf and Mickley (1998) also examined the concept of spirituality in nursing theories. One of their conclusions was that some theorists do not address the concept of spirituality (e.g., King, Peplau, Orem, & Orlando Pelletier). Others imply or embed the concept of spirituality within their theories as a subconcept (e.g., Levine, Johnson, Roy, Leininger, & Rogers). Furthermore, for some theorists spirituality is included as a major focus so that if the concept were removed from the theory, it would cause a significant theoretical shift (e.g., Neuman, Newman, Parse, & Watson). One important point that Martsolf and Mickley make is that spirituality is viewed differently by nurse theorists who have a reciprocal interaction worldview. This approach perceives people as multidimensional; and spirituality is seen as one dimension of a person, which interacts with other dimensions. Conversely, some theorists embrace the simultaneous action worldview where spirituality is viewed as "patterning focusing on inner experiences, feelings, values, etc." (p. 300). Martsolf and Mickley classify each nursing theory/model according to the theorist's worldview and the extent to which spirituality is addressed in the theory/model. Pesut's analysis of nine nurse theorists (Pesut, 2009b) took a different view. She examined theorists' writings from a position of theism (Christian perspective), humanism (universal spiritual dimension of personhood), and monism (universal consciousness with the nature of persons seen as energy). Pesut classified nursing theories into each of these three categories, and included the implications of each theory for nursing care. Other authors have also discussed the incorporation of spirituality into nursing theorists' work, for example, O'Brien (2011), Taylor (2002), and Wright (2005).

A review of each of the references mentioned in the previous paragraph leads to a more in-depth discussion. It is sufficient here to assert that the very foundation of how nursing is conceived by many nurse theorists includes some or significant focus on spirituality. As O'Brien (2011) states, "As more grand nursing theory, as well as theory of the middle range is generated, scholars anticipate that spirituality will be an important concept of interest. One example is the work of Judith Allen Shelly and Arline Miller, *Called to Care: A Christian Theology of Nursing* (1999)" (pp. 144–145). O'Brien goes on to say that the writings of theorists discussed in her book (Henderson, Abdellah, Travelbee, Neuman, Roy, Parse, Watson, and Paterson & Zderad) contain key words that are "related to patients' spiritual needs, including faith, worship, spiritual goals, spiritual values, transcendence, human soul, higher authority, and organized religion. Identifying the patient's understanding of these concepts is important for a nurse undertaking the practice of spiritual care" (p. 147).

Taylor (2002) points out that nurses use many theories that are external to the discipline of nursing, but such theories also support the inclusion of spiritual care for people experiencing health challenges. Examples cited by Taylor include grief theories, stress and coping theories, and crisis theories. There is ample support for a theoretical rationale advocating for the inclusion of spirituality into nursing practice.

The Positioning of Nurses

Nurses are the largest group of health care providers, have the most frequent contact with clients, and are involved with people at all points across the life span (Battey, 2012; Hoglund, 2013; Iacono, 2011; Kazemipour, Amin, & Pourseidi, 2012; Taylor, 2006). Clients in health care facilities usually have access to nurses on 24–7 basis. This is important, as it has been observed that it is during the late evening hours and night that clients are most vulnerable. It is during those times of the day that "support [including spiritual support] must be offered by a nurse because only that moment exists" (Iacono, 2011, p. 417). Thus, of all health care providers, nurses are seen to be the most accessible to those experiencing illness and other health-related crises.

Not only are nurses accessible to clients, but the nature and context of the nurse–client relationship is also conducive to providing spiritual care. Nurses encounter clients in their most private and intimate moments, and are focused on helping them deal with difficult life situations, such as pain, suffering, and illness. They do this by providing support, encouragement, and guidance (Creel, 2007; Hoglund, 2013; Hollywell & Walker, 2009; Hubbartt, Corey, & Kautz, 2012). As spirituality is often connected to illness and other significant life events, it is logical that nurses should be potential spiritual resources. As Ozbasaran and colleagues (2011) state, "Often, nurses encounter patients during 'rough parts of the trail' when spiritual care becomes one of the major components in holistic care" (p. 3103).

Nurses are often trusted by clients, creating a positive environment for conversations about matters, such as spirituality (Taylor, 2003). Nurses are seen as potential spiritual resources by clients (Highfield et al., 2000), but it is also the case, as confirmed by research, that nurses themselves consider spirituality as being integral to nursing care (Lundmark, 2006; Milligan, 2004; Stranahan, 2001; Taylor, 2002). Therefore, from this emic (or insider) perspective of nurses, there is clear rationale for the inclusion of spirituality into nursing practice. Nurses are also deemed to be the liaison people who are responsible for consistent care, including spiritual care (Baldacchino, 2006). In fact, there are some who believe that nurses *need* to focus on the spiritual needs of clients as the availability and extent of chaplaincy and pastoral care services declines (Battey, 2012).

As can be observed from the discussion, nurses are generally well positioned to be engaged with the spirituality of clients and their families, and, as such, nurses should be focusing on clients' spiritual needs and resources.

Reflection 3.5

Reflect on the notion of the nurse being the health care professional that is most accessible to clients. What factors contribute to the nurse being not only physically accessible to clients but also emotionally and spiritually accessible to them? How can one deal with factors that limit or restrain accessibility?

NURSING DIAGNOSTIC TAXONOMIES

The nursing process is a well-recognized tool in nursing practice, albeit there are some concerns regarding the use of the nursing process within the context of spiritual issues. Part of the nursing process involves the diagnosis of various client concerns, including spiritual concerns. Nursing diagnostic taxonomies (e.g., the North American Nursing Diagnosis Association-International [NANDA-I], 2011) include "spiritual distress" and "potential for enhanced spiritual well-being" as legitimate nursing diagnoses. Practice guidelines can also be found for such diagnoses. The NANDA-I is recognized internationally for its development of standardized terminology that is evidence based and that focuses on the safety and health care of people (Sessanna, Finnell, Underhill, Chang, & Peng, 2011).

A particular response to a client's needs may impact whether or not a health crisis will result in spiritual distress or spiritual growth (Timmins & Kelly, 2008). Obviously, nurses will want to promote spiritual growth and prevent spiritual distress as their norms. However, if such distress occurs, then the appropriate action is to alleviate such distress.

IMPORTANCE IN NURSING EDUCATION

Upon perusal of the nursing literature, it is found that there is much discussion not only about the lack of education in nursing on the spiritual dimension of practice, but also about the necessity of ensuring that such education is provided in both foundational nursing programs and continuing (or ongoing) nurse education programs. With respect to spirituality, education is proposed to encourage the growth of the nurse's own spirituality, to improve the nurse–client relationship, to improve attitudes toward spiritual care, and to improve competence and comfort in providing spiritual care (Cockell & McSherry, 2012; Highfield et al., 2000; Hoover, 2002; Musgrave & McFarlane, 2004; Narayanasamy, 1999; Wasner et al., 2005).

Various nursing education bodies endorse the importance of nursing education on the spiritual dimension of care. For example, the American Association of Colleges of Nursing (AACN, 2008, 2011) has developed an education framework for the education of nurses at both the undergraduate and graduate levels, which has outcomes related to the spiritual dimension of care. A holistic view of care is embedded in nursing curricula (AACN, 2008; Canadian Association of Schools of Nursing, 2015). In Canada, a national nursing framework includes guiding principles and essential components related to spirituality (Canadian Association of Schools of Nursing, 2015). Accreditation documents identify one of the goals of nursing education bodies is the assessment of the extent to which nursing programs reflect nursing professional standards and guidelines. This is the case in the United States: the Commission on Collegiate Nursing Education (2013) and the National League for Nursing Accrediting Commission Standards and Criteria (2016); and in Canada: the Canadian Association of Schools of Nursing (2014) Accreditation Standards.

If nursing education includes information about spirituality in the curriculum, then there needs to be a means by which nursing students and new graduates apply this knowledge into practice. Nurses in practice are expected to participate in the education of nursing students as part of their professional responsibilities, and are in a prime position to identify learning opportunities related to the spiritual dimension of care. Nurse managers also have a responsibility to ensure that nurses are delivering competent, holistic care, including spiritual care (Speck, 2005). Therefore, they have a responsibility to ensure that nurses are educated about such care. Nurse managers as well as practicing nurses need to create an environment conducive to the transfer of knowledge from theory about spiritual care to practice in spiritual care.

If nursing education frameworks, nursing curricula outcomes, and nursing education accreditation standards all reference and include spirituality and spiritual care, then it provides clear rationale for the inclusion of this concept into nursing education and practice.

Reflection 3.6

Reflect on your nursing education to date. What aspects of the nursing curriculum contained information related to the spiritual dimension of nursing practice? What were the topics of focus? How was the education delivered (e.g., a course, a class, a seminar, a workshop)? In your opinion, has this education been sufficiently extensive to contribute significantly to your sense of competency in attending to clients' spiritual issues and needs? If so, then in what ways? If not, then how can you facilitate your own education in this area of practice, and perhaps the education of your peers?

NURSING LEADERSHIP ROLE

The nursing profession is generating an increasingly important body of knowledge and insight into the relationship between spirituality and health/illness care (Hoffert, Henshaw, & Mvududu, 2007; Iranmanesh, Tirgari, & Cheraghi, 2011). In fact, according to Smith (2008), nursing as a profession is seen as the most advanced of all of the health care professions in terms of its focus on spirituality and spiritual care in practice. Swinton and McSherry (2006) agree when they state: "Indeed, of all the caring professions, nursing is probably the most advanced and forward thinking within this area of care . . . . [Nursing has offered] new, rich and challenging insights and clarifications in relation to this vital and sometimes contentious area of research and practice" (p. 801). This leadership role needs to continue and expand as nursing not only internally impacts its own profession in terms of the spiritual dimension of care, but also externally by positively influencing other helping professions.

If nurses contribute to the knowledge about spirituality and spiritual care through research, theory development, and practice implications, then nursing is validated as an evidence-based profession. Ties between nursing education, research, and practice will also be strengthened. Currently, there are some respectable scholars in nursing who have contributed much to the area of spirituality in nursing practice. Elizabeth Taylor, Verna Carson, Sr. Mary Elizabeth O'Brien, Wilfred McSherry, Aru Narayanasamy, Sheryl Reimer-Kirkham, Judith Shelly, Barbara Pesut, and Lorraine Wright are examples from an impressive list of such scholars. Research into these scholars will yield numerous articles and books devoted to the topic of spirituality in nursing practice, research, and education, which all serve to advance knowledge in this area.

NURSING ASSESSMENT TOOLS AND INTERVENTION MODELS

There have been many assessment tools developed by nurses for nursing practice and research. Examples include Stoll's (1979) Guidelines for Spiritual Assessment and the JAREL Spiritual Well-Being Scale (Hungelmann, Kenkel-Ross, Klassen, & Stollenwerk, 1996). Many more are identified in Chapter 5 on spiritual assessment.

Nurses have also developed models, theories, and frameworks for spiritual care. Examples of these include the Trinity Model (Wright, 2005), the Theory of Spiritual Care in Nursing Practice (Burkhart & Hogan, 2008), and the T.R.U.S.T. Model for Inclusive Spiritual Care (Barss, 2012). More are considered in Chapter 6 in the discussion on spiritual care.

The main point here is that such tools, models, and theories assist nurses in learning how to conduct research in the spiritual dimension of practice and how to educate nurses in this dimension of care, and also provide rationale and guidelines for spiritual care in practice settings. As research, education, and practice continue to develop, more such tools, models, and theories will become available for nursing in terms of embracing this vital aspect of nursing care.

PROFESSIONAL MANDATES

Codes of ethics for nurses have already been discussed as providing rationale for the inclusion of spirituality into nursing practice. In addition, other professional mandates require spiritual care to be included as part of health care (Hoffert et al., 2007). Examples include hospital/institutional accreditation organizations, such as the Joint Commission on Accreditation in the United States (Lemmer, 2010; Ruder, 2013). Although such accreditation organizations are not focused specifically on nurses, they do focus on the overall provision of health care relevant for nursing.

Other prominent health care organizations include information about spiritual care in their practice directives, and advocate for health care professional education on spirituality. In the United States, these organizations are the National Hospice and Palliative Care Organization and the Oncology Nursing Society; in Canada, the Canadian Hospice Palliative Care Association and the Canadian Association of Nurses in Oncology; and worldwide, the WHO. Professional associations from a variety of health care disciplines also endorse the inclusion of spiritual care in client care, such as the British Medical Association, the American Holistic Medical Association, and the International Federation of Social Workers.

Various health care policy documents also recognize the spiritual dimension of care. A significant one in Canada is the report by Romanow (2002), *Building on Values: The Future of Health Care in Canada.* Some organizations focus primarily on spirituality in health care, such as The Janki Foundation for Spirituality in Health Care, which have as two of their aims: "To provide an education forum for healthcare professionals by exploring how spirituality can be integrated into current working practices" [and] "To enhance understanding among patients and the public of the value of spirituality in healing and well-being" (The Janki Foundation for Spirituality in Health Care, 2016).

Professional associations focusing on nurses also promote spiritual care in practice. The ICN, the CNA, and the ANA have been previously referenced in the discussion on codes of ethics in nursing. Other documents published by these bodies also advocate for spiritual care, such as *Vision for the Future of Nursing* (ICN, 2007); *The Position Statement: Spirituality, Health and Nursing Practice* (CNA, 2010); and the book, *Nursing's Social Policy Statement: The Essence of the Profession* (ANA, 2003). The AHNA and parish nursing associations in both Canada and the United States also promote and educate about spiritual care in nursing. Some organizations, such as Nurses Christian Fellowship (an international organization), promote and educate nurses from a particular worldview, in their case: Christian.

As can be seen from these examples of professional mandates (and there are many more), spirituality is intended to be part of health care and nursing care. Because of such mandates, many agencies will have developed and/or adopted policies related to spiritual care for their particular agencies.

NURSING STANDARDS AND COMPETENCIES

Nursing education standards and competencies related to spiritual care have already been discussed. Nursing practice standards have implications for spiritual assessment and spiritual care (Lantz, 2007; McEwen, 2005; Pesut, 2009b): for example, the CNA's *Framework for the Practice of Registered Nurses in Canada* (CNA, 2015) and the ANA's *Nursing: Scope and Standards of Practice* (ANA, 2010). Specific groups within nursing also have standards relevant for spiritual assessment and care, for example, the Canadian Holistic Nursing Association (2009).

Competencies for spiritual care in nursing practice are discussed more thoroughly in Chapter 4. However, it should be noted here that both the United States and Canada have national nursing competencies focused on spiritual assessment and spiritual care of clients. The inclusion of a focus on the spiritual dimension of practice in both nursing standards and nursing competencies means that such a focus is not optional, or an "add-on" for nursing care, but such a focus needs to be integral to the practice of nursing.

SUMMARY OF RATIONALE

Overall, the discussion provides rationale for the inclusion of spirituality into nursing practice. There is ample guidance in the literature and in nurses' clinical wisdom to support this inclusion. As Mattison (2006) asks, "What do health care providers have to lose by integrating the spiritual dimension into care delivery and accessing a powerful intervention that can make a difference to patients" (p. 32)? To expand understanding and competency in articulating the rationale for the inclusion of spirituality into nursing practice, a thorough review of the resources identified for each rationale is recommended.

Reflection 3.7

Reflect on the many reasons for the inclusion of spirituality into nursing practice. Can you think of any additional reasons as to why spirituality should be included? How has your perspective been enriched by this discussion? Are you now more enthused and motivated to include the spiritual dimension in your own nursing practice?

CHALLENGES TO INCORPORATING SPIRITUAL CARE INTO NURSING PRACTICE, EDUCATION, AND RESEARCH

Although there is ample rationale for the inclusion of spirituality into nursing practice, education, and research, there are also challenges to such inclusion. Some would identify these challenges as "barriers," but the word "challenges" seems to have more potential for positive action with respect to exploring each challenge and ways to overcome it. Table 3.1 summarizes many of the challenges identified by nurses as existing within themselves and within their work environment. The challenges are discussed in the nursing literature complete with examples of supporting documentation.

Each challenge needs to be addressed by nurses. But because many of the challenges lie within the overall health care system/environment itself, they also need to be addressed by other health care professionals, health care managers, and government officials. Some challenges can be addressed by education in the area of spirituality in nursing and by conducting and/or considering research that would refute a challenge. For example, with respect to the challenge of "lack of time," in van Dover and Bacon's study (2001), it was found that nurses were providing spiritual care within a few hours of meeting the client/family. This suggests that spiritual care does not always require an in-depth knowledge of the person or situation, nor a long-term nurse–client relationship. Furthermore, with respect to time management, spirituality is so intricately connected to health and well-being that it can consume *more* time to *not* address it. For example, a client might initially present with considerable emotional distress and multiple physical ailments and complaints. After several medical tests, which generated normal results, more in-depth assessment might reveal that the "root" of the symptoms is related to a spiritual issue arising from a loss of meaning and purpose in life or some significant life event, or even guilt over an adulterous affair. Time and resources might be expended in addressing the emotional and physical complaints (and rightly so, as these would be very real to the client). However, if the spiritual issues are not dealt with, in a timely fashion, then the client's issues may never be fully addressed.

Table 3.1 Challenges to Spiritual Care

Challenges	References
Lack of awareness, uncertainty, comfort about own spirituality, and unresolved spiritual pain	McEwen (2005); Ruder (2013); Sweat (2011)
Inadequate preparation to provide spiritual care; lack of knowledge about spiritual assessment/care	Carr (2010); Jackson (2011); Lemmer (2010); Miller (2013)
Lack of confidence/comfort in spiritual assessment and providing spiritual care, including how to converse with clients about spirituality/religion; sense of/actual lack of competence	Jackson (2011); McEwen (2005); Miller (2013); Reimer-Kirkham, Pesut, Meyerhoff, & Sawatzky (2004); Taylor (2002)
Lack of time due to staff shortages, never-ending tasks, and so forth	Biro (2012); Burkhart & Hogan (2008); Swinton & McSherry (2006)
Institutional/workplace factors such as lack of support, and nonconducive environment	Burkhart & Hogan (2008); Carr (2008, 2010); McEwen (2005)
Confusion about concept of spirituality; spiritual needs versus psychosocial needs	Molzahn & Sheilds (2008); Narayanasamy & Owens (2001)
Confusion/uncertainty about role in spiritual assessment and care in relation to chaplain/pastoral care role	Carr (2010); McEwen (2005); Ruder (2013)
Health care system emphasis on physical/technical care/empirical science/economics	Carr (2008, 2010); Gilbert (2010); McSherry & Jamieson (2011); Miller (2013)
Spirituality of clients in a pluralistic society	Cockwell & McSherry (2012); Pesut (2009a, 2009b)
Differing spiritual beliefs/values of clients and nurses and appropriate action needed	Pesut (2009a, 2009c)
Ethical issues such as appropriateness of interventions, professional competency, boundaries	Pesut (2009a, 2009c)

(continued)

Table 3.1 Challenges to Spiritual Care (*continued*)

Challenges	References
Fear of being intrusive/proselytizing	McEwen (2005); Narayanasamy (2011); Pesut (2008)
Negative personal views of religion/religious people	National Health Service (NHS) Education for Scotland (2009)
Seeing spirituality/religion as "private" to client and therefore hesitant to explore same	Carson (1989)
Trend in society and health care toward secularism	Molzahn & Sheilds (2008)

Other challenges to incorporating spiritual care into nursing practice can be addressed through reflection on practice and from clinical experiences. For example, in addressing some of the challenges to spiritual care, Creel (2007) posed some thought-provoking questions for reflection by nurses relating to spiritual care: "How much education would it take to treat a person like a human being and not just a medical diagnosis? How much time would it take to smile and touch a person's hand while pushing the intravenous medicine? How much privacy would be needed to ask a person if they are afraid?" (p. 19).

Reflection 3.8

Reflect on the challenges to spiritual care as outlined in Table 3.1:

- Would you add any challenges to this list that you have encountered or that arise from your reflection?
- Which of these challenges have you encountered in your own nursing practice? How have you dealt with these challenges? Or, how might you deal with them?

This chapter has provided rationale for the inclusion of spirituality/religion into nursing practice. Such rationale can engender confidence in nurses as they endeavor to incorporate the spiritual dimension into their nursing practice. It can also provide the basis for advocacy for such inclusion in settings in which nurses practice.

The Bottom Line

- There is ample rationale for the inclusion of spirituality and spiritual care into nursing practice, education, and research.

- Being familiar with the rationale can facilitate personal inclusion of spirituality into one's nursing practice.

- The rationale for the inclusion of spirituality into nursing practice can be used to advocate for more attention to the spiritual dimension of nursing practice.

- Awareness of the challenges to spiritual care in nursing practice is one of the first steps in promoting spiritual care in one's own practice and also in advocating for spiritual care to be incorporated as an essential aspect of nursing practice in general.

- Challenges to incorporating spiritual care into nursing practice need to be seen as opportunities for growth in this area of practice as opposed to barriers that cannot be removed.

Taking It Further

1. Conduct a review of the nursing literature to examine for yourself the extent of articles and books on the spiritual dimension of nursing practice. You can use such search words as "spiritual," "spirituality," "religion," "spiritual care," "religious care," "spiritual assessment," and "spirit." Make a plan to read a number of the references each week to further your knowledge in this area of nursing care.

2. Create a "Movie Spirituality" group to search for and view movies that focus on some aspect of spirituality in the lives of the people featured in the movie. Watch a movie each week or month. Following the movie, discuss:

    a. Aspects of the movie that relate to spirituality

    b. Views of spirituality portrayed in the movie and how they are similar to or different from those of the people in the group who watch the movie

    c. The possible implications for nurses responding to any societal interest in spirituality as portrayed in the movies

3. Write your own ideas about the nature, values, and goals of nursing. How many of your ideas are related to some aspect of spirituality as discussed in this book? What are the implications for your nursing practice?

4. Review the literature related to the "art of nursing." What aspects of the discussion about this aspect of the nature of nursing relate to the provision of spiritual care? Compare and contrast the provision of spiritual care within a technological view of nursing and also within a view of nursing that sees it as a

healing art. Toward which view of nursing do you more heavily lean? How might viewing the nature of nursing as both a "science" and an "art" open up advanced possibilities with respect to attending to the spiritual dimension in nursing practice?

5. In your clinical practice, identify clients who you consider to be resilient. Have a conversation with them about the place of spirituality/religion in their lives. If it is important to the clients, then discuss with them how they perceive spirituality/religion to be of assistance to them in fostering resilience.

6. In a group setting, discuss each of the challenges to incorporating spirituality into nursing practice. Discuss how, or if, you would refute the challenge—as well as how you might address it. Who else, besides nursing, needs to be involved in addressing certain challenges and how might they be involved?

7. What personal characteristics do you possess that might impact on how you would converse with clients or colleagues about why spirituality is important to nursing practice? Which characteristics would be facilitative to such conversations, and which would be restricting? How can you address the characteristics that would restrict such conversations?

8. Research standards of practice for registered nurses in your own jurisdiction. Identify those that refer directly or indirectly to the spiritual and religious care of clients.

9. Research the practice specialty of parish nursing. Interview and spend some time with a parish nurse to broaden your perspective on the spiritual dimension of nursing practice in that context. How have these two activities broadened your perspective on this aspect of nursing care?

10. Interview a number of people in management positions in health care agencies. Inquire with respect to identifying agency policies that are related to the provision of spiritual care within their agency. What conclusions can you draw from this exercise?

11. Research the major nursing theories/models/frameworks presented in this chapter (see section on Nursing and Related Theorists). What specific aspects of these are related directly or indirectly to seeing clients and nursing as involving spiritual matters? What spiritual care nursing actions might be suggested in each theory/model/framework? Which are most helpful in terms of guidance for attending to the spiritual dimension of clients?

12. Review the two worldviews that Faucett (1993, 1995, as discussed in Martsolf & Mickley, 1998) discusses as being reflected in nursing theories and models, namely the reciprocal interaction worldview and the simultaneous action worldview. Identify how spirituality is reflected in each worldview. What are the implications for nursing practice?

13. Review the discussion of spirituality as a central concept in the theories/models of Neuman, Newman, Parse, and Watson in Martsolf and Mickley (1998). For each theory/model, develop case studies based on your area of nursing in which

some aspects of spirituality or religion are relevant for the client. Discuss these case studies with colleagues, including what spiritual care actions might be warranted and what might be the possible benefit of these actions.

14. Pesut (2013) has reflected on her experience as a scholar writing on the area of spirituality in nursing. She identifies three challenges within nursing that spirituality has attempted to address:

    a. To connect across differences in a globalized world

    b. To be "good" (p. 7) in a world of uncertain morality

    c. To find meaning in a disenchanted world

    Read Pesut's description of each of these challenges. What is your response to her ponderings? What are the implications for nursing as a profession?

15. Review the article by Pesut (2009a), which focuses on ontologies of nursing in an age of spiritual pluralism. Reflect on and discuss the following ideas present by Pesut as they pertain to nursing and to spiritual care in nursing:

    a. The secularization and sacralization within society

    b. The issue of ontological unity or diversity within nursing

    c. Ontology from the naturalistic/reductive and the holistic/unitary perspectives

    d. The issue of common ontology versus common ethics

16. Review the ICN *Code of Ethics* for Nurses (ICN, 2012):

    a. Identify phrases in each element of the code that relate directly or indirectly to spiritual or religious care.

    b. Study the standards of conduct that relate directly or indirectly to spiritual care under each of the elements in the code.

    c. Reflect on/discuss what each of these standards means to you personally.

    d. Reflect on/discuss how the standards can be applied to nursing practice so as to provide ethical spiritual care.

    e. Reflect on/discuss examples from nursing practice to identify ethical dilemmas and standards of conduct related to spiritual/religious care of clients. How might such dilemmas be resolved?

    f. Reflect on/discuss how nurses and nurse leaders can ensure that standards of conduct related to spiritual and religious care are translated into action? (Adapted from ICN, 2012, p. 6)

17. Review the code of ethics for nurses for nurses in your jurisdiction. Identify phrases and clauses that may be relevant to the spiritual/religious care of clients.

18. Review various professional mandates related to health, as referenced in the discussion in this chapter (see section on Professional Mandates). Identify material that may be relevant for spiritual and religious care of clients in these mandates.

19. Review the article by Cockell and McSherry (2012) in which they state: "Much has been learned about spiritual care over the last few years through a variety of research across contexts and countries. While there is much still to learn, enough is known to provide a solid evidence base [for including spiritual care in nursing practice]" (p. 966). Reflect on/discuss the following questions:

a. How can evidence-based information regarding spiritual care and nursing enable best practices to be developed?

b. How can the evidence regarding spiritual care and nursing address poor care delivery, the nurse's motivation to provide spiritual care, and the need for a nonmedicalized approach to care?

c. Which research tools might be appropriate to educate nurses about spiritual care and the delivery of spiritual care in your area of nursing practice?

d. What can be learned about spiritual care in oncology/palliative care that can be applied to your own practice setting?

e. How can clients be kept at the center of spiritual care so that spiritual care is relevant to them?

f. How can spiritual care departments/chaplains be of assistance in promoting and providing spiritual care and spiritual care education of nurses in your area of practice?

g. How can the seven activities for nurse managers who want to respond to the research on spiritual care in nursing (Cockell & McSherry, p. 966) be of assistance to you in your own nursing practice?

REFERENCES

American Association of Colleges of Nursing. (2008). *The essentials of baccalaureate education for professional nursing practice*. Retrieved from http://www.aacn.nche.edu/education-resources/BaccEssentials08.pdf

American Association of Colleges of Nursing. (2011). *The essentials of master's education in nursing*. Retrieved from http://www.aacn.nche.edu/education-resources/mastersessentials11.pdf

American Holistic Nurses Association. (2009). *What is holistic nursing?* Retrieved from http://www.ahna.org/AboutUs/WhatisHolisticNursing/tabid/1165/Default.aspx

American Nurses Association. (2003). *Nursing's social policy statement: The essence of the profession*. Silver Spring, MD: American Nurses Association.

American Nurses Association. (2010). *Nursing: Scope and standards of practice*. Silver Spring, MD: American Nurses Association.

American Nurses Association. (2011). *Code of ethics for nurses*. Retrieved from http://www.nursingworld.org/codeofethics

Baldacchino, D. (2006). Nursing competencies for spiritual care. *Journal of Clinical Nursing, 15*(7), 885–896. doi:10.1111/j.1365-2702.2006.01643.x

Baldacchino, D. (2011). Teaching on spiritual care: The perceived impact on qualified nurses. *Nurse Education in Practice, 11*(1), 47–53. doi:10.1016/j.nepr.2010.06.008

Barnum, B. S. (1996). *Spirituality in nursing: From tradition to new age*. New York, NY: Springer Publishing Company.

Barss, K. S. (2012). Building bridges: An interpretive phenomenological analysis of nurse educators' clinical experience using the T.R.U.S.T. Model for Inclusive Spiritual Care. *International Journal of Nursing Education Scholarship, 9*(1), 1–17. doi:10.1515/1548-923X.2389

Battey, B. W. (2012). Perspectives of spiritual care for nurse managers. *Journal of Nursing Management*, 20(8), 1012–1020. doi:10.1111/j.1365-2834.2012.01360.x

Becker, A. L. (2009). Ethical considerations of teaching spirituality in the academy. *Nursing Ethics*, 16(6), 697–706. doi:10.1177/0969733009342639

Biro, A. (2012). Creating conditions for good nursing care by attending to the spiritual. *Journal of Nursing Management*, 20(8), 1002–1011. doi:10.1111/j.1365-2834.2012.01444.x

Bonanno, G., Papa, A., & O'Neill, K. (2001). Loss and human resilience. *Applied and Preventive Psychology*, 10(3), 193–206.

Bonanno, G. A. (2004). Loss, trauma, and human resilience: Have we underestimated the human capacity to thrive after extremely aversive events? *American Psychologist*, 59(1), 20–28. doi:10.1037/0003-066X.59.1.20

Bonting, S. L. (2005). *Creation and double chaos: Science and theology in discussion*. Minneapolis, MN: Fortress Press.

Brady, M. J., Peterman, A. H., Fitchett, G., Mo, M., & Cella, D. (1999). A case for including spirituality in quality of life measurement in oncology. *Psycho-Oncology*, 8(5), 417–428. doi:10.1002/(SICI)1099-1611(199909/10)8:5<417::AID-PON398>3.0.CO;2-4

Burkhardt, M. A., & Nagai-Jacobson, M. G. (2002). *Spirituality: Living our connectedness*. Albany, NY: Delmar.

Burkhardt, M., & Nagai-Jacobson, M. (2005). Spirituality and health. In B. Dossey, L. Keegan, & C. Guzzetta (Eds.), *Holistic Nursing: A handbook for practice* (4th ed., pp. 168–172). Sudbury, MA: Jones & Bartlett.

Burkhart, L., & Hogan, N. (2008). An experiential theory of spiritual care in nursing practice. *Qualitative Health Research*, 18(7), 928–938. doi:10.1177/1049732308318027

Callister, L. C., Bond, A. E., Matsumura, G., & Mangum, S. (2004). Threading spirituality throughout nursing education. *Holistic Nursing Practice*, 18(3), 160–166.

Cameron, M. E. (2003). Legal and ethical issues: Our best ethical and spiritual values. *Journal of Professional Nursing*, 19(3), 117–118. doi:10.1016/S8755-7223(03)00067.X

Canadian Association of Schools of Nursing. (2014). *Accreditation program standards*. Retrieved from http://www.casn.ca/wp-content/uploads/2014/12/2014-FINAL-EN-Accred-standards-March-311.pdf

Canadian Association of Schools of Nursing. (2015). *National education framework: Baccalaureate*. Retrieved from http://www.casn.ca/wp-content/uploads/2014/12/FINAL-BACC-Framwork-FINAL-SB-Jan-2016.pdf

Canadian Holistic Nurses Association. (2009). *Standards of practice*. Retrieved from http://www.chna.ca/standards-of-practice

Canadian Nurses Association. (2008). *Code of ethics for registered nurses*. Retrieved from https://www.cna-aiic.ca/~/media/cna/page-content/pdf-fr/code-of-ethics-for-registered-nurses.pdf?la=en

Canadian Nurses Association. (2010). *Position statement: Spirituality, health and nursing practice*. Retrieved from https://www.cna-aiic.ca/~/media/cna/page-content/pdf-en/ps111_spirituality_2010_e.pdf?la=en

Canadian Nurses Association. (2015). *Framework for the practice of registered nurses in Canada*. Retrieved from https://www.cna-aiic.ca/~/media/cna/page-content/pdf-en/framework-for-the-pracice-of-registered-nurses-in-canada.pdf?la=en

Carr, T. (2008). Mapping the processes and qualities of spiritual nursing care. *Qualitative Health Research*, 18(5), 686–700. doi:10.1177/1049732307308979

Carr, T. J. (2010). Facing existential realities: Exploring barriers and challenges to spiritual nursing care. *Qualitative Health Research*, 20(10), 1379–1392. doi:10.1177/1049732310372377

Carson, V. B. (1989). *Spiritual dimensions of nursing practice*. Philadelphia, PA: Saunders.

Chung, L. Y. F., Wong, F. K. Y., & Chan, M. F. (2007). Relationship of nurses' spirituality to their understanding and practice of spiritual care. *Journal of Advanced Nursing*, 58(2), 158–170. doi:10.1111/j.1365-2648.2007.04225.x

Clarke, J. (2009). A critical view of how nursing has defined spirituality. *Journal of Clinical Nursing*, 18(12), 1666–1673. doi:10.1111/j.1365-2702.2008.02707.x

Cockell, N., & McSherry, W. (2012). Spiritual care in nursing: An overview of published international research. *Journal of Nursing Management, 20*(8), 958–969. doi:10.1111/j.1365-2834.2012.01450.x

Cohen, M. Z., Holley, L. M., Wengel, S. P., & Katzman, M. (2012). A platform for nursing research on spirituality and religiosity: Definitions and measures. *Western Journal of Nursing Research, 34*(6), 795–817. doi:10.1177/0193945912444321

Commission on Collegiate Nursing Education. (2013). *Standards for accreditation of baccalaureate and graduate nursing programs.* Retrieved from http://www.aacn.nche.edu/ccne-accreditation/stan dards-Amended-2013.pdf

Creel, E. (2007). The meaning of spiritual nursing care for the ill individual with no religious affiliation. *International Journal for Human Caring, 11*(3), 14–21.

Curlin, F. A., Chad, J., Roach, B. S., Gorawara-Bhat, R., Lantos, J. D., & Chin, M. H. (2005). When patients choose faith over medicine: Physician perspectives on religiosity-related conflict in the medical encounter. *Archives of International Medicine, 165*(1), 88–91. doi:10.1001/archinte.165.1.88

Daaleman, T. P., Cobb, A. K., & Frey, B. B. (2001). Spirituality and well-being: An exploratory study of the patient perspective. *Social Science & Medicine, 53*(11), 1503–1511. doi:10.1016/S0277 -9536(00)00439-1

Davie, G. (1994). *Religion in Britain since 1945: Believing without belonging.* Oxford, England: Blackwell.

Fahrenwald, N. L., Bassett, S. D., Tschetter, L., Carson, P. P., White, L., & Winterboer, V. J. (2005). Teaching core nursing values. *Journal of Professional Nursing, 21*(1), 46–51. doi:10.1016/j.profnurs .2004.11.001

Frankl, V. E. (1985). *Man's search for meaning: An introduction to logotherapy.* New York, NY: Washington Square Press.

Gilbert, P. (2010). Seeking inspiration: The rediscovery of the spiritual dimension in health and social care in England. *Mental Health, Religion & Culture, 13*(6), 533–546. doi:10.1080/13674676.2 010.488422

Green, S., & Harkness, J. (1997). *ITP Nelson Canadian Dictionary of the English language: An encyclopedic reference.* Scarborough, ON, Canada: Thomson.

Hexem, K. R., Mollen, C. J., Carroll, K., Lanctot, D. A., & Feudtner, C. (2011). How parents of children receiving pediatric palliative care use religious, spiritual, or life philosophy in tough times. *Journal of Palliative Medicine, 14*(10), 39–44. doi:10.1089/jpm.2010.0256

Highfield, M. E. F., Taylor, E. J., & Amenta, M. O. (2000). Preparation to care: The spiritual care education of oncology and hospice nurses. *Journal of Hospice & Palliative Nursing, 2*(2), 53–63.

Hoffert, D., Henshaw, C., & Mvududu, N. (2007). Enhancing the ability of nursing students to perform a spiritual assessment. *Nurse Educator, 32*(2), 66–72. doi:10.1097/01.NNE.0000264327.17921.b7

Hoglund, B. A. (2013). Practicing the code of ethics, finding the image of God. *Journal of Christian Nursing, 30*(4), 228–233. doi:10.1097/CNJ.0b013e3182a18d40

Hollywell, C., & Walker, J. (2009). Private prayer as a suitable intervention for hospitalized patients: A critical review of the literature. *Journal of Clinical Nursing, 18*(5), 637–651. doi:10.1111/j.1365 -2702.2008.02510.x

Hoover, J. (2002). The personal and professional impact of undertaking an education module on human caring. *Journal of Advanced Nursing, 37*(1), 79–86. doi:10.1046/j.1365-2648.2002.02051.x

Horton, K., Tschudin, V., & Forget, A. (2007). The value of nursing: A literature review. *Nursing Ethics, 14*(6), 716–740. doi:10.1177/0969733007082112

Hubbartt, B., Corey, D., & Kautz, D. D. (2012). Prayer at the bedside. *International Journal for Human Caring, 16*(1), 42–46.

Hufford, D. J., Fritts, M. J., & Rhodes, J. E. (2010). Spiritual fitness. *Military Medicine, 175*(8S), 73–87. doi:10.7205/MILMED-D-10-00075

Hungelmann, J., Kenkel-Rossi, E., Klassen, L., & Stollenwerk, R. (1996). Focus on spiritual well-being: Harmonious interconnectedness of mind-body-spirit—use of the JAREL spiritual well-being scale. *Geriatric Nursing, 17*(6), 262–266. doi:10.1016/S0197-4572(96)80238-2

Iacono, M. V. (2011). *Colleagues in caring: Pastoral care at the bedside. Journal of PeriAnesthesia Nursing, 26*(6), 416–419. doi:10.1016/j.jopan.2011.09.003

International Council of Nurses. (2007). *Vision for the future of nursing.* Retrieved from http://www
.icn.ch/who-we-are/icns-vision-for-the-future-of-nursing

International Council of Nurses. (2012). *The ICN code of ethics for nurses.* Retrieved from http://www
.icn.ch/images/stories/documents/about/icncode_english.pdf

Iranmanesh, S., Tirgari, B., & Cheraghi, M. A. (2011). Developing and testing a spiritual care questionnaire in the Iranian context. *Journal of Religion & Health, 51*(4), 1104–1116. doi:10.1007/
s10943-011-9458-8

Jackson, C. (2011). Addressing spirituality: A natural aspect of holistic care. *Holistic Nursing Practice,
25*(1), 3–7. doi:10.1097/HNP.0b013e3182002b9d

Jowett, B. (1871). *The dialogues of Plato* (Vol. 1). Oxford, England: Clarendon Press.

Karairmak, O. (2004). The role of spirituality in psychological counseling. *Turkish Psychological Counseling and Guidance Journal, 22*, 45–55.

Kazemipour, F., Amin, S. A., & Pourseidi, B. (2012). Relationship between workplace spirituality
and organizational citizenship behavior among nurses through mediation of affective organizational commitment. *Journal of Nursing Scholarship, 44*(3), 302–310. doi:10.1111/j.1547-5069
.2012.01456.x

Lantz, C. M. (2007). Teaching spiritual care in a public institution: Legal implications, standards of
practice and ethical obligations. *Journal of Nursing Education, 46*(1), 33–38.

Lemmer, C. M. (2010). Reflections on teaching "Spirituality in the Healthcare Environment." *Journal of Holistic Nursing, 28*(2), 145–149. doi:10.1177/0898010109350770

Lind, B., Sendelback, S., & Steen, S. (2011). Effects of a spirituality training program for nurses on
patients in a progressive care unit. *Critical Care Nurse, 31*(3), 87–90. doi:10.4037/ccn2011372

Lundberg, P. C., & Kerdonfag, P. (2010). Spiritual care provided by Thai nurses in intensive care
units. *Journal of Clinical Nursing, 19*(7–8), 1121–1128. doi:10.1111/j.1365-2702.2009.03072.x

Lundmark, M. (2006). Attitudes to spiritual care among nursing staff in a Swedish oncology clinic.
Journal of Clinical Nursing, 15(7), 863–874. doi:10.1111/j.1365-2702.2006.01189.x

MacDonald, D. A. (2011). Studying spirituality scientifically: Reflections, considerations, recommendations. *Journal of Management, Spirituality & Religion, 8*(3), 195–210. doi:10.1080/14766086.201
1.599145

Maj, M. (2010). Forward. In P. J. Verhagen, H. M. van Praag, J. J. López-Ibor Jr., J. L. Cox, &
D. Moussaoui (Eds.), *Religion and psychiatry: Beyond boundaries* (pp. xiii–xiv). Hoboken, NJ:
Wiley.

Martsolf, D. S., & Mickley, J. R. (1998). The concept of spirituality in nursing theories: Differing
world-views and extent of focus. *Journal of Advanced Nursing, 27*(2), 294–303. doi:10.1046/
j.1365-2648.1998.00519.x

Mattison, D. (2006). The forgotten spirit: Integration of spirituality in health care. *Nephrology News
& Issues, 20*(2), 30–32.

McCord, G., Gilchrist, V. J., Grossman, S. D., King, B. D., McCormick, K. F., Oprandi, A. M., . . . Srivastava, M. (2004). Discussing spirituality with patients: A rational and ethical approach. *Annals
of Family Medicine, 2*(4), 356–361. doi:10.1370/afm.71

McEwen, M. (2005). Spiritual nursing care: State of the art. *Holistic Nursing Practice, 19*(4), 161–168.

McSherry, W., & Jamieson, S. (2011). An online survey of nurses' perceptions of spirituality and spiritual care. *Journal of Clinical Nursing, 20*(11–12), 1757–1767. doi:10.1111/j.1365-2702.2010.03547.x

McSherry, W., & Jamieson, S. (2013). The qualitative findings from an online survey investigating
nurses' perceptions of spirituality and spiritual care. *Journal of Clinical Nursing, 22*(21–22), 3170–
3182. doi:10.1111/jocn.12411

Meehan, T. C. (2012). Spirituality and spiritual care from a careful nursing perspective. *Journal of
Nursing Management, 20*(8), 990–1001. doi:10.1111/j.1365-2834.2012.01462.x

Miller, P. (2013). Thoughts on spiritual care. *Journal of Christian Nursing, 30*(3), 137. doi:10.1097/
CNJ.0b013e318299163a

Milligan, S. (2004). Perceptions of spiritual care among nurses undertaking postregistration education. *International Journal of Palliative Nursing, 10*(4), 162–171. doi:10.12968/ijpn.2004.10.4
.12792

Miner-Williams, D. (2006). Putting a puzzle together: Making spirituality meaningful for nursing using an evolving theoretical framework. *Journal of Clinical Nursing, 15*(7), 811–821. doi:10.1111/ j.1365-2702.2006.01351.x

Moberg, D. O. (2008). Spirituality and aging: Research and implications. *Journal of Religion, Spirituality & Aging, 20*(1–2), 95–134. doi:10.1080/15528030801922038

Molzahn, A. E., & Sheilds, L. (2008). Why is it so hard to talk about spirituality? *Canadian Nurse, 104*(1), 25–29.

Musgrave, C. F., & McFarlane, E. A. (2004). Israeli oncology nurses' religiosity, spiritual well-being, and attitudes towards spiritual care: A path analysis. *Oncology Nursing Forum, 31*(2), 321–327. doi:10.1188/04.ONF.321-327

Narayanasamy, A. (1999). Learning spiritual dimensions of care from a historical perspective. *Nurse Education Today, 19*(5), 386–395. doi:10.1054/nedt.1999.0325

Narayanasamy, A. (2011). Commentary on Chan MF (2009): Factors affecting nursing staff in practicing spiritual care. *Journal of Clinical Nursing,* 19 2128–2136. *Journal of Clinical Nursing, 20*(5–6), 915–916. doi:10.1111/j.1365-2702.2010.03653.x

Narayanasamy, A., & Owens, J. (2001). A critical incident study of nurses' responses to the spiritual needs of their patients. *Journal of Advanced Nursing, 33*(4), 446–455. doi:10.1046/j.1365-2648 .2001.01690.x

National Health Service (NHS) Education for Scotland. (2009). *Spiritual care matters: An introductory resource for all NHS Scotland staff.* Edinburgh, Scotland: National Health Service. Retrieved from http://www.nes.scot.nhs.uk/media/3723/spiritualcaremattersfinal.pdf

North American Nursing Diagnosis Association-International. (2011). *Nursing diagnoses: Definitions and classification 2012-2014.* Indianapolis, IN: Wiley-Blackwell.

O'Brien, M. E. (2011). *Spirituality in Nursing: Standing on holy ground* (4th ed.). Sudbury, MA: Jones & Bartlett.

Oldnall, A. (1996). A critical analysis of nursing: Meeting the spiritual needs of patients. *Journal of Advanced Nursing, 23*(1), 138–144. doi:10.1111/j.1365-2648.1996.tb03145.x

Olson, J. K., Paul, P., Douglass, L., Clark, M. B., Simington, J., & Goddard, N. (2003). Addressing the spiritual dimension in Canadian undergraduate nursing education. *Canadian Journal of Nursing Research, 35*(3), 94–107.

Ozbasaran, F., Ergul, S., Temel, A. B., Aslan, G. G., & Coban, A. (2011). Turkish nurses' perceptions of spirituality and spiritual care. *Journal of Clinical Nursing, 20*(21–22), 3102–3110. doi: 10.1111/j.1365-2702.2011.03778.x

Pesut, B. (2003). Developing spirituality in the curriculum: Worldviews, intrapersonal connectedness, interpersonal connectedness. *Nursing Education Perspectives, 24*(6), 290–294. doi:10.1043/1094 -2831(2003)024<0290:DSITCW>2.0.CO;2

Pesut, B. (2008). Spirituality and spiritual care in nursing fundamentals textbooks. *Journal of Nursing Education, 47*(4), 167–173. doi:10.3928/01484834-20080401-05

Pesut, B. (2009a). Ontologies of nursing in an age of spiritual pluralism: Closed or open worldview? *Nursing Philosophy, 11*(1), 15–23. doi:10.1111/j.1466-769X.2009.00420.x

Pesut, B. (2009b). Care of the spirit: Passing the mantle from institutional religion to institutional health care. *Touchstone, 27*(1), 16–25. Retrieved from http://touchstonecanada.ca/wp-content/up loads/2013/08/Jan-2009-Article2.pdf

Pesut, B. (2009c). Incorporating patients' spirituality into care using Gadow's ethical framework. *Nursing Ethics, 16*(4), 418–428. doi:10.1177/0969733009104606

Pesut, B. (2013). Nursings' need for the idea of spirituality. *Nursing Inquiry, 20*(1), 5–10. doi:10.1111/ j.1440-1800.2012.00608.x

Pesut, B., Fowler, M., Reimer-Kirkham, S., Taylor, E. J., & Sawatzky, R. (2009). Particularizing spirituality in points of tension: Enriching the discourse. *Nursing Inquiry, 16*(4), 337–346. doi:10.1111/ j.1440-1800.2009.00462.x

Pesut, B., Fowler, M., Taylor, E. J., Reimer-Kirkham, S., & Sawatzky, R. (2008). Conceptualizing spirituality and religion in Healthcare. *Journal of Clinical Nursing, 17*(21), 2803–2810. doi:10.1111/ j.1365-2702.2008.02344.x

Post, S. G., Puchalski, C. M., & Larson, D. B. (2000). Physicians and patient spirituality: Professional boundaries, competency, and ethics. *Annals of Internal Medicine, 132*(7), 578–583. doi:10.7326/0003-4819-132-7-200004040-00010

Reimer-Kirkham, S., Pesut, B., Meyerhoff, H., & Sawatzky, R. (2004). Spiritual caregiving at the juncture of religion, culture, and state. *Canadian Journal of Nursing Research, 36*(4), 148–169.

Reimer-Kirkham, S., Pesut, B., Sawatzky, R., Cochrane, M., & Redmond, A. (2012). Discourses of spirituality and leadership in nursing: A mixed methods analysis. *Journal of Nursing Management, 20*(8), 1029–1038. doi:10.1111/j.1365-2834.2012.01480.x

Reimer-Kirkham, S., Sharma, S., Pesut, B., Sawatzky, R., Meyerhoff, H., & Cochrane, M. (2011). Sacred spaces in public places: Religious and spiritual plurality in health care. *Nursing Inquiry, 19*(3), 202–212. doi:10.1111/j.1440-1800.2011.00571.x

Reinert, K. G., & Koenig, H. G. (2013). Re-examining definitions of spirituality in nursing research. *Journal of Advanced Nursing, 69*(12), 2622–2634. doi:10.1111/jan.12152

Ribaudo, A., & Takahashi, M. (2008). Temporal trends in spiritual research: A meta-analysis of journal abstracts between 1944 and 2003. *Journal of Religion, Spirituality & Aging, 20*(1–2), 16–28. doi:10.1080/15528030801921972

Romanow, R. J. (2002). *Building on values: The future of health care in Canada.* Retrieved from http://publications.gc.ca/collections/Collection/CP32-85-2002E.pdf

Ross, L. (2006). Spiritual care in nursing: An overview of the research to date. *Journal of Clinical Nursing, 15*(7), 852–862. doi:10.1111/j.1365-2702.2006.01617.x

Ross, L., & McSherry, W. (2010). Considerations of the future of spiritual assessment. In W. McSherry & L. Ross (Eds.), *Spiritual assessment in healthcare practice* (pp. 161–171). Keswick, England: M&K Publishing.

Ruder, S. (2013). Spirituality in nursing: Nurses' perceptions about providing spiritual care. *Home Healthcare Now, 31*(7), 356–367. doi:10.1097/NHH.0b013e3182976135

Sampson, C. (1982). *The neglected ethic: Religious and cultural factors in the care of patients.* Toronto, ON, Canada: McGraw-Hill.

Sessanna, L., Finnell, D., & Jezewski, M. A. (2007). Spirituality in nursing and health-related literature: A concept analysis. *Journal of Holistic Nursing, 25*(4), 252–262. doi:10.1177/0898010107303890

Sessanna, L., Finnell, D. S., Underhill, M., Chang, Y., & Peng, H. (2011). Measures assessing spirituality as more than religiosity: A methodological review of nursing and health-related literature. *Journal of Advanced Nursing, 67*(8), 1677–1694. doi:10.1111/j.1365-2648.2010.05596.x

Sharma, S., Reimer-Kirkham, S., & Fowler, M. (2012). Emergent non-religious spiritualities. In M. Fowler, S. Reimer-Kirkham, R. Sawatzky, & B. Johnson (Eds.), *Religion, religious ethics, and nursing* (pp. 285–300). New York, NY: Springer Publishing Company.

Smith, A. R. (2009). Nursing and spirituality: What happened to religion? *Journal of Christian Nursing, 26*(4), 216–222. doi:10.1097/01.CNJ.0000361243.35944.69

Smith, S. (2008). Toward a flexible framework for understanding spirituality. *Occupational Therapy in Health Care, 22*(1), 39–54. doi:10.1080/J003v22n01_04

Speck, P. (2005). The evidence base for spiritual care. *Nursing Management, 12*(6), 28–31. doi:10.7748/nm2005.10.12.6.28.c2038

Stanhope, M., Lancaster, J., Jessup-Falcioni, H., & Viverais-Dresler, G. A. (2011). *Community health nursing in Canada* (2nd ed.). Toronto, ON, Canada: Elsevier.

Stern, J., & James, S. (2006). Every person matters: Enabling spirituality education for nurses. *Journal of Clinical Nursing, 15*(7), 897–904. doi:10.1111/j.1365-2702.2006.01663.x

Stoll, R. I. (1979). Guidelines for spiritual assessment. *American Journal of Nursing, 79*(9), 1574–1577. doi:10.1097/00000446-197909000-00041

Stranahan, S. (2001). Spiritual perceptions, attitudes about spiritual care, and spiritual care practices among nurse practitioners. *Western Journal of Nursing Research, 23*(1), 90–104. doi:10.1177/01939450122044970

Sweat, M. T. (2011). What are the gaps in spiritual care? *Journal of Christian Nursing, 28*(2), 112. doi:10.1097/CNJ.0b013e31820ccaff

Swinton, J. (2001). *Spirituality and mental health care: Rediscovering a 'forgotten' dimension*. London, England: Jessica Kingsley.

Swinton, J. (2005). Forward. In M. Cobb (Ed.), *The hospital chaplain's handbook: A guide for good practice* (pp. vii–ix). Norwich, England: Canterbury Press.

Swinton, J., & McSherry, W. (2006). Editorial: Critical reflections on the current state of spirituality-in-nursing. *Journal of Clinical Nursing, 15*(7), 801–802. doi:10.1111/j.1365-2702.2006.01687.x

Taylor, E. J. (2002). *Spiritual care: Nursing theory, research, and practice*. Upper Saddle River, NJ: Prentice-Hall.

Taylor, E. J. (2003). Nurses caring for the spirit: Patients with cancer and family caregiver expectations. *Oncology Nursing Forum, 30*(4), 585–590. doi:10.1188/03.ONF.585-590#sthash.mB6BlJpe.dpuf

Taylor, E. J. (2006). Prevalence and associated factors of spiritual needs among patients with cancer and family caregivers. *Oncology Nursing Forum, 33*(4), 729–735. doi:10.1188/06.ONF.729-735#sthash.sYYu7J84.dpuf

Taylor, E. J. (Ed.). (2012). *Religion: A clinical guide for nurses*. New York, NY: Springer Publishing Company.

The Janki Foundation for Spirituality in Health Care. (2016). *Aims of the Foundation*. Retrieved from http://www.jankifoundation.org/about_us/aims_of_foundation.jsp

Timmins, F., & Kelly, J. (2008). Spiritual assessment in intensive and cardiac care nursing. *Nursing in Critical Care, 13*(3), 124–131. doi:10.1111/j.1478-5153.2008.00276.x

Timmins, F., & McSherry, W. (2012). Spirituality: The Holy Grail of contemporary nursing practice. *Journal of Nursing Management, 20*(8), 951–957. doi:10.1111/jonm.12038

Tisdell, E. J. (2006). Spiritual, cultural identity, and epistemology in culturally responsive teaching in higher education. *Multicultural Perspectives, 8*(3), 19–25. doi:10.1207/s15327892mcp0803_4

Tyler, I. D., & Raynor, J. E. (2006). Spirituality in the natural sciences and nursing: An interdisciplinary perspective. *The ABNF Journal, 17*(2), 63–66.

Unruh, A. M. (2007). Spirituality, religion, and pain. *Canadian Journal of Nursing Research, 39*(2), 66–86.

Van Dover, L. J., & Bacon, J. M. (2001). Spiritual care in practice: A close-up view. *Nursing Forum, 36*(3), 18–28. doi:10.1111/j.1744-6198.2001.tb00245.x

Wasner, M., Longaker, C., Fegg, M. J., & Borasio, G. D. (2005). Effects of spiritual care training for palliative care professionals. *Palliative Medicine, 19*(2), 99–104. doi:10.1191/0269216305pm995oa

World Health Organization. (2006). A cross-cultural study of spirituality, religion, and personal beliefs as components of quality of life. *Social Science & Medicine, 62*(6), 1486–1497. doi:10.1016/j.socscimed.2005.08.001

World Health Organization. (2016). Definition of palliative care. Retrieved from http://www.who.int/cancer/palliative/definition/en

Wright, K. B. (1998). Professional, ethical and legal implications for spiritual care in nursing. *Journal of Nursing Scholarship, 30*(1), 81–83. doi:10.1111/j.1547-5069.1998.tb01241.x

Wright, L. M. (2005). *Spirituality, suffering, and illness: Ideas for healing*. Philadelphia, PA: F. A. Davis.

4

Competencies for Spiritual Assessment and Care

In order to appropriately incorporate spiritual assessment and care into practice, nurses need the requisite professional competency (Pesut, 2009a). Yet, it is widely reported in the nursing literature that nurses generally feel unprepared to assess clients' spirituality or to provide spiritual care. This is primarily due to inadequate education with respect to this dimension of care (McSherry, 2006; Ross, 2006; van Leeuwen, Tiesinga, Post, & Jochemsen, 2006). There are calls for nursing to prepare nurses to be more competent in this area (Ruder, 2013). A sense of confidence and competence within nurses to attend to the spiritual dimension of care is acquired through a variety of means. These include increasing one's knowledge base in the area, honing of one's skills in assessing and intervening to meet clients' spiritual needs, and engaging in and reflecting upon one's spirituality and spiritual development. Education in such areas has been noted to have a positive impact on competencies (van Leeuwen, Tiesinga, Middel, Post, & Jochemsen, 2008). Certain professional and personal attributes traditionally found in nurses contribute to competence in this area, as well.

This chapter focuses on competencies needed to incorporate spirituality into nursing practice. As these are operationalized within the nurse–client relationship as well as the nursing process, comments about this relationship and the nursing process are made. Examples of key attributes noted to be conducive to spiritual assessment and care are identified, and some are explored further. Communication skills that are essential to developing competency are also summarized. The nurse as a spiritual being is also discussed.

Competencies are integral to nursing practice and usually accompany standards of practice. Standards for educating nurses about spiritual care are present in both educational and practice contexts in that they are part of the accreditation criteria for institutions (Lantz, 2007). Competencies are one means by which such standards can be achieved. Conversely, adhering to the standards of practice increases competency. Just as nurses need certain competencies to be able to provide physical and emotional assessment and care, they also need competencies for spiritual assessment and care. In fact, competency for spiritual caregiving has been linked to competency in technical/ physical or emotional caregiving. Competent physical and emotional care can contribute to comfort for both body and spirit. As Carr (2008) maintains, if nurses cannot properly care for a client's body, then they cannot comfort the spirit.

THE CONCEPT OF COMPETENCY

What is a competency? The Canadian Nurses Association (CNA, 2008) states that a competency is "the integrated knowledge, skills, judgment and attributes required of a registered nurse to practice safely and ethically in a designated role and setting. (Attributes include, but are not limited to attitudes, values and beliefs.)" (p. 23). Van Leeuwen and Cusveller (2004) describe competencies as "complex sets of skills used in a professional context, i.e. the clinical nursing process. Being competent depends on the correct assessment of a clinical situation and on the ability to implement knowledge and skill in the right way at the right moment" (p. 236). McMullan and colleagues (2003) add to the description in stating that competency and competencies are "person-oriented, referring to the person's underlying characteristics and qualities that lead to an effective and/or superior performance in a job" (p. 285). From these descriptions, it can be seen that nursing competencies not only involve knowledge and skills, but also reference personal attributes and the therapeutic use of self.

Competencies can be stated in very specific terms so that individual nurses can assess their personal levels of competency. For example, for entry-level registered nurses, four competencies given by the Association of Registered Nurses of Newfoundland and Labrador (ARNNL, 2013) that relate to the spiritual dimension of practice are the following:

- Provides nursing care to meet palliative care or end-of-life care needs (e.g., pain and symptom management, psychosocial and spiritual support and support for significant others, p. 12)

- Demonstrates consideration of the spiritual and religious beliefs and practices of clients (p.13)

- Engages clients in an assessment of the following: physical, emotional, spiritual, cultural, cognitive, developmental, environmental and social needs (p. 9)

- Accepts and provides care for all clients, regardless of gender, age, health status, lifestyle, beliefs, and health practices (p. 14)

Nursing codes of ethics assume spirituality to be an obligation of care. These codes also address the issue of competency. For example, the International Council of Nurses (ICN, 2012) *Code of Ethics* states: "The nurse uses judgement regarding individual competence when accepting and delegating responsibility" (p. 4). The CNA (2008) *Code of Ethics* also states: "Nurses practice within the limits of their competence. When aspects of care are beyond their level of competence, they seek additional information or knowledge, seek help from their supervisor or a competent practitioner" (p. 18). Similarly, the American Nurses Association (ANA, 2015) *Code of Ethics* states: "Nurses are responsible for assessing their own competence. When the needs of the patient are beyond the qualifications or competencies of the nurse, that nurse must seek consultation and collaboration from qualified nurses, other health professionals, or other appropriate resources" (p. 16). Framed within the context of spiritual nursing care, the nurse would need to not only maintain competence in this area, but also recognize when the spiritual issues and concerns of clients are beyond his or her competency. In such cases, a consultation or referral to a competent spiritual care provider is warranted. Thus, in all three of these *Codes of Ethics* mentioned, it is apparent that competencies are intricately connected to ethical nursing practice.

Logical questions that emerge from the discussion so far are: What are the specific competencies needed for spiritual assessment and care? What specific knowledge, attributes, and skills do nurses need? Although a number of studies that indicate that competencies necessary for spiritual care are underdeveloped (McSherry, 2006; Ross, 2006; van Leeuwen et al., 2006), there has been some advancement in delineating appropriate and relevant competencies for spiritual assessment and care.

COMPETENCIES FOR SPIRITUAL ASSESSMENT AND CARE

Van Leeuwen and Cusveller (2004) conducted a literature review to determine nursing competencies needed for adequate spiritual care, creating a nursing competency profile. Six main competencies were identified in three different domains (pp. 241–244).

- Domain A: Awareness and use of self

  a. Competency A1: "Nurses handle their own values, convictions and feelings in their professional relationships with patients of different beliefs and religions" (p. 241). Inherent in this competency is respect for the clients' beliefs; examination of one's own spirituality and any possible or actual impact on care; and the examination of personal limitations plus any appropriate action regarding same—including referral to a professional spiritual care provider.

  b. Competency A2: "The nurse addresses the subject of spirituality with patients from different cultures in a caring manner" (p. 241). Active listening, acceptance of the client, compassion, empathy, authenticity, sincerity, accessibility, and the use of communication skills are all relevant aspects to this competency.

- Domain B: Spiritual dimensions of nursing

  a. Competency B3: "The nurse collects information about the patient's spirituality and identifies the patient's need" (p. 242). Key aspects of this competency include spiritual assessment and the identification of the client's spiritual needs (the focus of Chapter 5 in this book).

  b. Competency B4: "The nurse discusses with patients and team members how spiritual care is provided, planned and reported" (p. 242). Examples of key activities under this competency include the reporting of aspects of a client's spirituality; the planning and coordination of the best spiritual care for clients; and the consultation with or referral to a professional spiritual care provider.

  c. Competency B5: "The nurse provides spiritual care and evaluates it with the patient and team members" (p. 243). Inherent in this competency are such activities as supporting the client's spiritual practices; monitoring the client's spiritual expressions as nursing care is provided; conversing with clients about spiritual matters/needs; providing spiritual care interventions; and evaluating the spiritual care given.

- Domain C: Assurance of quality and expertise

    a. Competency C6: "The nurse contributes to quality assurance and improving expertise in spiritual care in the organization" (p. 244). Examples of activities associated with this competency include facilitating colleagues in the provision of spiritual care; recommending policies regarding spiritual care; and implementing projects to improve spiritual care.

An important point stressed by van Leeuwen and Cusveller (2004) is the importance of the working environment for nurses in terms of them being able to demonstrate their competencies associated with spiritual care. For each domain, van Leeuwen and Cusveller's article also provides clinical vignettes, which outline situations regarding each competency in which nurse behaviors are appropriate (Table 3, pp. 241–244). Referral to the article and a review of the clinical vignettes are beneficial for further discussion and illustration of each competency.

Van Leeuwen, Tiesinga, Middel, Post, and Jochemsen (2009) later developed and tested an instrument called the Spiritual Care Competency Scale (SCCS), which was deemed to be suitable for measuring nursing competency in spiritual care. This scale has 27 items with questions about spiritual care competencies derived from the key behaviors described in the nursing competency profile. The level of competence is assessed using a Likert scale. Examples of some items in the scale under the title "Personal support and patient counselling" (p. 2868), deemed by van Leeuwen and colleagues (2009) to be the "heart of spiritual care" (pp. 2862–2863), include the following:

- I can provide a patient with spiritual care.

- I can evaluate the spiritual care that I have provided in consultation with the patient and in the disciplinary/multidisciplinary team.

- I can give a patient the information about spiritual facilities within the care institution (including spiritual care, meditation center, religious services).

- I can help a patient continue his or her daily spiritual practices (including providing opportunities for rituals, prayer, meditation, reading the Bible/Quran, listening to music).

- I can attend to a patient's spirituality during the daily care (e.g., physical care).

- I can refer members of a patient's family to a spiritual advisor/pastor, if they ask me and/or if they express spiritual needs. (van Leeuwen et al., 2009, p. 2868)

A reference to this competency scale is recommended in order to measure your own competence with respect to providing spiritual care.

Baldacchino is a nurse educator who has studied competencies for spiritual care. She explored the main nursing competencies for spiritual care in a sample of nurses who were working in institutions in Malta: a primarily Christian population (Baldacchino, 2006). Four main competency foci were identified with examples of competencies for each focus provided. These are depicted in Table 4.1.

Table 4.1 Competencies and Examples

Main Competency Focus	Examples of Competencies
"The role of the nurse as a professional" (Baldacchino, 2006, p. 889) [and] the role of the nurse as an individual person" (p. 890)	Provision of holistic care; referral to spiritual care professional if warranted; meeting clients' spiritual needs; self-awareness of own spirituality including own spiritual beliefs/values
"Delivery of spiritual care by the nursing process" (Baldacchino, 2006, p. 890)	Assessment of spiritual needs/problems; organization of nursing care based on a trustful nurse–client relationship; effective use of communication skills; provision of a quiet environment; facilitating spiritual/ religious coping; instilling hope in the future; assisting with finding meaning and purpose; referral to spiritual care professional; evaluation of spiritual care
"Nurses' communication with patients, inter-disciplinary team and clinical/ educational organizations" (Baldacchino, 2006, p. 892)	Communication within the health care team including spiritual care professionals; coordination of client care
"Safeguarding ethical issues in care" (Baldacchino, 2006, p. 893)	Documentation of client progress; maintaining privacy, confidentiality; seeking informed consent from client; respecting client's choices; advocating for clients

Refer to Baldacchino's article for a complete discussion of each of the competencies, including the nurses' perceptions of their own levels of competence in each area. As can be seen from Table 4.1, many of the competencies Baldacchino identified are similar to those elaborated upon by van Leeuwen and Cusveller (2004). Such competencies can serve as a guide to practice in the area of spiritual care.

Reflection 4.1

Review the various competencies for spiritual assessment and care as identified by van Leeuwen and Cusveller (2004) and by Baldacchino (2006). For each of the competencies identified, rate your perception of your own competency using a Likert scale of 1 to 5, with 1 being "not at all competent" and 5 being "very competent." For those competencies in which you rated "high" in competency, reflect upon those factors that may have contributed to your sense of competence. For those competencies where you rated "low," what do you need to do in order to increase such competencies?

ATTRIBUTES FOR SPIRITUAL ASSESSMENT AND CAREGIVING

As mentioned earlier, attributes are included in competencies, and are important in the provision of spiritual care. In fact, Kevern (2012) suggests that, when it comes to spiritual care, placing emphasis on the nurse's character (including attributes) is just as important as identifying and attending to a client's spiritual needs. The CNA (2008) identifies the nurse's attitudes, values, and beliefs to be part of such attributes. If the nurse does not have a positive attitude toward spirituality/spiritual care, then this will impact that nurse's competency in this area of care. If the nurse has a sense of curiosity, then he or she will be curious about the place of spirituality/religion in the client's life, how it is impacted and/or how it impacts the illness or suffering experience. Similarly, what a nurse personally believes about spirituality, religion, and spiritual care can also impact the level of competency that will be achieved. For example, if the nurse believes that spiritual assessment and care are to be provided only by spiritual care professionals, then he or she might not seek competency in this area of care. And if the nurse values his or her own spirituality, then he or she will more likely attend to the client's spirituality.

In the discussion on specific nursing behaviors, some attributes have been identified that accompany select competencies. Table 4.2 identifies just some of these. The sample references provided at the end of the table attest to the level of agreement as to the identified attributes for spiritual care.

Table 4.2 Attributes for Spiritual Care

Personal/character attributes	Kind, loving, concerned, compassionate, nurturing, trustworthy, humble, respectful, caring, accepting, open, understanding, gentle, polite, receptive, approachable, nonjudgmental, authentic, genuine, honest, sensitive, curious
Interpersonal attributes	Holistic focus, client-centered, good listener, empathetic, able to be present with clients, able to effectively use communication skills, able to recognize and respond to clients as a person, intuitive
Spiritual intelligence attributes	Adequate inner resources, positive self-concept, unselfish giving, high moral character, personal transcendence
Self-reflection attributes	Able to reflect on self, client, and one's practice, including one's values, attitudes, beliefs, prejudices, assumptions, and motivations

Sources: Biro (2012), Brooks et al. (2005), Carr (2008, 2010), Chism and Magnan (2009), Cockell and McSherry (2012), Crain (1994), Creel (2007), Cusveller (2013), Iacono (2011), Kaur, Sambasivan, and Kumar (2013), Kumar (2004), McSherry and Jamieson (2013), Miner-Williams (2006), National Health Service (NHS) Education for Scotland (2009), Narayanasamy (2004), Reimer-Kirkham et al. (2004), Rew (1989), Sawatzky and Pesut (2005), and Sellers (2001).

Reflection 4.2

Reflect on the attributes in Table 4.2. Which of the attributes do you feel that you possess? Which do you judge to be more closely related to your personality? Which have you learned and how have you learned them?

As can be seen from these examples of attributes, the vast majority of them are general attributes that are helpful in developing and maintaining competence in multiple dimensions of caregiving. They are also attributes connected to "good nursing" (Biro, 2012, p. 1002) generally. In fact, in a study by McSherry and Jamieson (2013), nurses did not see spiritual care as separate from fundamental care provided by nurses. Nurses, by virtue of their individual personalities, may possess variable intensities of these attributes. However, many attributes can be intentionally fostered by reflection and deliberate action on the part of the nurse. For example, Rew (1989) identifies a number of exercises (e.g., listening to music, progressive relaxation, and guided imagery) intended to promote one's receptivity to intuition and to spiritual experiences. Moreover, some people are, by nature, blessed to be good communicators; for others, effective use of communication skills can be learned and developed.

It is interesting to note that many of the attributes identified in the nursing literature as being conducive to spiritual care are also those identified by clients as important. For example, in an ethnographic research study by Sellers (2001), adult participants identified the following attributes as being important to them in receiving spiritual care: caring, presence, compassion, active listening, a good sense of humor, individualized and personalized nursing care, understanding the lived experience of the person, unconditional regard, honesty, and sensitivity.

Not all attributes can be discussed at length in this chapter, but the attributes of presence, caring, and listening have been chosen for further in-depth discussion due to the foundational nature of such attributes for effective spiritual assessment and care.

Presence

The ability to be fully "present" to the client is critical for effective spiritual assessment and care. In fact, Burkhardt and Nagai-Jacobson (2002) state: "Spiritual care begins with presence" (p. 86), describing presence as "the most essential element of spiritual care giving" (p. 1). Presence is also recognized as a means to providing spiritual care and support to clients (Brooks et al., 2005). In some nursing contexts, presence is the only intervention that nurses can offer (Osterman & Schwartz-Barcott, 1996). Meyer (2000) sees presence as a gift that nurses can give to clients. Some nurse scholars see presence as an intuitive attribute; whereas others see it from a developmental perspective as a skill to be learned with professional maturity. Still others see presence as a process that can be taught through role-modeling and formal teaching (Rankin & DeLashmutt, 2006). Benner (1984) describes "presencing" as one of the eight competencies within the expert nurse's role. Benner's research offers that presence can involve touch, having person-to-person contact between nurse and client, and allowing the client to ventilate feelings without the nurse feeling the need to verbalize in response. Presence, then, is the essence of using oneself therapeutically and indicates to clients that the nurse cares about and shares in their situation. The concept of presence views the nurse–client relationship as more mutual and egalitarian, rather than a hierarchical view of this relationship. Presence can be "lost" if the focus is only on technological interventions.

The concept of presence can be difficult to describe, but several authors have attempted to examine the concept and how it can be operationalized in nursing practice. Doona, Chase, and Haggerty (1999) describe and discuss six features of presence: "uniqueness, connecting with the patient's experience, sensing, going beyond the scientific data, knowing (what will work and when to act), and being with the patient" (p. 57). Participants in a study by Reimer-Kirkham and colleagues (2004) describe presence within the context of the spiritual dimension of care as including the creation of "sacred spaces through subtle but intentional movement towards a discussion of things spiritual" (p. 159). Zerwekh (1997) states: "Presencing requires deliberate focused attention, receptivity to the other person, and persistent awareness of the other's shared humanity. The practice of presence results in growth of both nurse and patient" (p. 261). Sellers (2001) maintains: "Being present requires nurses to recognize the uniqueness and value of each person, focus on being with rather than doing for the person, and exhibit genuineness, honesty, respect and sensitivity" (p. 245). Rankin and DeLashmutt (2006) describe presence as being in communion with clients, describing this communion as "the willingness to be unknowing, available, and open and to risk the investment of self in another" (p. 287). Eliopoulos (2004) identifies active listening, exploring comments made by the client, and being with the client (even silently) as reflecting presence, with availability of the nurse being central, both physically and emotionally. Eliopoulos sees presence as characterized by intentionality on the part of the nurse—having an attitude or state of mind that focuses on clients and that wants to be of assistance to them. It is going beyond performing tasks to making heart-to-heart connections with clients. As can be seen from these descriptions, presence is intricately connected to other attributes known to be conducive to spiritual assessment and care. It is also intricately connected to the nurse–client relationship. In fact, Rankin and DeLashmutt (2006) describe presence as, in essence, a healing relationship characterized by "soul-to-soul/ spirit-to-spirit communion" (p. 286) that meets the client's holistic needs. As Ranking and DeLashmutt put it, "Without a relationship, there can be neither the manifestation of spirituality nor presence" (p. 285). Presence is also connected to the spirituality of the nurse. A nursing student aptly put this connection when stating, "We achieve nursing presence by giving our whole self to the patient. Spirituality is a component of our personality, and if we are missing an aspect of our personality, how can we be totally giving of ourselves?" (Rankin & DeLashmutt, p.285).

Osterman and Schwartz-Barcott (1996) describe four "ways of being" (p. 24) present with clients, some of which are much better than others:

- The nurse is physically present with the client, but due to some factor within the nurse, he or she is not focused upon the client or the relationship but is self-absorbed (e.g., the nurse may be anxious about some aspect of care). In this situation, there is little or no interpersonal exchange between the nurse and the client, albeit the client *can* feel reassured just that "someone is there."

- The nurse is partially present with the client in the sense that there is not only a physical presence but also a focus on a task relevant to the client—but the nurse is not directly focused on the client. For example, the nurse may focus on some technical aspect of care such as checking an intravenous but does not really acknowledge the client. There is little or no interpersonal exchange, but the nurse's dealing with the technical aspect of care can serve to reduce the client's stress.

- The nurse is fully present with the client physically (e.g., making eye contact and perhaps leaning toward the client) and psychologically (e.g., actively listening and responding). The nurse is using the self, being empathetic, caring and open. There is a reciprocal interpersonal exchange in the context of a meaningful relationship.

- The nurse is present in a transcendent manner, described as "spiritual presence." In this way of being the nurse feels a sense of "oneness" with the client as he or she shares in the client's suffering. The client feels less alone and at peace as "connection" with the nurse is experienced.

Reflection 4.3

- What helps you to be present in the moment? How is when you are alone different from when you are in the midst of much activity?
- Recall an experience in which you felt that you were truly present with another person. How would you describe what this sense of presence looked like and felt like? What helped you to be present with this person?
- Recall an experience in which you felt that you were unable to be authentically present with another person. What factors limited your ability to be present? What feelings did you have in this situation?
- Reflect on the four ways of being present with clients presented by Osterman and Schwartz-Barcott (1996). Which is most characteristic of your practice? How can you aspire to "be more present" for clients in ways that are meaningful and healing for them?

Adapted from Burkhardt & Nagai-Jacobson (2002, p. 96)

The impact of being fully present with clients can be seen in the following account of a nurse–client encounter from a client's perspective:

There was this nurse . . . I don't remember her name but I can see her face. It was one of those nights when I just couldn't settle down. I had too much going on between my ears. Boy, your thoughts can run away with you sometimes, especially when you don't know what's happening 'cause you've never been through this before. This cancer is an ugly thing. Well, it's the middle of the night and I put my light on . . . and this nurse came in, and she must have stayed with me for about an hour. She just sat down and asked me how I was doing . . . and we went from there. We'd talk about everything. I'd tell her some of my story and she'd tell me some about her life. Then, every once in awhile, we'd get around to some of the things that were bothering me. I had about four or five things going on that were really eating my lunch, and over the course of the hour we talked about them all. She talked. I talked. I listened, she listened. I had questions. I'd never been through anything like this before. She had some answers, but she didn't mind saying she didn't have an answer either. She could tell me what usually happened, make it easier for me to go into the unknown. Yes, I remember that nurse for sure. I think most nurses are like a part of heaven. (Burkhardt & Nagai-Jacobson, 2002, p. 95)

In this scenario, we see the nurse present with the client. The nurse was present when the client needed her, not necessarily when she scheduled time for him. Presence was instrumental in this client disclosing to the nurse his concerns—which constitutes a testimony to the power of this competency. Nurses should strive toward such ways of being with clients.

Caring

Caring is a concept foundational to nursing itself. It is an attribute identified by many authors and practitioners as being conducive to effective spiritual care. Caring involves an affective or feeling component as well as a service or doing component (Castaneda, Habert, Witt, Younker, & Crigger, 2007). In other words, "caring about" a client (i.e., being affectively responsive toward the client) leads to "caring for" a client (i.e., acting) in a far richer way than if only "caring for" the client is present. An important point to make with respect to caring—as with any attribute really—is that the client needs to *experience* such from the nurse in order for there to be a therapeutic benefit.

Based on Chapman's five love languages (Chapman, 1995), Castaneda and colleagues (2007) propose the following descriptions of caring (p. 90). These five ways of caring are provided in Table 4.3, along with some examples of each provided by Castaneda and colleagues.

Although not all caring behaviors of the nurse may fit precisely within the structure of Chapman's five love languages, the framework does have value in terms of reflecting on caring actions.

Reflection 4.4

Reflect on the descriptors of caring as based on Chapman's five love languages (Table 4.3).

- Which of the five "languages" would be your preferred way to experience and receive caring from others?

(continued)

Reflection 4.4 (*continued*)

- Which would be your preferred way(s) to provide care for others?
- Observe how clients respond to the various expressions of caring that you give them according to the five love languages. What does this say about their primary love language(s)?
- In reflecting on the examples of each "language," which of these examples do you feel most reflects your way of caring for clients? Are there any languages that you would like to better incorporate into your practice? If so, then how might you develop this ability?

Some authors describe caring from particular worldviews, each of which provides alternate frameworks for caring. For example, Dameron (2012) describes caring by a nurse who would look at a Christian worldview as encompassing many of the traits of secular caring nursing theories. Additionally, from this worldview the origin of caring for such nurses would be rooted in the example of Jesus Christ and his teachings for a theory of caring. A good question to ask is: Does my own personal spirituality and/or worldview impact how I perceive caring for clients, and if so, how?

Table 4.3 **Ways of Caring**

Descriptor	Examples
Words of affirmation	Listening and giving encouraging words; conveying empathy in a genuine manner; accepting client; explaining things to client
Quality time	Providing undivided attention; spending time being with client; being accessible; allowing client to express feelings; being open and communicating effectively
Giving/receiving gifts	Meeting the client's needs; being present with the client; giving clients the gift of time
Acts of service	Showing love through actions based on the client's preferences and wishes; good and timely physical care
Physical touch	Gentle, loving, and appropriate use of touch to show comfort and bring security to the client

What options does a nurse have when dealing with a client who may not wish to enter into a caring relationship with the nurse? One nurse in a study by Carr (2008) provides a good response to this question: accept the person where he or she is and convey that acceptance—respecting however the client wishes to respond at that time. Such acceptance and respect *can* lead to a deeper relationship at a later time. In a somewhat similar situation, in clinical contexts where clients are unconscious or otherwise cannot communicate with the nurse, then the nurse can still approach such clients with a caring attitude demonstrated by respect for them and concern about their comfort, well-being, and dignity. The key is basically recognizing and promoting their sense of personhood (Carr, 2010).

Listening

The importance of listening in spiritual assessment and care cannot be overemphasized. Listening attentively to clients is one of the most important attributes required in exploring and responding to the spiritual dimension of clients. As Taylor (2007) states, "It is impossible to provide a healing response to a patient when you have not first heard his or her spiritual pain. Not only is listening a prerequisite for a healing response, it *is* a healing response" (p. 25). As such, listening, in itself, is an intervention. A nurse in the study by Carr (2008) describes the importance of listening when stating, "It doesn't really matter what you do or what you say. The important thing is that you're there [listening and being receptive]" (p. 694). Another nurse in this same study said, "the less you say, the more you do" (p. 694). Burkhardt and Nagai-Jacobson (2002) similarly stress the importance of listening: "Attentive listening and focused presence are the heart of caring for the spirit, both for ourselves [as nurses] and others" (p. 322). Some examples of the features of intentional listening described by Burkhardt and Nagai-Jacobson include the following:

- Paying attention to verbal and nonverbal cues indicating a spiritual concern
- Listening with one's whole being
- Using silence effectively
- Noting congruence/incongruence in clients' words and nonverbal expressions
- Using communication skills appropriately

The outcome of such listening is that clients share their stories, are understood, acknowledged and validated, and are encouraged to express all feelings—both positive and negative—as well as to pay attention to their own spirituality. Possible barriers to such listening on the part of the nurse include discomfort with the topic of spirituality/religion, distractions in the clinical environment, and time pressures (Burkhardt & Nagai-Jacobson, 2002). Duff (1994) stresses the importance of listening by citing an example of a nurse who does *not* listen to the client and therefore can miss the client's spiritual distress: "Not long ago a patient was heard to say that he did not understand why God would allow him to be afflicted with cancer. The nurse quickly stated that he shouldn't worry because the staff at the hospital would take good care of him" (p. 30).

The manner in which a nurse listens is important. Nurses need to listen to the verbal expressions of clients and then, in their responses to the clients, appropriately convey that the client has been heard and understood. They also need to listen to emotional nonverbal expressions and then respond to such emotions. Listening for aspects of the client's spirituality must be done with intentionality and with a willingness to notice and explore subtle cues. Egan and Schroeder (2009) state:

> Full listening means listening actively, listening accurately, and listening for meaning (p. 101). . . . Empathetic listening centers on the kind of attending, observing and listening—the kind of "being with"—needed to develop an understanding of clients and their worlds. . . . Helpers must put aside their own concerns to be fully with their clients. . . . Empathetic listening leads to empathetic understanding, which leads to empathetic responding. (p. 103)

For example, a client may be discussing with the nurse the impact of his or her illness on his or her feelings and behavior toward his or her family. If the nurse is listening empathetically and truly understanding the client's situation, then the nurse can provide an empathetic response such as: "It sounds as if you are feeling hopeless that the situation with your family can improve because of how long this suffering has gone on." The client then feels understood and "heard" and will likely further discuss the situation with the nurse. The Chinese character for "to listen" illustrates just how the nurse should listen to clients. This character and its components are shown in Figure 4.1.

As can been seen in this figure, the intent of listening is to listen with our ears, to listen with our eyes, to listen with our heart, and to listen with our whole being. The focus on the client is the most important thing and the client should be the only focus for listening. This type of listening is full and comprehensive.

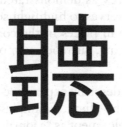

耳: ear

王 : the most important thing

十 : many, much, a lot

目 : eye (罒)

一 : one (only focus)

心 : heart

Figure 4.1 Chinese character for "to listen."

Reflection 4.5

As you read about the nature of listening and the manner in which nurses need to listen, reflect upon your own ability to listen to clients. What factors—internal and environmental—impact your ability to listen in such a manner? Where do you need to improve so as to enhance your ability to listen? And what do you need to do to make such improvements?

Taylor (2007) identifies the following targets as being important to listen for in terms of conversing with clients about spirituality in particular (pp. 29–31):

- Spiritual themes present in the conversation such as " . . . the incessant need for attention, respect, love; betrayal or victimization; inadequacy or failure; struggle or supremacy against the odds; abandonment; and so forth" (p. 29). Spiritual themes can shape a client's identity, ideas about their meaning of life, their values, and their response to illness or other adversity.

- The client's feelings as expressed by such indicators as voice tone, shifts in emotion, and bodily expression. Listening for primary feelings—feelings beneath the expressed feelings—is critical. For example, a client may be expressing anger but the primary feeling beneath the anger may be fear. It is particularly important to listen for negative feelings.

- Where the client is placing energy as demonstrated by a quickening or slower pace in the conversation, which serves to highlight some aspect of the conversation; a stronger or quieter voice in places in the conversation; a tearing of the eyes; or looking away when speaking. Such behavior or indicators will reveal what is meaningful to the client.

- Metaphors used by the client to describe experience that may help identify feelings and spiritual concerns of the client. Examples given by Taylor include a description of their spiritual development as "a journey" (p. 31); describing prayer as "like talking to the ceiling" (p. 31); and describing an experience that is spiritually challenging as "like someone threw me into a pit and left me" (p. 31).

- The dominant mode in the client's talk. For example, some clients express themselves "visually (e.g., 'I recognized' . . . or 'I see' . . .), [others] auditorily (e.g., 'I could tell that' . . . or 'I hear what you're saying' . . .), [while others express themselves] . . . kinesthetically (e.g., 'I felt . . . ' or 'I get what you're saying'", p. 31). Once the dominant mode is recognized, then nurses can connect better to clients by responding using the same mode—"matching the language of the client."

Taylor (2007) also identifies key questions that nurses need to keep in mind while listening for spiritual concerns:

- "What are the deepest feelings? What spiritual needs are being exposed?" (p. 31)

- "How is the patient describing his/her experience? How does this process inform me?" (p. 31)

- "Why is the patient telling me this and why now? Why does the patient want me to know this?" (p. 31)

Finally, Taylor (2007) discusses guidelines offered by spiritual care experts as to how to listen to and hear clients:

- Be curious! Want to hear the patient

- Be authentic

- View the patient as a fellow human on a journey called life

- Trust the patient

- Let the patient set the rules for the conversation

- Offer the patient safety as you listen

- Do not interrupt

- Keep your story to yourself

- Maintain neutrality as you listen

- Allow silence to do its work

- Avoid worrying about what to say after the patient has finished talking

- Use body language to convey your interest in listening

- Spend at least half to three-quarters of your time listening

- Use questions only when necessary

- Take comfort in the three strikes rule [Taylor describes this rule as meaning that a person will typically give you three opportunities to hear them] (pp. 32–36)

Most of the guidelines that Taylor presents are relevant for listening to *any* concern of the client, not just spiritual concerns. Reference to Taylor is recommended for in-depth discussion of these guidelines.

Reflection 4.6

- Reflect on clinical situations where you "heard" any of the five "targets" for listening for spiritual concerns as identified by Taylor (2007). How did you convey

(continued)

Reflection 4.6 (continued)

that you had listened so that the client knew that you had heard and understood him or her? What areas do you feel that you need to "listen for" more effectively?
* Try to listen for spiritual concerns in your clinical practice this week—not only keeping in mind the targets for listening but also the guidelines provided by Taylor (2007)—including responding to clients in such a way that they know you have truly listened to them. What was the resulting impact on you—and on the client?

THE NURSE–CLIENT RELATIONSHIP

Spiritual assessment and care occurs within the context of the nurse–client relationship and this relationship is the vehicle by which spiritual care is provided (Biro, 2012; Mok, Wong, & Wong, 2010; van Leeuwen et al., 2006). It is also within the nurse–client relationship that competencies are operationalized. Indeed, developing a therapeutic relationship is a competency in and of itself. A beneficial interpersonal relationship between nurses and clients is also closely related to desirable personal attributes of the nurse, for example, genuineness, honesty, and compassion. However, there *are* also skills that can be learned by the nurse, which are helpful in developing interpersonal relationships— such as the skill of listening or conveying empathy. And no matter where the nurse begins in terms of personal competency in such skills, there is always room for further development. In fact, it is imperative that a nurse's interpersonal skills be periodically reviewed and examined to ensure quality care. It is also imperative to realize that the basic structure of the therapeutic nurse–client relationship is where such interpersonal skills emerge and are applied.

Pesut (2006) raises an important issue with respect to the nurse–client relationship— that of power relations. The fact that the nurse–client relationship is asymmetrical is an important point to remember when it comes to the provision of spiritual care. There *is* a power imbalance, with the client being in the vulnerable position within the relationship. The client's vulnerability needs to be considered in terms of the provision of ethical care. However, in spite of the power imbalance within the relationship, nurses should still strive for a partnership perspective for the relationship—as such has been repeatedly promoted in this book. The importance of the client's "expertise" on his or her own life and situation cannot be overemphasized, for the client's perception and resources are critical in the area of spiritual assessment and care. Yet, nurses, by virtue of their education and experience, can also bring "expertise" to the relationship. Viewed in this way, the nurse–client relationship becomes one of mutuality. As Pesut (2006) states:

Nurses can view patients as subjects who need to be influenced toward some particular spiritual endpoint [such as objective criteria that characterize spiritual well-being], or nurses can view patients within a perspective of mutuality, acknowledging that many patients bring significant spiritual expertise and capacity. As nurses hold a position of trust with potentially vulnerable patients, it is vital to question where our care might be experienced as spiritual coercion. (p. 131)

As such, careful consideration of the possible misuse of a nurse's position of trust and power is critical in spiritual care.

COMMUNICATION

The interpersonal relationship between the nurse and the client is made possible through communication. Communication is not only an essential part of spiritual care, but, in a sense, is also spiritual care itself. Various communication skills and their importance have already been alluded to throughout this chapter. In this section, a brief review of these and other communication skills is provided. The purpose of such communication skills is to facilitate client self-disclosure as well as to enable the nurse to seek to understand the client, to convey that understanding, and also to convey information, support, and encouragement to the client (Egan & Schroeder, 2009).

Egan and Schroeder (2009) identify several communication skills that are useful in working with clients (Box 4.1). These skills can be quite helpful for the nurse to use in spiritual assessment and care.

Box 4.1 *Communication Skills for Spiritual Assessment and Care*

"Visibly tuning in" (p. 95) to clients is akin to being present with clients, a concept already discussed in this chapter (see section on Presence). Nonverbal behavior such as body language, eye contact, and facial expressions are part of this skill, as is using silence therapeutically.

"Probing" (p. 150) refers not only to the use of open-ended and close-ended questions, but also to statements and short prompts. Short prompts are statements that encourage the client to continue talking, such as "I see," "Yes," or "Go on." They can also refer to nonverbal behaviors such as nodding one's head.

"Information sharing" (p. 199) can be a quite helpful skill in, among other things, normalizing what the client is experiencing. For example, a nurse may say, "The research shows that a common question people ask in health crises is 'Why is this happening to me?'" and go on to then probe whether the client is asking such questions.

"Immediacy" (p. 205) conveys to the client the nurse's experience or perspective of what is happening in the relationship with the client, or what is happening in the "here and now" of the conversation. For example, a nurse might say, "I noticed when you talked about the sense of alienation that you feel from God in the midst of this suffering that you looked very sad and close to tears."

"Confrontation" (p. 210) is a skill that involves challenging clients with respect to consequences of persisting in dysfunctional or unhealthy behaviors and/or

---

(continued)

Box 4.1 *Communication Skills for Spiritual Assessment and Care (continued)*

pointing out discrepancies between the client's words and behaviors. For example, a nurse may say, "You say that religion and God are not important to you, but you still seem to want to engage in religious practices to provide hope and comfort at this time."

"Empathetic highlights" (p. 193) can be quite helpful in conveying to the clients that you have heard and understood them. An example of such a response has been given in the discussion on listening, but another example of such a response is: "You sound as if you are feeling hurt because your connections with family have changed since your illness. But you also seem to feel abandoned by them."

"Summarization" (p. 161) can be a very helpful skill that provides focus, direction, and challenge in the conversation as main points are highlighted. For example, a nurse might say, "Let me see if I have understood what you have said so far. It sounds as if you feel that you have lost meaning in your life because your accident has resulted in so many losses—your job, coaching hockey, etc. Further, what you understood about your faith has also been shaken." Egan and Schroeder also point out the fact that it is sometimes better for the nurse to facilitate the *client* pulling together the major points in his or her story.

"Self-disclosure" (p. 201) can be a helpful skill if it is used carefully. It is particularly important with this skill that the nurse redirects back to the client after self-disclosing. An example of appropriate self-disclosure is: "I remember when my father died, I felt disconnected not only to myself, but to others and to God. I wonder if you have such feelings?"

Taylor has published a book that focuses on talking to clients about spirituality including many practical examples of the skills needed for conversations (Taylor, 2007). Her book is recommended for her in-depth discussion of practical ways to engage in such conversations.

Reflection 4.7

Reflect on the communication skills discussed in this section. How familiar are you with each communication skill and the appropriate use of each? Where do you need to improve?

Nonverbal communication is important to observe in clients; and awareness by the nurse of the use of nonverbal communication is similarly critical. The nonverbal communication of the client is important in providing a window into his or her spirituality. Specifically, the skill of touch as nonverbal communication from nurse to client is especially important to consider in spiritual care. Nurses touch clients constantly in the delivery of nursing care (procedural touch). Nonprocedural touch, or caring touch, is also important as it conveys support and nurtures spiritual health (Taylor, 2002). While touch can be a powerful intervention, the nurse must be cognizant of the factors that determine how a client might respond to touch—and act accordingly. For example, clients who have had people in their lives touch them in aggressive ways may not respond in a positive way to being touched. Some cultural groups may also feel that touching their bodies is an undesirable invasion of their personal space. The timing of a touch, the place where it is done, the body part touched, and the permission of the client are all important considerations for appropriate use of this nonverbal skill (Taylor, 2002).

THE PERSONAL SPIRITUALITY/RELIGIOSITY OF THE NURSE

The personal spirituality of the nurse is important to consider in looking at the place of spirituality in nursing practice. Many authors who write in the area affirm this position (e.g., Chung, Wong, & Chen, 2007; Dossey & Keegan, 2000; Ruder, 2013). Further, Taylor, Highfield, and Amenta (1999) identify the nurse's sense of his or her own spirituality as the best single predictor of a positive attitude toward the integration of spirituality into nursing practice. Similarly, Meyer (2003) identifies the personal spirituality of the nurse as being the strongest predictor of the nurse's perceived ability to provide spiritual care. Such an attitude is conducive to providing effective spiritual care in one's practice (Chan et al., 2006). Nurses with a strong sense of personal spiritual well-being also have a more positive attitude toward spiritual care (Musgrave & McFarlane, 2004; Stranahan, 2001; Swinton & McSherry, 2006). Cockell and McSherry (2012) in their review of published international research on spiritual care in nursing found that nurses need to meet their own spiritual needs in terms of providing quality care to clients. The nursing literature has many references to the fact that nurses who are aware of their own spirituality are better able to attend to the spiritual needs of clients, are more comfortable and confident in providing spiritual care, and are more able to create a positive spiritual environment (e.g., Baldacchino, 2010; Chan, 2009; Grant, 2004; Miner-Williams, 2006; Taylor et al., 1999; Unruh, Versnel, & Kerr, 2002). In fact, Wasner, Longaker, Fegg, and Borasio (2005) identify the nurses' awareness of their own spirituality and spiritual beliefs and how these might impact care as *necessary* for the recognition of others' spirituality. As Callister, Bond, Matsumura, and Mangum (2004) say:

> A nurse provides the best spiritual care when she or he is aware of her or his own religious and spiritual frame of reference and does not allow it to intrude on that of the patient but rather can use his or her own spirituality as a resource on behalf of the patient. (p. 163)

Some nursing scholars have written about how their own spiritual positioning influences their practice (e.g., Chan, 2011; Cusveller, 2013; Lee, 2006; Pesut, 2009b).

Nurse self-awareness is a theme in nursing education programs that focuses on the study of the spiritual dimension of care (Delashmutt, 2007; Grant, 2004; McEwen, 2005; van Leeuwen et al., 2006). Such educational programs increase awareness of one's own spirituality. For example, Delashmutt (2007) implemented a clinical experience for nursing students that included readings and discussions focused on spirituality. The nursing students became more aware of their own spirituality as a result of this experience and were able to appreciate the fact that "if one is to enter into true communion with the self of their clients, then they, by necessity, needed to know themselves spiritually" (Meisenhelder, 2006, p. 186). Reflection on what values, beliefs, and practices one holds is considered part of competent nursing care, including spiritual care (van Leeuwen & Cusveller, 2004). In this book, the reality of the connection between one's own spirituality and one's nursing practice is addressed in the many reflections and directives provided for reflection on personal beliefs, values, and practices regarding spirituality/spiritual care as well as the actual or anticipated impact on client care.

An illustration of the importance of self-awareness to the ability to provide spiritual care is found in a recent conversation with a nurse who related that she "can't have anything to do with religion when it comes to patients." As this was discussed further, she related experiences that she encountered while growing up as the child of a religious leader. Without discounting the legitimacy and impact of these experiences, the question arises as to how this nurse will then respond to a client who has particular spiritual or religious needs. If this nurse is self-aware, then she can hopefully lay her biases aside, and attend to the client's needs. Without self-awareness, she may avoid any and all conversation with a client about spirituality or religion, even if it is important to the client to have such a conversation.

The concept of "the wounded healer" is important to consider in discussing the nurse's own spirituality. Nouwen (1979) maintains that woundedness in a helper can be a source of healing and life for others. Sweat (2010) supports this idea when she states:

> Instead of following the fixer model of giving spiritual care, we may need to see ourselves as fellow pilgrims who share in the struggles and sufferings of our patients. We can't cure everything, but we can care and come alongside our patients and offer companionship . . . . We also have a tendency to deny our own story. However, our struggles and problems may not be only for us to learn from, but also to help others. If we deny our story, we may be denying healing to others. (p. 74)

Of course, caution must be taken that our own woundedness enters into the nurse–client relationship in an appropriate manner. One inappropriate approach would be if the nurse "worked through" such spiritual woundedness in the context of his or her relationship with clients. Self-awareness and a commitment to ethical practice will be safeguards against such a situation from occurring.

Not only does the nurse's own spirituality impact client care, but the spirituality of the nurse is reciprocally impacted by caring for clients. For example, one way that nurses can be personally impacted by the care that they provide is in being stimulated to examine their own beliefs and practices. For example, when faced with a person who is dying and who is experiencing comfort and peace because of what that person believes will happen after death, a nurse can then reflect on what he or she personally believes about life, death, and life after death. When encountering clients who feel peaceful and healthy in the midst of adverse events in their lives because of their belief that God is with them, helping them, a nurse who has a similar faith can be strengthened in his or her belief about God's presence (or be stimulated to reflect on the existence of God). When working with a client whose life has been forever changed as a result of an accident, a nurse can be stimulated to reflect on what he or she values most as well as to realize one's own vulnerability. Spiritual care can also impact nurses in a manner so as to increase their spiritual well-being. If spiritual well-being is increased, then the nurse is more likely to provide beneficial spiritual care (Burkhart & Schmidt, 2012). When faced with clients who are very resilient in the face of great adversity, a nurse can be stimulated to appreciate life and significant people in that nurse's life (Taylor & Amenta, 1994).

One issue related to the spiritual dimension of care is the sharing of one's spiritual/religious beliefs and perspectives with clients, an issue related to ethical care. Van Leeuwen and Cusveller (2004) state:

> [Nurses] . . . will always bring their own personal "frames of reference" to bear on practice, including the spiritual care provided. This means that there is room for a nurse's personal convictions when providing spiritual care, in terms of talking about faith in the same way they talk about other things . . . in a professional manner. (p. 236)

General guidelines for nurse self-disclosure have been developed, for example, Egan and Schroeder (2009). However, Taylor (2011) and Winslow and Wehtje-Winslow (2007) identify guidelines that are important for appropriate nurse self-disclosure about spiritual and religious beliefs in particular. These guidelines protect the client and ensure that care is ethical. The five guidelines provided by Winslow and Wehtje-Winslow indicate that health care professionals should do the following:

1. Seek a basic understanding of patients' spiritual needs, resources, and preferences (p. S63).

2. Follow the patient's expressed wishes regarding spiritual care (p. S64).

3. Neither prescribe spiritual practices nor urge patients to relinquish religious beliefs or practices (p. S64).

4. Seek to understand their own spirituality (p. S65).

5. Participate in spiritual care consonant with their professional integrity.

In an earlier work, Taylor (2002) identified guidelines for nurse self-disclosure about spiritual and religious beliefs that are additional to the five just presented:

1. "Establish nurse–client boundaries" (p.71). Helpful aspects that the nurse can consider in this regard are what the purpose of the self-disclosure might be, and if the disclosure will enhance the relationship with the client.

2. "Practice existential advocacy" (p. 72), which involves balancing respect for the autonomy of clients with the recognition that the nurse has expertise that he or she can offer to the client.

3. "Examine your motivation" (p. 72), especially determining if the disclosure is to meet the nurse's needs.

4. "Strive for symmetry in client relationships" (p. 72), which involves nurses encountering clients " . . . from a shared woundedness" (p. 72).

5. "Respond in ways that strengthen nurse–client relationships" (p. 73), such as with empathy and acceptance.

6. "Observe the Golden Rule" (p. 73). A helpful question that nurses can ask themselves with respect to this guideline is: "If I were in this client's situation, would I want to hear my nurse say what I want to say now" (p. 73)?

7. "Offer responses that reflect a common ground" (p. 73), for example, sharing universal spiritual beliefs and ideas.

Taylor (2011) poses questions that nurses can ask of themselves with respect to sharing their spiritual or religious beliefs with clients, such as, "Why do I *need* to share my beliefs?" and, "What might I be gaining from sharing?" (p. 202). Taylor cautions against proselytizing on the part of the nurse, as this does not respect a client's spiritual positioning, and takes advantage of the vulnerability of the client—a bilateral breach of ethical practice.

Reflection 4.8

- Are you aware of your own woundedness? How have you used your woundedness in your work with clients? What has been the impact for both you and the client?
- Have you ever disclosed your personal spiritual or religious beliefs with clients? Under what circumstances did this occur and what was the outcome of the disclosure? What guidelines (if any) for self-disclosure did you follow?
- Have you witnessed any inappropriate sharing of spiritual or religious beliefs by your peers? What was the impact on the client?

Nurses are impacted by clients. As Remen, quoted in Remen and Rabow (2007), stated, "The expectation that we can be immersed in suffering or loss daily and not be touched by it is as unrealistic as expecting to be able to walk through water without getting wet" (p.4). Hoglund (2013) writes about the issue of clients who impact the nurse at the very core of his or her being in a negative manner. Such clients

> may be viewed as objectionable—offensive, unpleasant, even unworthy of care. Such patients or families can elicit negative feelings and perceptions. Nurses have the potential to experience anger, frustration, disgust, or revulsion toward the demands of an encounter with an objectionable patient or family. (p. 229)

Examples given by Hoglund include caring for perpetrators of horrific acts toward another person, intoxicated people who have neglected themselves, defiant teens whose actions have seriously hurt or even killed others, clients who have quite poor personal hygiene, and rude or demanding clients. Adhering to nursing codes of ethics in such situations is important, for example, respecting "the inherent dignity, worth, unique attributes, and human rights of all individuals" (ANA, 2015, p. 1). Moreover, Hoglund (2013) identifies her own positioning as a Christian as being important to enable her to care for such clients. She adheres to a worldview that sees all people as made in the image of God and as being of incredible worth. This is an example where the spiritual positioning of the nurse can impact client care in a positive way. Hoglund also supports the practice of commendations as particularly helpful in such situations, an intervention rooted in family therapy that empowers clients. Commendations are verbal statements that are distinguished from compliments in that compliments are one-time observations whereas commendations are related to patterns of behavior over time. In providing commendations, the nurse needs to focus on client strengths, looking for opportunities to comment on same to clients (Wright & Leahey, 2009). This type of intervention is in keeping with a strength-based approach to nursing practice. Hoglund (2013) gives an example of a commendation given to a mother who cared for her critically ill daughter: "You are doing a good job of encouraging your daughter. Your patience and persistence in supporting her is to be commended" (p. 232). Hoglund identifies several benefits of commendations:

- They are empowering for both clients and nurses.

- They help nurses "create a milieu of compassionate and respectful care in very difficult situations" (p. 232).

- They "allow the patient and family to reframe their experiences and circumstances in a different light, which, in turn enhances patient/family resilience and strengths" (Wright & Leahey, 2009, p. 232).

- They "foster new ideas and new possibilities for patient and family participation in care and healing" (p. 232).

- They foster positive nurse–client relationships.

One crucial way to deal with the impact of clients on a nurse's personhood is in caring for the self. Because of the nature of nursing and the environment within which it occurs, there is the potential for nurses to feel drained, fatigued, and burned out. Such feelings can deplete not only the physical, social, and emotional self, but also the spiritual self. Codes of ethics place importance on the self-care of the nurse. For example, the ANA (2015) *Code of Ethics* states: "The nurse owes the same duties to self as to others, including the responsibility to . . . preserve wholeness of character and integrity, maintain competence, and continue personal and professional growth" (p. 19). Self-care is important for nurses because it helps them to provide effective spiritual care for clients (Barnum, 2011; Murphy & Walker, 2013; Taylor, 2007). As McCarver (2011) states of herself as a nurse who experienced an illness: "As I learned how to respond to the spiritual needs of my soul I discovered I was being equipped to meet the spiritual needs of my patients' souls" (p. 86). Mauk and Schmidt (2004) and Bay, Ivy, and Terry (2010) identify ways to promote spiritual wellness in particular: meditation; prayer; progressive relaxation; worship in a faith community; listening to music; reading poetry; positive affirmations such as meditating on spiritually inspiring writings; spiritual journaling; connecting to nature; obtaining spiritual support from a mentor or faith community; and deriving spiritual energy from the practice of nursing—particularly if the practice is viewed as a "calling" and not merely a "job." Other activities might include engaging in some creative work such as painting or knitting. Not all of these activities will be relevant for every nurse. The key point here is the importance of nurses engaging in activities that nurture their own personal spirituality.

Reflection 4.9

Do you intentionally engage in activities that nurture your spirituality? What are these and how do they protect you from burnout? If you feel that you need to devote more attention to self-care, then what concrete plan can you develop and follow? What obstacles might you encounter in executing your plan and how might you deal with these? Follow your plan and identify any differences that you have noted in your own spiritual well-being. Also identify any impact on client care in general; and on the spiritual needs of clients in particular.

THE NURSING PROCESS AND SPIRITUAL ASSESSMENT AND CARE

The nursing process of assessment, planning, implementation, and evaluation is a well-known process within nursing. A perusal of the nursing literature will reveal multiple references to "spiritual assessment," "planning spiritual care," "spiritual nursing diagnoses," and "spiritual interventions." This abundance of references attests to the popularity of the nursing process in attending to the spiritual dimension of care. It is also within this nursing process that the competencies and attributes for spiritual care are operationalized. A few comments about the nursing process are in order inasmuch as the following two chapters in this book are framed within this process.

First of all, although the nursing process *begins* with assessment, assessment is actually ongoing throughout the nursing process. Every encounter with a client should be a new opportunity for assessment. Secondly, the process of conducting a spiritual assessment can, in and of itself, be an intervention. As clients reflect on questions asked during any discussion of spiritual issues, they can come to new realizations, which will be helpful in dealing with whatever situation they are experiencing. Thirdly, although the process is a nursing process, each stage should include the client as an active partner. This means that the client is not merely the recipient of assessment, planning, implementation, and evaluation, but is actively involved throughout. The client brings his or her expertise to the process just as much as the nurse does.

Pesut and Sawatzky (2006) present an excellent discussion of problems associated with a *prescriptive* view of the nursing process when it comes to the spiritual dimension of care. Such a view assumes that spirituality is a universal concept with a normative frame against which a person's spiritual condition can be uncovered and/or judged. Casarez and Engebretson (2012) maintain that in this approach the nurse would set goals for the client, in essence, seeking to "modify the spirituality . . . " (p. 2102) of the client. Yet, the goals and outcomes of spiritual care are intricately connected to how clients understand spirituality for themselves. Pesut and Sawatzky ask some thought-provoking questions:

Does the spiritual dimension of persons have a normative component, or is it purely a subjective experience that cannot be judged? Further, if it has a normative component, is that component universally agreed upon or does it have the potential to differ between patients and health care providers? What if a nurse diagnoses depression leading to spiritual risk of a patient, who frames the situation as a 'dark night of the soul' leading to spiritual growth? Whose perspective prevails and under what conditions? (p. 130)

Pesut and Sawatzky also maintain that the common language of a prescriptive nursing process approach may not be understood by clients. Not all clients accept that they have a spiritual dimension or are able to conceptualize spirituality constructions. This may be for multiple reasons, for example, cognitive impairment. Again, Pesut and Sawatzky propose some thought-provoking questions in this regard:

If spirituality is dependent on a functioning intellect does that mean that those who are cognitively impaired have less spirituality? Also, our preoccupation with meaning and purpose in the context of spirituality may be a product of a society where we have the luxury of focusing on such things. Would those living in poverty, who expend most of their energy simply surviving, be as concerned with individual meaning and purpose, and if not, does that mean they are less spiritual? (p. 131)

A third point that Pesut and Sawatzky make with respect to a prescriptive view of the nursing process is that such a view assumes that the spiritual dimension of persons should be influenced by nurses toward some desirable outcome. A key issue here is whether nurses *should* influence clients and when might that influence become coercive. The nurse can impose his or her own belief system in setting goals for the client, which could be viewed as coercive. An example given by Casarez and Engebretson (2012) is when a nurse prays with a client when that client did not request same. As Pesut and Sawatzky state, "Even if we believe that we can influence patients in the realm of the spiritual, we have to ask ourselves whether it is ethically appropriate to do so" (p. 132). A personalized question relates to this point:

Imagine yourself on an acute care oncology unit having just received a diagnosis of terminal cancer. Would you desire your nurse, a relative stranger, to perform a complete spiritual assessment on you and to formulate a plan of care that would entail intervening in your life toward some predefined spiritual end? (p. 132)

A final point that Pesut and Sawatzky make is that a prescriptive view of the nursing process assumes that nurses are competent to assess and intervene in the spiritual dimension of care. That is, the nurse goes beyond the client's subjective view of spirituality and the nurse is competent to assess that client's spirituality so as to intervene appropriately. A key issue here is with respect to education so as to ensure competencies, to determine what competencies are needed, and to propose how they are obtained. The nursing role in the literature is portrayed as making judgments regarding the spirituality of clients, but are nurses competent to do so? Pesut and Sawatzky again pose questions for consideration:

[W]hat nursing competency is required to perform [a spiritual assessment] and to intervene accordingly? How does a nurse ensure that he or she has enough knowledge about spirituality to assess competently and completely? . . . What body of knowledge is given to [nursing] students in [spiritual assessment] and how confident can we be that two educated nurses would arrive at similar assessments? What about the existential aspects of spirituality related to purpose, meaning and connectedness? What body of knowledge do we provide to educate nurses in this area? (p. 132)

Pesut and Sawatzky conclude that a prescriptive view of the nursing process "extends the nursing role beyond appropriate professional boundaries, making it ethically problematic" (p. 133). Instead, a *descriptive* view of the nursing process (Varcoe, 1996) is suggested as more desirable. Such a view is described by Pesut and Sawatzky as "descriptive in that it describes what the nurse does in response to the desires of the patient in relation to the spiritual. Spiritual interventions such as listening, respect and establishing trust are described as ways to make room for the spirituality of patients" (p. 132). A review of Pesut and Sawatzky's article is beneficial for a more in-depth discussion of spirituality and the nursing process.

Reflection 4.10

Reflect on your own conceptualization and use of the nursing process:

- Do you see yourself as "expert" or do you value a true partnership between you and the client? If the latter, how is this operationalized in your practice? If the former, how can moving to a partnership stance improve your nursing practice?
- Reflect on the four points made by Pesut and Sawatzky (2006) with respect to a prescriptive view of the nursing process when it comes to the spiritual dimension of care compared to a descriptive view of this process. Which view do you currently hold of the nursing process? What opportunities might having a descriptive view of this process provide when it comes to spiritual assessment and care?

The competencies discussed in this chapter position the nurse well in incorporating spirituality/religion into nursing practice. Reflection on same is important to create awareness of one's own positioning with respect to each of the competencies. A nurse's goal should be to continually improve and develop expertise in each of the competencies that are noted to be conducive to spiritual assessment and care.

The Bottom Line

- Competencies are critical to effective and appropriate spiritual assessment and care.

- There are competencies and attributes that have been identified that are conducive to effective and appropriate spiritual assessment and care. Nurses should strive to acquire them.

- Presence, listening, and caring are foundational nursing attributes/competencies for spiritual assessment and care.

- Competencies and attributes are operationalized within a therapeutic nurse–client relationship.

- Effective use of communication skills is critical to the nurse's effective and appropriate spiritual assessment and care.

- The personal spirituality of the nurse is important in terms of its impact on spiritual assessment and care.

Taking It Further

1. Review the article by van Leeuwen and Cusveller (2004). Note the competency profile that is organized around the three domains, in particular the vignettes indicating situations in which the nurse behaviors attached to each competency are appropriate (Table 3). Reflect on your own vignettes that pertain to some aspect of spiritual or religious care. Then formulate which competencies are relevant for each of your vignettes. If any of these vignettes are current in your practice, act on these competences, noting the outcome for both the client and yourself.

2. Review the SCCS (van Leeuwen et al., 2009). Rate yourself in terms of the listed competencies in the scale:

   a. What are your reflections on the completion of this scale and the analysis of your score? Were you surprised by your score on any of the items and why?

   b. Do you feel that there are aspects of spirituality in nursing not included in the scale? If so, what are such aspects? Write an item or items related to these aspects and add to the scale.

   c. How competent are you at this point in terms of providing spiritual care? What factors have contributed to this competence—or lack thereof?

   d. Which areas might you need to further develop competence and what do you need to do to increase your competence?

   e. Revisit the SCCS at varying points in your future practice to determine if you are increasing your competence in the spiritual dimension of care.

   f. How might you use this scale in promoting spiritual care in the clinical setting?

3. Write a job description for a nurse, which includes spiritual assessment and care competencies. If that description is generated in the context of a group of peers/colleagues, then compare your lists. Discuss the rationale for each of the competencies listed.

4. Write your own list of nursing competencies that you think are important for spiritual assessment and care, including indicators of such competencies. Compare this list with those identified in the nursing literature.

5. Interview a number of clients and ask them what qualities, characteristics, and attitudes they would deem to be important for nurses to have in terms of attending to their spiritual needs. How might their responses inform your nursing practice?

6. Conduct a literature review on the concepts of "presence" and "caring." How does this review expand your perception of these concepts? How can it inform your nursing practice?

7. Review Karl's identification of the three sources of the ability to be present with clients (Karl, 1992) and reflect on the following questions:

    a. Why is being present to and with clients so important in spiritual assessment and care?

    b. Why is it difficult to establish and maintain presence?

    c. What conditions facilitate the ability to be present for and with clients?

8. Review the article by Doona and colleagues (1999) on the concept of nursing presence, in particular the six key features of presence that are identified in the article (p. 57). Reflect on these six features, noting instances where these have been present in your nursing practice. How does this reflection inform the sense of your own ability to be present to and with clients?

9. Review an article by Rankin and DeLashmutt (2006) focused on spirituality and nursing presence. In this article, Rankin and DeLashmutt make the following comments about spirituality, the nurse–client relationship, and nursing presence:

    Relationship is a prerequisite to the manifestation of presence and spirituality. Presence is the revelation of holism in action that cannot exist outside of communion. Spirituality is a way of being and experiencing that shapes and impacts nursing presence (p. 287).

    a. Reflect on this statement: How does it inform your understanding of the relationship between spirituality, the nurse–client relationship, and presence?

    b. Review the depiction of elements involved in experiencing spirituality and presence in the nurse–client relationship in this article (pp. 285–287). How does the visual aid depicted enable you to be more aware of spirituality and nursing presence? How might you use this aid to encourage the development of presence within yourself and your peers/colleagues?

10. Review Table 5 in the article by Highfield, Taylor, and Amenta (2000) regarding nurses' descriptions of how clients influenced the spirituality of the nurse. Can you identify with any of these descriptions? If so, how does the spiritual examination and spiritual self-development caused by contact with clients impact your nursing practice?

11. Discuss with your nursing peers/colleagues the idea of nursing as a "calling" and nursing as a "job." Also, discuss the creation of balance between work and a lifestyle outside of one's work in terms of developing oneself as a holistic

human being. What insights arise from this discussion? How can they be helpful in informing your nursing practice?

12. Chung and colleagues (2007) completed a study on the relationship of nurses' own spirituality to their understanding and practice of spiritual care. Review the 27 items in the Nurses' Spirituality and Delivery of Spiritual Care Scale (NS-DSC) developed for this study (Table 1, p. 163). On a scale of 1 to 5, with 1 being "not at all characteristic of me" and 5 being "very characteristic of me," rate yourself on each item. What insights did you gain related to your own spirituality in completing this scale? What are the implications for your nursing practice?

13. Describe in writing three stories about your nursing practice that involved the spiritual dimension of care and that made a difference not only in the client's life but also your own. Reflect on your stories. What aspects of spirituality and spiritual care are present in each story? What themes do you notice? For each story, how did the impact on you inform your nursing practice (Hudacek, 2008)?

14. To increase your awareness of your own spiritual self, complete the following exercise:

    a. Write a two- or three-line epitaph denoting what is important or significant about your life.

    b. Write a brief reflection on completing this epitaph, including your feelings and perception of how well it describes you.

    c. Share the epitaph with someone for verification/modification based on his or her knowledge of you.

    d. If done as a group exercise) discuss and share your epitaph and reactions to same with peers/colleagues (adapted from Beckman, Boxley-Harges, Bruick-Sorge, & Salmon, 2007).

15. Reflect on your own spiritual history and how your past experiences, education, and upbringing impact how you think and feel about issues related to spirituality and religion. How does your spiritual history affect how you recognize and respond to your own spiritual needs? What attitudes are highlighted in reflection on your history that might prevent you from caring for yourself spiritually? How can you integrate your spiritual history into your life in a healthy and appropriate way in order to develop your spiritual self?

16. Reflect on situations of crisis in your past (recent or distant) that resulted in spiritual distress or unresolved feelings, such as loss or guilt. How might these impact your ability to listen to clients dealing with similar situations or crises? How might they impact your ability to engage in spiritual assessment and spiritual care? What do you need to do in order to explore and deal with your own woundedness and pain? How might this resolution positively impact your ability to listen and to provide spiritual care (Sweat, 2011)?

17. Review the study by Bay and colleagues (2010) of the impact of spiritual retreats on nurses' spiritual well-being, in particular noting an outline of a two, one-day retreats (p. 130):

a. Might you be able to use this outline to plan a similar retreat for nurses, especially given the fact that Bay and colleagues identified nurses' spiritual well-being to be enhanced by the retreats?

b. What might you change in the outline so that the retreat would best suit your context of practice and why?

c. How might you evaluate the impact of the retreat on nurses' spiritual well-being?

REFERENCES

American Nurses Association. (2015). *Code of ethics for nurses with interpretative statements.* Retrieved from http://www.nursingworld.org/codeofethics

Association of Registered Nurses of Newfoundland and Labrador. (2013). *Competencies in the context of entry-level registered nurse practice 2013-18.* Retrieved from https//www.arnnl.ca/competencies-context-entry-level-registered-nurse-practice-2013-18-2013

Baldacchino, D. (2006). Nursing competencies for spiritual care. *Journal of Clinical Nursing, 15*(7), 885–896. doi:10.1111/j.1365-2702.2006.01643.x

Baldacchino, D. (2010). *Spiritual care: Being in doing.* Marsa, Malta: Preca Library.

Barnum, B. S. (2011). *Spirituality in nursing: The challenges of complexity* (3rd ed.). New York, NY: Springer Publishing Company.

Bay, P. S., Ivy, S. S., & Terry, C. L. (2010). The effect of spiritual retreat on nurses' spirituality: A randomized controlled study. *Holistic Nursing Practice, 24*(3), 125–133. doi:10.1097/HNP.0b013e3181dd47dd

Beckman, S., Boxley-Harges, S., Bruick-Sorge, C., & Salmon, B. (2007). Five strategies that heighten nurses' awareness of spirituality to impact client care. *Holistic Nursing Practice, 21*(3), 135–139. doi:10.1097/01.HNP.0000269150.80978.c3

Benner, P. (1984). *From novice to expert: Excellence and power in clinical nursing practice.* Menlo Park, CA: Addison-Wesley.

Biro, A. (2012). Creating conditions for good nursing care by attending to the spiritual. *Journal of Nursing Management, 20*(8), 1002–1011. doi:10.1111/j.1365-2834.2012.01444.x

Brooks, D., Henry, J., LeBlanc, J., McKenzie, G., Nagy, T., Tallon, H., . . . Flegel-Desautels, C. (2005). Incorporating spirituality into practice. *Canadian Nurse, 101*(6), 22–24.

Burkhardt, M. A., & Nagai-Jacobson, M. G. (2002). *Spirituality: Living our connectedness.* Albany, NY: Delmar.

Burkhart, L., & Schmidt, W. (2012). Measuring effectiveness of a spiritual care pedagogy in nursing education. *Journal of Professional Nursing, 28*(5), 315–321. doi:10.1016/j.profnurs.2012.03.003

Callister, L. C., Bond, A. E., Matsumura, G., & Mangum, S. (2004). Threading spirituality throughout nursing education. *Holistic Nursing Practice, 18*(3), 160–166.

Canadian Nurses Association. (2008). *Code of ethics for registered nurses.* Retrieved from https://www.cna-aiic.ca/~/media/cna/page-content/pdf-fr/code-of-ethics-for-registered-nurses.pdf?la=en

Carr, T. (2008). Mapping the processes and qualities of spiritual nursing care. *Qualitative Health Research, 18*(5), 686–700. doi:10.1177/1049732307308979

Carr, T. J. (2010). Facing existential realities: Exploring barriers and challenges to spiritual nursing care. *Qualitative Health Research, 20*(10), 1379–1392. doi:10.1177/1049732310372377

Casarez, R. L. P., & Engebretson, J. C. (2012). Ethical issues of incorporating spiritual care into clinical practice. *Journal of Clinical Nursing, 21*(15–16). doi:10.1111/j.1365-2702.2012.04168x

Castaneda, L., Habert, B., Witt, P., Younker, D., & Crigger, N. (2007). Are we speaking the same language? *Journal of Christian Nursing, 24*(2), 88–93. doi:10.1097/01.CNJ.0000265573.27834.1f

Chan, M. F. (2009). Factors affecting nursing staff in practicing spiritual care. *Journal of Clinical Nursing, 19*(15–16), 2128–2136. doi:10.1111/j.1365-2702.2008.02690.x

Chan, M. F., Chung, L. Y., Lee, A. S., Wong, W. K., Lee, G. S., Lau, C. Y., . . . Ng, J. W. S. (2006). Investigating spiritual care perceptions and practice patterns in Hong Kong nurses: Results of a cluster analysis. *Nurse Education Today, 26*(2), 139–150. doi:10.1016/j.nedt.2005.08.006

Chan, Z. C. Y. (2011). How has liberation theology influenced my practice? *International Journal of Nursing practice, 17*(4), 330–335. doi:10.1111/j.1440-172X.2011.01946.x

Chapman, G. (1995). *The five love languages: How to express heartfelt commitment to your mate.* Chicago, IL: Northfield.

Chism, L. A., & Magnan, M. A. (2009). The relationship of nursing students' spiritual care perspectives to their expressions of spiritual empathy. *Journal of Nursing Education, 48*(11), 597–605. doi:10.3928/01484834-20090716-05

Chung, L. Y. F., Wong, F. K. Y., & Chan, M. F. (2007). Relationship of nurses' spirituality to their understanding and practice of spiritual care. *Journal of Advanced Nursing, 58*(2), 158–170. doi:10.1111/j.1365-2648.2007.04225.x

Cockell, N., & McSherry, W. (2012). Spiritual care in nursing: An overview of published international research. *Journal of Nursing Management, 20*(8), 958–969. doi:10.1111/j.1365-2834.2012.01450.x

Crain, A. (1994). Why are you doing this for me? A student nurse cares enough to help a patient regain self-respect. *Journal of Christian Nursing, 11*(2), 4–8.

Creel, E. (2007). The meaning of spiritual nursing care for the ill individual with no religious affiliation. *International Journal for Human Caring, 11*(3), 14–21.

Cusveller, B. (2013). A Calvinist account of nursing ethics. *Nursing Ethics, 20*(7), 762–770. doi:10.1177/0969733012473010

Dameron, C. M. (2012). Presence. *Journal of Christian Nursing, 29*(4), 201. doi:10.1097/CNJ.0b013e31826804cc

Delashmutt, M. B. (2007). Students' experience of nursing presence with poor mothers. *Journal of Obstetric, Gynecologic & Neonatal Nursing, 36*(2), 183–189. doi:10.1111/J.1552-6909.2007.00135.x

Doona, M. E., Chase, S. K., & Haggerty, L. A. (1999). Nursing presence: As real as a Milky Way bar. *Journal of Holistic Nursing, 17*(1), 54–70. doi:10.1177/089801019901700105

Dossey, B., & Keegan, L. (2000). Self-assessment: Facilitating healing in self and others. In B. M. Dossey, L. Keegan, & C. Guzzetta (Eds.), *Holistic nursing: A handbook for practice* (3rd ed., pp. 361–374). Gaithersburg, MD: Aspen.

Duff, V. (1994). Spiritual distress: Deciding to care. *Journal of Christian Nursing, 11*(1), 29–31.

Egan, G., & Schroeder, W. (2009). *The skilled helper: A problem-management and opportunity-development approach to helping, first Canadian edition.* Toronto, ON, Canada: Nelson.

Eliopoulos, C. (2004). Spiritual care: Not just the domain of clergy. *Director, 12*(4), 252–253.

Grant, D. (2004). Spiritual interventions: How, when, and why nurses use them. *Holistic Nursing Practice, 18*(1), 36–41.

Highfield, M. E. F., Taylor, E. J., & Amenta, M. O. (2000). Preparation to care: The spiritual care education of oncology and hospice nurses. *Journal of Hospice & Palliative Nursing, 2*(2), 53–63.

Hoglund, B. A. (2013). Practicing the code of ethics, finding the image of God. *Journal of Christian Nursing, 30*(4), 228–233. doi:10.1097/CNJ.0b013e3182a18d40

Hudacek, S. S. (2008). Dimensions of caring: A qualitative analysis of nurses' stories. *Journal of Nursing Education, 47*(3), 124–129. doi:10.3928/01484834-20080301-04

Iacono, M. V. (2011). Colleagues in caring: Pastoral care at the bedside. *Journal of PeriAnesthesia Nursing, 26*(6), 416–419. doi:10.1016/j.jopan.2011.09.003

International Council of Nurses. (2012). *The ICN Code of Ethics for Nurses.* Retrieved from http://www.icn.ch/images/stories/documents/about/icncode_english.pdf

Karl, J. C. (1992). Being there: Who do you bring to practice? In D. Gault (Ed.), *The presence of caring in nursing* (pp. 1–13). New York, NY: National League for Nursing.

Kaur, D., Sambasivan, M., & Kumar, N. (2013). Effect of spiritual intelligence, emotional intelligence, psychological ownership and burnout on caring behaviour of nurses: A cross-sectional study. *Journal of Clinical Nursing, 22*(21–22), 3192–3202. doi:10.1111/jocn.12386

Kevern, P. (2012). Who can give "spiritual care?" The management of spiritually sensitive interactions between nurses and patients. *Journal of Nursing Management, 20*(8), 981–989. doi:10.1111/j.1365-2834.2012.01428.x

Kumar, K. (2004). Spiritual care: What's worldview got to do with it? *Journal of Christian Nursing*, *21*(1), 24–28. doi:10.1097/01.CNJ.0000262275.10582.66

Lantz, C. M. (2007). Teaching spiritual care in a public institution: Legal implications, standards of practice and ethical obligations. *Journal of Nursing Education*, *46*(1), 33–38.

Lee, E. A. D. (2006). Finding your model of caring practice: Articulating my theory gave me greater satisfaction with my practice. *Journal of Christian Nursing*, *23*(3), 14–19.

Mauk, K. L., & Schmidt, N. K. (Ed.). (2004). *Spiritual care in nursing practice*. Philadelphia, PA: Lippincott Williams & Wilkins.

McCarver, P. K. (2011). Nursing . . . focused on tasks or people? *Journal of Christian Nursing*, *28*(2), 85–87. doi:10.1097/CNJ.0b013e31820b93ae

McEwen, M. (2005). Spiritual nursing care: State of the art. *Holistic Nursing Practice*, *19*(4), 161–168.

McMullan, M., Endacott, R., Gray, M. A., Jasper, M., Miller, C. M. L., Scholes, J., & Webb, C. (2003). Portfolios and assessment of competence: A review of the literature. *Journal of Advanced Nursing*, *41*(3), 283–294. doi:10.1046/j.1365-2648.2003.02528.x

McSherry, W. (2006). The principal components model: A model for advancing spirituality and spiritual care within nursing and health care practice. *Journal of Clinical Nursing*, *15*(7), 905–917. doi:10.1111/j.1365-2702.2006.01648.x

McSherry, W., & Jamieson, S. (2013). The qualitative findings from an online survey investigating nurses' perceptions of spirituality and spiritual care. *Journal of Clinical Nursing*, *22*(21–22), 3170–3182. doi:10.1111/jocn.12411

Meyer, C. (2000). Providing spiritual care: A mutual journey of discovery. *Kansas Nurse*, *75*(10), 1–3.

Meyer, C. L. (2003). How effectively are nurse educators preparing students to provide spiritual care? *Nurse Educator*, *28*(4), 185–190.

Miner-Williams, D. (2006). Putting a puzzle together: Making spirituality meaningful for nursing using an evolving theoretical framework. *Journal of Clinical Nursing*, *15*(7), 811–821. doi:10.1111/j.1365-2702.2006.01351.x

Mok, E., Wong, F., & Wong, D. (2010). The meaning of spirituality and spiritual care among the Hong Kong Chinese terminally ill. *Journal of Advanced Nursing*, *66*(2), 360–370. doi:10.1111/j.1365-2648.2009.05193.x

Murphy, L. S., & Walker, M. (2013). Spirit-guided care: Christian nursing for the whole person. *Journal of Christian Nursing*, *30*(3), 144–152. doi:10.1097/CNJ.0b013e318294c289

Musgrave, C. F., & McFarlane, E. A. (2004). Israeli oncology nurses' religiosity, spiritual well-being, and attitudes towards spiritual care: A path analysis. *Oncology Nursing Forum*, *31*(2), 321–327. doi:10.1188/04.ONF.321-327

Narayanasamy, A. (2004). The puzzle of spirituality for nursing: A guide to practical assessment. *British Journal of Nursing*, *13*(19), 1140–1144. doi:10.12968/bjon.2004.13.19.16322

National Health Service (NHS) Education for Scotland. (2009). *Spiritual care matters: An introductory resource for all NHS Scotland staff*. Retrieved from http://www.nes.scot.nhs.uk/media/3723/spiritualcaremattersfinal.pdf

Nouwen, H. J. M. (1979). *The wounded healer: Ministry in contemporary society*. New York, NY: Image Books.

Osterman, P., & Schwartz-Barcott, D. (1996). Presence: Four ways of being there. *Nursing Forum*, *31*(2), 23–30. doi:10.1111/j.1744-6198.1996.tb00490.x

Pesut, B. (2006). Fundamental or foundational obligation? Problematizing the ethical call to spiritual care in nursing. *Advances in Nursing Science*, *29*(2), 125–133.

Pesut, B. (2009a). Incorporating patients' spirituality into care using Gadow's ethical framework. *Nursing Ethics*, *16*(4), 418–428. doi:10.1177/0969733009104606

Pesut, B. (2009b). Care of the spirit: Passing the mantle from institutional religion to institutional health care. *Touchstone*, *27*(1), 16–25. Retrieved from http://touchstonecanada.ca/wp-content/uploads/2013/08/Jan-2009-Article2.pdf

Pesut, B., & Sawatzky, R. (2006). To describe or prescribe: Assumptions underlying a prescriptive nursing process approach to spiritual care. *Nursing Inquiry*, *13*(2), 127–134. doi:10.1111/j.1440-1800.2006.00315.x

Rankin, E. A., & DeLashmutt, M. B. (2006). Finding spirituality and nursing presence: The student's challenge. *Journal of Holistic Nursing*, 24(4), 282–288. doi:10.1177/0898010106294423

Reimer-Kirkham, S., Pesut, B., Meyerhoff, H., & Sawatzky, R. (2004). Spiritual caregiving at the juncture of religion, culture, and state. *Canadian Journal of Nursing Research*, 36(4), 148–169.

Remen, N. R., & Rabow, M. R. (2007). The healer's art: Sharing grief and honoring loss. *AAHPM Bulletin*, Fall 2007, 4–5. Retrieved from http://www.ishiprograms.org/wp-content/uploads/pro grams-medical_educators-publications_5_21250082.pdf

Rew, L. (1989). Intuition: Nursing knowledge and the spiritual dimension of persons. *Holistic Nursing Practice*, 3(3), 56–68. doi:10.1097/00004650-198905000-00010

Ross, L. (2006). Spiritual care in nursing: An overview of the research to date. *Journal of Clinical Nursing*, 15(7), 852–862. doi:10.1111/j.1365-2702.2006.01617.x

Ruder, S. (2013). Spirituality in nursing: Nurses' perceptions about providing spiritual care. *Home Healthcare Now*, 31(7), 356–367. doi:10.1097/NHH.0b013e3182976135

Sawatzky, R., & Pesut, B. (2005). Attributes of spiritual care in nursing practice. *Journal of Holistic Nursing*, 23(1), 19–33. doi:10.1177/0898010104272010

Sellers, S. C. (2001). The spiritual care meanings of adults residing in the Midwest. *Nursing Science Quarterly*, 14(3), 239–248. doi:10.1177/08943180122108355

Stranahan, S. (2001). Spiritual perceptions, attitudes about spiritual care, and spiritual care practices among nurse practitioners. *Western Journal of Nursing Research*, 23(1), 90–104. doi:10.1177/01939450122044970

Sweat, M. T. (2010). Can I give spiritual care when my spiritual life is in shambles? *Journal of Christian Nursing*, 27(2), 74. doi:10.1097/CNJ.0b013e318d049a7

Sweat, M. T. (2011). What are the gaps in spiritual care? *Journal of Christian Nursing*, 28(2), 112. doi:10.1097/CNJ.0b013e31820ccaff

Swinton, J., & McSherry, W. (2006). Editorial: Critical reflections on the current state of spirituality-in-nursing. *Journal of Clinical Nursing*, 15(7), 801–802. doi:10.1111/j.1365-2702.2006.01687.x

Taylor, E. J. (2002). *Spiritual care: Nursing theory, research, and practice*. Upper Saddle River, NJ: Prentice-Hall.

Taylor, E. J. (2007). *What do I say? Talking with patients about spirituality*. Philadelphia, PA: Templeton Press.

Taylor, E. J. (2011). Spiritual care: Evangelism at the bedside? *Journal of Christian Nursing*, 28(4), 194–202. doi:10.1097/CNJ.0b013e31822b494d

Taylor, E. J., & Amenta, M. (1994). Midwifery to the soul while the body dies: Spiritual care among hospice nurses. *The American Journal of Hospice and Palliative Medicine*, 11(6), 28–35. doi:10.1177/104990919401100608

Taylor, E. J., Highfield, M. F., & Amenta, M. (1999). Predictors of oncology and hospice nurses' spiritual care perspectives and practices. *Applied Nursing Research*, 12(1), 30–37. doi:10.1016/S0897-1897(99)80156-6

Unruh, A. M., Versnel, J., & Kerr, N. (2002). Spirituality unplugged: A review of commonalities and contentions, and a resolution. *Canadian Journal of Occupational Therapy*, 69(1), 5–19. doi:10.1177/000841740206900101

vanLeeuwen, R., & Cusveller, B. (2004). Nursing competencies for spiritual care. *Journal of Advanced Nursing*, 48(3), 234–246. doi:10.1111/j.1365-2648.2004.03192

vanLeeuwen, R., Tiesinga, L. J., Middel, B., Post, D., & Jochemsen, H. (2008). The effectiveness of an educational programme for nursing students on developing competence in the provision of spiritual care. *Journal of Clinical Nursing*, 17(20), 2768–2781. doi:10.1111/j.1365-2702.2008.02366.x

vanLeeuwen, R., Tiesinga, L. J., Middel, B., Post, D., & Jochemsen, H. (2009). The validity and reliability of an instrument to assess nursing competencies in spiritual care. *Journal of Clinical Nursing*, 18(20), 2857–2869. doi:10.1111/j.1365-2702.2008.02594.x

vanLeeuwen, R., Tiesinga, L. J., Post, D., & Jochemsen, H. (2006). Spiritual care: Implications for nurses' professional responsibility. *Journal of Clinical Nursing*, 15(7), 875–884. doi:10.1111/j.1365-2702.2006.01615.x

Varcoe, C. (1996). Disparagement of the nursing process: The new dogma. *Journal of Advanced Nursing, 23*(1), 120–125. doi:10.1111/j.1365-2648.1996.tb03144.x

Wasner, M., Longaker, C., Fegg, M. J., & Borasio, G. D. (2005). Effects of spiritual care training for palliative care professionals. *Palliative Medicine, 19*(2), 99–104. doi:10.1191/0269216305pm995oa

Winslow, G. R., & Wehtje-Winslow, B. J. (2007). Ethical boundaries of spiritual care. *Medical Journal of Australia, 186*(10, Suppl.), S63–S66.

Wright, L. M., & Leahey, M. (2009). *Nurses and families: A guide to family assessment and intervention* (5th ed.). Philadelphia, PA: F. A. Davis.

Zerwekh, J. V. (1997). The practice of presencing. *Seminars in Oncology Nursing, 13*(4), 260–262. doi:10.1016/S0749-2081(97)80022-8

5

Spiritual Assessment

The first four chapters in this book have provided the necessary background for considering the inclusion of spirituality into nursing practice. The topics discussed in those chapters are intricately connected to the focus of this chapter and the next chapter. For example, the focus of Chapters 1 and 2, namely how spirituality and religion are conceptualized, springboards into an exploration of *what* is being assessed and what interventions are appropriate. Similarly, much of the rationale for spirituality in nursing practice discussed in Chapter 3 (see section on Rationale for Spirituality in Health Care and Nursing) parallels the rationale for the inclusion of spiritual assessment and care into practice. And finally, the competencies discussed in Chapter 4 (see section on Competencies for Spiritual Assessment and Care) are relevant for spiritual assessment (in this chapter), just as they are for providing spiritual care (in the next chapter).

Accurate and sensitive spiritual assessment is key to addressing a client's spiritual needs in an appropriate and effective manner. It is also essential to holistic care as the spiritual dimension should be included in that care. Better client outcomes can be achieved if a client's spiritual needs are met. Spiritual assessment contributes to accountability in terms of what nurses are doing in the realm of spiritual care. It also provides a foundation for research on the spiritual dimensions of nursing practice. Spiritual assessment is mandated by various nursing documents (e.g., codes of ethics, and standards and competencies of practice) and by health care organizations (e.g., the Joint Commission on the Accreditation of Health Care Organizations [JCAHCO]). Spiritual assessment also provides a means not only to converse with clients about their spirituality but also to converse with other members of the health care team about essential client care. It can also be helpful in advance care planning, particularly with advance directives, in which such an assessment can identify clients' beliefs, wishes, values, and preferences that might otherwise remain unidentified and unknown (Chrash, Mulich, & Patton, 2011; Draper, 2012; Fitchett, 1993a; Fitchett & Handzo, 1998; Hodge, 2006; Katerberg, 1997; Massey, Fitchett, & Roberts, 2004).

Nursing has contributed much to the area of spiritual assessment. Nurses have developed spiritual well-being scales, such as the JAREL Spiritual Well-Being Scale (JAREL SWBS; Hungelmann, Kenkel-Rossi, Klassen, & Stollenwerk, 1996). They have also developed guidelines for spiritual assessment, such as Stoll's (1979) Guidelines for

Spiritual Assessment. Models for spiritual assessment have been developed by nurses, for example, the ASSET (actioning spirituality and spiritual care in education and training) model (Narayanasamy, 1999) and the model developed by Hawley and Taylor (2003). Other theorists include spiritual assessment in their nursing models as part of their models (Barss, 2012). Several nurses have developed a collection of questions to be used in spiritual assessment, such as those by Larson (2003). And protocols have been developed to guide nurses in not only spiritual assessment but also with respect to the other stages of the nursing process, for example, the Spiritual Wellness in Older Adult Protocol (Leetun, 1996) and the Spiritual Needs Protocol (Sumner, 1998).

DEFINITION/DESCRIPTION OF SPIRITUAL ASSESSMENT

Reference has already been made to explain how spirituality is defined/described and how the definitions of spirituality determine how spiritual assessment is conceptualized. For example, if spirituality is framed in Judeo-Christian terms, then it follows that a definition of spiritual assessment from such a conceptualization would include reference to Judeo-Christian concepts. This would also be the case for any spiritual assessment tool derived from that worldview. Fitchett (1993a) points out that the word "assessment" itself needs to be examined. For example, in nursing a "needs" assessment is both a noun and a verb as there is both a "content" aspect to assessment (i.e., information or data) and a "process" aspect to assessment (i.e., how one conducts the assessment). As such, assessment can also have both subjective and objective components.

There are a number of definitions and descriptions of spiritual assessment in the health care literature, and a few examples are given here for consideration. Burkhardt and Nagai-Jacobson (2002) describe spiritual assessment as taking stock of one's life and situation and becoming aware of one's deepest core. Fitchett (1993a) does not make any distinction between spirituality and religion (including religiosity, faith, and belief) for the purpose of assessment; depending on the client's worldview, either of these will need to be assessed. A description of spiritual assessment is provided by Fitchett and Handzo (1998):

> Spiritual assessment is the process of discerning the spiritual needs and resources of persons in various contexts where spiritual care is offered (p. 790). The aim of spiritual assessment is not to exhaust the complexity or mystery of the spiritual dimension of life. The aim is to organize observations about peoples' spiritual beliefs, behaviors, and relationships in ways that enhance caregiving. (p. 791)

Hodge (2006) defines spiritual assessment as "the process of gathering, analyzing, and synthesizing spiritual and religious information into a specific framework that provides the basis for, and gives direction to, subsequent practice decisions" (p. 318).

THE FOCUS OF SPIRITUAL ASSESSMENT

A key question with respect to spiritual assessment is just *what* is being assessed. In Chapter 1, a number of definitions of spirituality were given (see section on Defining Spirituality), and each definition could spawn an accompanying assessment guide. Key themes were also identified that are associated with spirituality. Again, spiritual assessment tools could be developed to focus on such themes. Spirituality was also presented in terms of worldview, and distinctive assessment tools could be developed for each of the major worldviews today. However, if one peruses the health care literature, one will find that there *are* key specific and common components related to spirituality and religion that can be the focus for quality spiritual assessment. Some examples of foci for spiritual assessment include the following:

- Whether spirituality/religion is part of a person's worldview and whether it is considered relevant to health
- Willingness to converse about and address spiritual dimension
- How spirituality is conceptualized
- Religious affiliation, commitment, beliefs, values, practices, rituals, needs, and impact on illness
- Spiritual beliefs, values, practices, rituals, needs, and impact on illness
- History of spiritual/religious experiences
- Relationships with other people and the quality of the relationships
- Issues of shame, guilt, and forgiveness
- Relationship and style of interacting with God, Supreme Being, or other indicators of the sacred things
- Expressions of spirituality (music, art, nature, etc.)
- Sources of hope and strength
- Connection to and involvement with a faith community, if supported by that community, and how
- Spiritual/religious coping strategies, including how one is impacted by illness
- Sources of support, including spiritual/religious sources (Burkhardt & Nagai-Jacobson, 2002; Darden, 2005; Fetzer Institute, 1999; Harris, Allen, Dunn, & Parmelee, 2013; JCAHCO, 2016; Pesut, Fowler, Reimer-Kirkham, Taylor, & Sawatzky, 2009; Treloar, 2001)

Reflection 5.1

Reflect on the examples of the assessment foci. Are there other aspects of spirituality that you would see as important to assess? If so, what would these be? Formulate one question that you would ask to assess each of these foci.

THE "HOW" OF SPIRITUAL ASSESSMENT

When assessing the spirituality of clients, the rationale for inquiry is important to present to the client. The rationale itself can facilitate client disclosure. Taylor (2011) provides some examples of how this rationale can be presented:

> Your health care team knows that the beliefs and values people have, whether religious or not, influence the decisions they make about the care they want to get. Given this, it would help us if we could learn from you how your spiritual or religious views might affect your _____ decision now (p. 198)? . . . [Or] We know that people often cope with difficult times like this by finding comfort in their spiritual beliefs or practices. If there are beliefs or practices that might have an impact on your health, it would be helpful for your health care providers to know. (p. 198)

Barss (2012) also stresses the importance of clearly communicating the relevance of spiritual inquiry to clients and gives an example of how to do so: "As part of offering holistic care, we would like to be aware of anything you consider to be important in relation to the spiritual aspect of your care" (p. 29). She also advocates for inviting clients to "self-define the nature of 'the spiritual'" (p. 29). Barss recommends using language that is more directly related to spiritual needs that are relevant to the client. For example, phrases such as "finding hope" or "making meaning" (p. 29) in relation to the current challenges that the client is experiencing might be helpful. Barss developed a model to assist nurses in the spiritual assessment of clients called the T.R.U.S.T. Model for Spiritual Assessment and Care (p. 30). Barss suggests: "At the appropriate time in the ensuing conversation (in a nonlinear, nonintrusive, client-centered manner), the initial questions [of the T.R.U.S.T. model] need to be addressed" (pp. 29–30). Examples of the rationale for spiritual inquiry that have been used in my own practice include: "Religion and spirituality are known to be helpful resources for people experiencing _____. Is religion or spirituality important to you and if so, how?" and "Many people draw on spiritual or religious resources during times of illness and suffering. Is this true for you as well, and if so, can you tell me more about that?"

Reflection 5.2

Develop two or three statements that you might use in your own nursing practice to explain to clients the rationale for spiritual inquiry. Use these in your practice this coming week. Which were most effective in encouraging the client to disclose? What changes in these statements might you make, if any?

As can be seen from the earlier list of assessment foci, there are quite a few areas that can be explored in a spiritual assessment. Not all areas or foci need to be assessed with each client. Pesut and colleagues (2009) suggest that a foundational spiritual assessment should begin with an inquiry into whether the client's worldview includes spirituality, and if spirituality is seen by the client as relevant to his or her health. If the client responds in the affirmative, then the nurse can proceed from this basic inquiry. For example, if the client responded with a statement such as: "Well, I am not religious but I do consider myself to be spiritual," then the nurse can proceed to ask, "What does spirituality mean to you?" and then continue to explore the client's spiritual beliefs and how they are relevant to his or her life, illness, or whatever situation the client is facing. If the client responds with a statement such as: "Well, to me my spirituality and my religion are one and the same," then the nurse can explore the client's religious commitment, beliefs, values, and any rituals important for him or her that are associated with his or her religion.

Taylor (2001) and Fitchett and Handzo (1998) also advocate for a brief initial assessment followed by more in-depth assessment depending on the client's responses. Hodge (2006) identifies conditions under which a more in-depth assessment is warranted:

- When it is important or relevant to the client, such as when some verbal or non-verbal indication of spiritual concern is present

- Whether it respects the client's autonomy in that the client indicates a desire for further exploration and gives consent for the same

- Whether the clinician is competent to conduct a more in-depth assessment in a culturally sensitive way

- Whether such an assessment is relevant to the client's health and also to the care to be delivered, as is the case when the client's beliefs may impact decisions about care

Although asking questions is an appropriate methodology in assessing the spiritual dimension of clients, nurses need also to be aware of cues that clients provide that may have spiritual or religious overtones and that might stimulate the use of such questions. In fact, Burkhart and Hogan (2008) identify certain client cues as the first step toward spiritual care, noting that such cues can be particularly present during times of crisis. Clients can give verbal cues. For example, clients may make a comment about God, religion, or spiritual or religious concerns, talk about what is meaningful in their lives, what makes them happy, and to what or to whom they are connected (e.g., their families). Some cues can be very subtle and may not only be manifested in what clients do or do not say, but also by nonverbal conduct. For example, in the context of a conversation pertaining to spirituality, clients' affect (e.g., joy, or, conversely, distress) and behavior might suggest spiritual connection or concern. Cues can also be environmental. For example, clients may have religiously oriented objects in their room or on their person. And finally, cues can be found in relationships. For example, clients may receive visitors from their faith community, who may have a positive impact on them. Key listening skills and careful observation skills are critical in picking up on such cues (Miner-Williams, 2006; Narayanasamy, 1991). One important point is the importance of verifying cues with clients to confirm a spiritual relevance to clients. For example, clients may have a Bible on the bedside table; it can be there for them to read and as a source of substantive comfort and strength; or it can be there merely as a symbol of good luck. Carson (2008) provides a list of important observations that are related to clients' verbalizations, nonverbal behavior, interpersonal relationships, and environment (p. 134). Reference to this list is recommended.

Reflection 5.3

Pay particular attention to the immediate environment of the clients that you encounter this week. Are there any cues to the clients' spirituality present? If so, how might you begin a conversation about spirituality with the clients utilizing such cues?

Clients' stories can also be particularly important as they can provide a window into the clients' spirituality. In fact, Browning (2008) indicates that listening to a person's story is one of the most important ways to show respect to clients. Not only is it important to pay attention to the content of the story, but focus on the client's affect and nonverbal behaviors in the telling of the story is also critical.

Draper (2012) explores four overlapping approaches to spiritual assessment. A summary of these approaches and accompanying features is presented in Table 5.1. A review of Draper's article for an in-depth discussion with respect to each approach, including its strengths and limitations, is recommended.

As can be seen from this discussion, the "how to" of spiritual assessment involves listening to clients, observing cues to their spirituality, and directly inquiring about aspects of spirituality. Perhaps the two most important methodologies for nurses to conduct a spiritual assessment in many health care contexts today are to assess the client's spirituality as part of an initial general history taking (a brief assessment) and to then continue with the assessment in an ongoing fashion in further interactions with the client. If nurses have an arsenal of questions pertinent to spiritual assessment at their disposal, then they can pick and choose questions that fit with the client's conversation

Table 5.1 **Approaches to Spiritual Assessment**

Generic	Occurs during routine encounters with clients; is open-ended; often occurs as an initial assessment of spiritual and/or religious needs; seeks to identify spiritual or religious resources; various spiritual assessment tools can be used in this assessment; is the most widely used approach in nursing practice.
Quantitative	Often derived from and developed for research purposes; various spiritual assessment scales are used to measure specific constructs of spirituality.
Qualitative	Includes biographical and narrative approaches focusing on the unique spiritual journey of the person; is widely applicable in clinical settings.
Domain	Seeks to assess spirituality in relation to overlapping domains such as the physical, emotional, family, and community domains.

at the time. Assessing the spiritual dimension in this manner does not need an inordinate amount of time, something that Larson (2003) noted in her own practice. Where more in-depth assessment and examination of spiritual issues are warranted, referral to a pastoral care professional or chaplain may be in order.

SPIRITUAL ASSESSMENT TOOLS/MODELS

The use of spiritual tools and models has already been referenced in this chapter. Tools and models are helpful as they provide a framework for the "what" of spiritual assessment. They are particularly valuable for nurses who are novices in the area of spiritual assessment. As experience and competence increase, nurses can adapt a model or tool to suit their own particular practice context, or even develop their own tool or model. However, as Swinton and Narayanasamy (2002) maintain, although such tools and models can direct nurses to the content to be assessed in a spiritual assessment as well as provide guidelines for the assessment, the real success of spiritual assessment lies in the sensitivity and empathy of nurses in the process of conducting the assessment.

A perusal of the health care literature will reveal that spiritual assessment tools have been developed for multiple ages and contexts of practice. For example, there are distinct tools that are suitable for assessing older adults, others for clients suffering from cancer, and yet others for clients with chronic illnesses, and so on. Spiritual assessment tools can be administered formally, for example, by giving a client a spiritual tool to independently complete or by working through such a tool with the client. They can also be used informally within any naturally occurring conversation with the client. These tools can be lengthy, as in the case of Fitchett's (1993a) 7×7 Model; or they can be quite brief, as in the case of Kumar's four questions for spiritual assessment (Kumar, 2004). Rubrics for spiritual assessment have been developed, with the assumption that clinicians can develop pertinent and specific questions to examine elements of the rubric. An example is Battey's rubric, BVMGR, focusing on beliefs, values, meanings, goals, and relationships (Battey, 2012). Tools have also been developed for conducting research in the area of spirituality/religion. Some of these research tools are also adaptable for use in clinical practice.

There are far too many spiritual assessment tools and models to include in this book. Table 5.2 gives some distinctive examples of spiritual assessment/spiritual well-being scales. Table 5.3 gives examples of tools comprising questions to be asked of clients. Further examination of these tools is recommended by consulting the references provided.

SPIRITUAL ASSESSMENT SCALES

Spiritual assessment scales are traditionally used for research purposes. However, some, such as Ellison's Spiritual Well-Being Scale (SWBS), may be adapted for use in clinical contexts. Some tools are focused on clients dealing with particular health problems, for example, the Remuda Spiritual Assessment Questionnaire (RSAQ) targeted for persons experiencing an eating disorder (The Free Library, 2014). Others have subscales measuring various aspects of spirituality, for example, Ellison's SWBS. Some tools have been translated and used with diverse cultural groups distinct from those for which the tool was originally developed. For example, the SWBS, developed in the

Table 5.2 **Spiritual Assessment Scales/Questionnaires**

Scales/Questionnaires	References
Spiritual Well-Being Scale (SWBS)	Ellison (1983)
Self-Transcendence Scale (STS)	Reed (1991)
Serenity Scale (SS)	Roberts and Aspy (1993)
Spiritual Transcendence Scale (STS)	Piedmont (1999)
Spiritual Assessment Scale (SAS)	Howden (1992)
Spiritual Involvement and Belief Scale (SIBS)	Hatch, Burg, Naberhaus, and Hellmich (1998)
Daily Spiritual Experience Scale (DSE)	Underwood and Teresi (2002)
Spiritual Attitude and Involvement List (SAIL)	de Jager Meezenbroek et al. (2012)
Spiritual Health Scale (Short Form)	Hsiao, Chiang, Lee, and Han (2013)
Spiritual Health & Life Orientation Measure (SHALOM)	Fisher (2010)
Religious Involvement Inventory	Hilty and Morgan (1985)
JAREL Spiritual Well-Being Scale (JAREL SWBS)	Hungelmann et al. (1996)
The Spiritual Needs Scale	Flannelly, Galek, and Flannelly (2006)
The Spiritual Meaning Scale (SMS)	Fetzer Institute (1999)
Intrinsic Religious Motivation Scale (RMS)	Hoge (1972)
Brief Religious Coping Scale (Brief RCOPE)	Pargament, Smith, Koenig, and Perez (1998)
The Spirituality Scale (SS)	Delaney (2005)

(continued)

Table 5.2 **Spiritual Assessment Scales/Questionnaires (*continued*)**

Scales/Questionnaires	References
Geriatric Spiritual Well-Being Scale (GSWS)	Dunn (2008)
World Health Organization Quality of Life-Spirituality, Religiousness and Personal Beliefs (WHOQOL-SRPB) Questionnaire	World Health Organization Quality of Life-Spirituality, Religiousness and Personal Beliefs Group (2006)

United States, has been translated and used with a Muslim population in Jordan (Musa & Pevalin, 2012). Some tools have a spirituality subscale as part of a larger tool. For example, the Mental, Physical & Spiritual Well-being Scale (MPS) has a spirituality subscale (Vella-Brodrick & Allen, 1995).

An important point with respect to the use of spiritual assessment scales in clinical practice is that they should never be used alone and be "a substitute for the intentional presence and attentive listening that is so basic to soul-to-soul encounter" (Burkhardt & Nagai-Jacobson, 2002, p. 322). Draper (2012) concurs with this when he indicates that instruments and guidelines should never sideline spiritual assessment models that focus on deep human relationships. Such relationships characterize the journeys nurses take with clients who are searching for meaning in illness, dying, or bereavement. If scales are used in clinical settings, the interaction between the nurse and the client greatly enhances assessment. For example, if the client scores high on a spiritual assessment scale, then the nurse can discuss these strengths, thereby affirming them. If the client scores low on a spiritual assessment scale, further discussion can also occur. In this way, if the questions accompanying the scale open up further discussion, scales are most effective in such clinical contexts (Burkhardt & Nagai-Jacobson, 2002).

A specific example of a spirituality scale is the SWBS (Ellison, 1983) in Box 5.1. Spirituality scales are typically in a Likert format: the SWBS is a 20-item scale. The SWBS has two subscales: a 10-item scale related to religious well-being (RWB), and a 10-item scale related to existential well-being (EWB). It has been established as a valid and reliable tool, and has been hailed by Delaney (2005) as "the most widely used instrument to assess spirituality as well as the one most frequently referred to and applied in studies examining spirituality" (p. 147). The SWBS can be used as a brief subjective assessment of spiritual well-being. It can be read to clients, including children, and a retrospective version of the scale has been developed for use with children who are able to read (Life Advance, 2009). Although the tool has been criticized for its Judeo-Christian bias, for example, its use of the word "God," (Fulton & Carson, 1995), instructions can be provided to respondents to interpret the word "God" as "higher power" in whatever sense this is meaningful to the respondent (Life Advance). The SWBS can also be used in clinical contexts in that it can point clinicians to general areas relative to spirituality/religion that can be explored (Life Advance). In this way, it can be used as an aid to discussion about spirituality.

Box 5.1 SWB Scale

For each of the following statements, circle the choice that best indicates the extent of your agreement or disagreement as it describes your personal experience:

1. I don't find much satisfaction in private prayer with God.	SA	MA	A	D	MD	SD
2. I don't know who I am, where I came from, or where I'm going.	SA	MA	A	D	MD	SD
3. I believe that God loves me and cares about me.	SA	MA	A	D	MD	SD
4. I feel that life is a positive experience.	SA	MA	A	D	MD	SD
5. I believe that God is impersonal and not interested in my daily situations.	SA	MA	A	D	MD	SD
6. I feel unsettled about my future.	SA	MA	A	D	MD	SD
7. I have a personally meaningful relationship with God.	SA	MA	A	D	MD	SD
8. I feel very fulfilled and satisfied with life.	SA	MA	A	D	MD	SD
9. I don't get much personal strength and support from my God.	SA	MA	A	D	MD	SD
10. I feel a sense of well-being about the direction my life is headed in.	SA	MA	A	D	MD	SD

(continued)

Box 5.1 SWB Scale (continued)

11. I believe that God is concerned about my problems.	SA	MA	A	D	MD	SD
12. I don't enjoy much about life.	SA	MA	A	D	MD	SD
13. I don't have a personally satisfying relationship with God.	SA	MA	A	D	MD	SD
14. I feel good about my future.	SA	MA	A	D	MD	SD
15. My relationship with God helps me not to feel lonely.	SA	MA	A	D	MD	SD
16. I feel that life is full of conflict and unhappiness.	SA	MA	A	D	MD	SD
17. I feel most fulfilled when I'm in close communion with God.	SA	MA	A	D	MD	SD
18. Life doesn't have much meaning.	SA	MA	A	D	MD	SD
19. My relation with God contributes to my sense of well-being.	SA	MA	A	D	MD	SD
20. I believe there is some real purpose for my life.	SA	MA	A	D	MD	SD

A, agree; D, disagree; MA, moderately agree; MD, moderately disagree; SA, strongly agree; SD, strongly disagree; SWB, spiritual well-being.

Reflection 5.4

- Complete the SWBS for yourself. Notice how difficult or easy it was for you to respond to the items. Did you tend to score higher or lower in terms of spiritual well-being? What insights, if any, did you gain from this exercise?
- Examine Ellison's SWBS. What items in the tool, if any, might you be hesitant to discuss with a client; and why? Reflect on the tool's usefulness in your clinical practice. Could you use it as it is presented, that is, by giving it as is to a client to complete? If not, how might you adapt it for use?

QUALITATIVE SPIRITUAL ASSESSMENT TOOLS

Qualitative spiritual assessment tools generally have questions that the nurse can use when talking with clients. Although such tools can be used in an interview format, they may best be seen as prompts to be used in informal conversations with clients, and then explored in more depth as warranted (Carpenito-Moyet, 2004; Jackson, 2004). One or two questions in the tool can serve as a "bridge" to talking about spirituality. For some tools, their developers have provided guides for professionals to utilize in inquiring about and observing signs of spiritual needs, for example, Stoll (1979) and Narayanasamy (2004). Examples of qualitative tools are found in Table 5.3.

Stoll's (1979) Guidelines for Spiritual Assessment (presented in Box 5.2) have been widely used in spiritual assessment within nursing and beyond. They have also been adapted in a variety of ways. For example, Kerrigan and Harkulich (1993) adapted Stoll's guidelines for use in a specific nursing context: long-term care. Their adapted tool uses open-ended questions that residents could answer in a story-telling manner, along with a checklist of common answers to facilitate documentation (pp. 48–49). Stoll's tool explores four aspects related to spirituality/religion. The questions pertaining to each of the four areas can be incorporated into an overall general nursing history, or used in informal conversations with clients. Although the tool is rooted in the Judeo-Christian worldview, it can be adapted for use by clients who do not subscribe to this worldview. For example, Stoll's tool explores the person's relationship with "God" or "Deity." Stoll suggests that if a person does not believe in God, the nurse can ask the person what he or she would determine his or her highest value to be. Another example is with respect to questions pertaining to religion. If the person does not identify with a particular religion, then he or she can be asked about spirituality and spiritual practices. Stoll (1979, pp. 1574–1577) provides illustrations of the major themes in the guidelines as well as clinical examples in her article describing the tool. These guidelines are given in Box 5.2.

Fitchett (1993b) evaluated Stoll's tool and noted the following observations about it:

- It is multidimensional, focusing on both beliefs and practices.

- It has a functional and dynamic conception of spirituality elaborating on meaning of life as perceived by the person responding to the questions.

- It can be used with nonreligious people.
- It attends to the connection between beliefs/practices and health.
- It is simple and easy to use.
- It does not require an inordinate amount of time to use.

Table 5.3 Qualitative Spiritual Assessment Tools

Tools	References
Guide to Assessing Spiritual Needs	Davidhizar, Bechtel, and Juratovac (2000)
Spiritual Assessment Instrument	Stoddard and Burns-Haney (1990)
HOPE: Model of Spiritual History Taking	Anandarajah and Hight (2001)
Guidelines for Spiritual Assessment	Stoll (1979)
Spiritual Wellness Reflective Questions	Espeland (1999)
Spiritual Assessment Guiding Questions	Jackson (2004)
Five Basic Spiritual Assessment Questions	Carpenito-Moyet (2004)
Four Questions for Spiritual Assessment	Kumar (2004)
Brief Spiritual Assessment Model	Hodge (2006)
Spiritual Needs Assessment/Spiritual Life Review	Kearns (2002)
S.P.I.R.I.T. Tool	Maugens (1996)
FICA Spiritual Assessment Tool	Puchalski and Romer (2000)
BVMGR Spiritual Assessment Tool	Battey (2012)
Spiritual Assessment Form	Hay (1989)

Box 5.2 *Stoll's (1979) Guidelines for Spiritual Assessment*

A. Concept of God or Deity

1. Is religion or God significant to you? If yes, can you describe how?

2. Is prayer helpful to you? What happens when you pray?

3. Does a God or deity function in your personal life? If yes, can you describe how?

4. How would you describe your God or what you worship?

B. Sources of Hope and Strength

1. Who is the most important person to you?

2. To whom do you turn when you need help? Are they available?

3. In what ways do they help?

4. What is your source of strength and hope?

C. Religious Practices

1. Do you feel your faith (or religion) is helpful to you? If yes, would you tell me how?

2. Are there any religious practices that are important to you?

3. Has being sick made any difference in your practice of praying? Your religious practices?

4. What religious books or symbols are helpful to you?

D. Relation Between Spiritual Beliefs and Health

1. What has bothered you most about being sick (or what is happening to you)?

2. What do you think is going to happen to you?

3. Has being sick (or what has happened to you) made any difference in your feelings about God or the practice of your faith?

4. Is there anything that is especially frightening or meaningful to you now?

Reflection 5.5

- Complete Stoll's questions for yourself. What insights, if any, did you obtain from this exercise?
- Examine Stoll's guidelines. What is the potential for their use in your clinical practice? Would you change any of the language in the tool to best suit your context of practice? If so, what would these changes be?

(continued)

Reflection 5.5 **(continued)**

- Use questions from Stoll's guidelines (or the questions that you adapted) in your clinical practice this coming week. How did they provide a window into the client's spirituality? What was the impact on the client and on yourself?
- Reflect on the differences in the process of completing Stoll's tool and that for Ellison's SWBS in terms of your understanding of your own spiritual health. Which do you think might be more helpful in clinical practice in terms of understanding the client's spirituality?

REVIEWS OF SPIRITUAL ASSESSMENT/SPIRITUAL ASSESSMENT TOOLS

There have been a number of reviews that evaluate the state of spiritual assessment and of spiritual assessment tools reported in the health care literature. For example, de Jager Meezenbroek and colleagues (2012) reviewed 10 tools that address spirituality as a universal human experience. Draper (2012) conducted an integrated review of "the current 'state of the art' in relation to spiritual assessment, focusing on quantitative, qualitative and generic approaches" (p. 970) to measuring spirituality. This review considered a number of spiritual assessment instruments. Monod and colleagues (2011) identified and reviewed 35 instruments used to measure spirituality in clinical research. In the same year, Sessanna, Finnell, Underhill, Chang, and Peng (2011) reviewed tools reported in nursing and health-related literature that were being used to evaluate spirituality as more than just religiosity. They concluded that such measures were "grossly lacking" (p. 1677). Kilpatrick and colleagues (2005) reviewed nursing research journals (from 1995 to 1999) to ascertain the extent to which spirituality/religiousness measures were included in the research referenced in those journals. As a result of their review, they called for greater inclusion of such measures in order to contribute to the scientific information about the role of spirituality/religion in nursing care. An earlier review by Fitchett (1993b) includes an annotated bibliography of 28 published models of spiritual assessment, including five models that had been developed by nurses. An examination of these reviews is recommended for an expansive discussion.

GUIDELINES FOR EVALUATING SPIRITUAL ASSESSMENT TOOLS

Nurses can develop their own assessment tools, or they can use tools developed by others, such as the tools presented in this chapter. Lengthy assessment tools, such as Fitchett's (1993a) 7×7 Model, may not be appropriate for many nursing contexts. Tools that require clients to complete the assessment on their own may also not be appropriate. Some institutions adapt spiritual assessment tools that have already been developed, whereas others develop their own for use by health care professionals within their institutions. If nurses are using tools that have been developed externally, then the question remains as to how *do* nurses decide which tool might be most effective in their practice?

Various criteria can be used to evaluate the suitability of a given spiritual assessment tool or model. The following questions give some examples of possible criteria (Draper, 2012; Fitchett, 1993a; Fitchett & Handzo, 1998; Gow, Watson, Whiteman, & Deary, 2011; Timmins & Kelly, 2008; Weston, quoted in Fitchett, 1993a):

- Is the tool valid and reliable?

- Is the tool suitable for the target population (age, gender, faith group, health status)?

- Is the tool simple and clear?

- Is the tool suitable for the clinical setting?

- Are a diversity of spiritual/religious beliefs and attitudes addressed in the tool?

- Is the tool safe, adaptable, easy to use, nonintrusive, and inclusive?

- Does the tool utilize wording and language such that clients are encouraged to participate?

- Does the tool highlight key dimensions of spirituality/religion?

- Is the tool useful in providing direction for planning and implementing care?

- Does the tool include both spiritual and religious dimensions?

- Does the tool address both the substantive (what people believe) and the functional (how beliefs impact life)?

- Does the tool assume continuity or change in spiritual life?

- Does the tool assume that the spiritual dimension and other dimensions of the person influence one another?

- Does the tool distinguish between spiritual and psychosocial aspects of life?

- Is the tool in a format suitable for the practice context?

- Does the tool lend itself to a partnership stance with clients?

- What conceptualization of spirituality is inherent in the tool?

- Does the tool have explicit or implicit norms against which the person is assessed?

SPIRITUAL NEEDS

Spiritual needs can provide an organizing framework for spiritual assessment. A nurse can develop questions that address each of the major spiritual needs. However, it is paramount that nurses also ask clients what *they* perceive their spiritual needs to be (McSherry & Watson, 2002). In taking a spiritual needs approach to spiritual assessment, the nurse is identifying behaviors and comments of the client that suggest that one or more spiritual needs are not being met. For example, an illness might impact a client's ability to meet his or her spiritual needs due to the incapacitation and vulnerability experienced at such a time. There are many references in the health care literature that suggest that clients' spiritual needs are not adequately addressed in most health care institutions, which can result in poorer health outcomes.

It is important to be cautious about interpreting the word "need" as a "deficit." A better way to conceptualize a "need" is as a normative requirement for all people that may be altered in some way by illness or some other significant life event. Spiritual needs are needs that are intricately connected to a person's developmental level, so when the spiritual dimension of the client is assessed, the client's developmental level is an important context for that assessment.

Spiritual needs are present in all people, regardless of their worldview (Carroll, 2001; Hermann, 2007; Walter, 2002)—a perspective that is prominent and recurring in the health care literature. For example, Agostino (1988) quotes Billinger (1960, p. 49) in describing spiritual needs as the "deepest requirements of the self, which, if met, make it possible for the person to function with a meaningful identity and purpose, so that in all stages of life that person may relate to reality with hope" (Agostino, 1988, p. 80). Monod and colleagues (2011) describe spiritual needs in a similar manner as "something required or wanted by an individual to find a purpose and meaning in life" (p. 1346). Wright (1998) identifies spiritual needs as "essential components of spirituality that require development or reinforcement throughout life" (p. 81). A list of spiritual needs that have been identified in the health care literature (Eliopoulos, 2005; Fish & Shelly, 1988; Galek, Flannelly, Vane, & Galek, 2005; Greenstreet, 1999; Lemmer, 2010; Narayanasamy, 1991; Taylor, 2002) indicates the primary spiritual needs that nurses will encounter in their practice:

- The need for meaning and purpose in life, and in life events
- The need for love and relatedness (also termed the need to be loved unconditionally and give love; the need for love and harmonious relationship)
- The need for forgiveness (giving and receiving)
- The need for hope (present and future) and strength
- The need for spiritual/religious practices and rituals
- The need for transcendence
- The need for beauty
- The need for creativity
- The need for continuity in the past
- The need to worship and connect to God or a higher power
- The need for gratitude
- The need for expression of faith, personal beliefs, and values
- The need for trust
- The need for preparation and acceptance of death

It is important to note that spiritual needs may be interconnected to one another. For example, the need for love is intricately connected to the need for meaning and purpose in that many people find meaning and purpose in loving relationships (Narayanasamy, 2004). Similarly, when transcendent meaning is discovered, hope and sustenance for one's spirit is provided (Emblen & Pesut, 2001).

THE NEED FOR MEANING AND PURPOSE

The need for meaning and purpose is widely recognized as a spiritual need in the health care literature. In fact, it is the most commonly occurring theme in the nursing literature focused on spirituality (Clarke, 2006). Willard (1998) captures this well by describing meaning as "a kind of spiritual oxygen . . . that enables our souls to live" (p. 386). Travelbee (1971), an early nurse theorist, included meaning as a central part of her theory, emphasizing the nurse's role in helping clients develop meaning.

What provides meaning and purpose for each individual varies depending on his or her worldview, which points to the importance of individualized assessment (Clarke, 2006). For example, if a client is a committed Christian, he or she may find prime meaning and purpose in being intricately connected to God. Other sources of meaning include close relationships with family and friends, work, pursuing creative endeavors, commitment to "a cause," and so on (Burkhardt & Nagai-Jacobson, 2002).

The need for meaning and purpose refers not only to finding meaning and purpose in life generally, but also in life events. For example, many people will search for a reason in their illness or suffering. That illness and suffering can result in a sense of meaninglessness and then spiritual distress can occur. Finding meaning in that suffering can alleviate such distress (Emblen & Pesut, 2001; Galek et al., 2005; Greenstreet, 1999; Narayanasamy, 1991). New meaning and purpose can be attained, leading to spiritual growth. When loss of meaning and purpose in life occurs in people who are experiencing illness or bereavement, nurses can function as catalysts to help them regain or find new meaning and purpose (Chan, Ng, Ho, & Chow, 2006; Narayanasamy, 1991). For example, many self-help groups and support groups have been started by people who have experienced some event in life. Their response to the life event was to create a support group—thereby generating and deriving some meaning out of the life event.

A well-known example that demonstrates the importance of finding meaning in suffering is the life and work of Viktor Frankl. Frankl was a Jewish psychiatrist who was interned in concentration camps during the World War II. Based on his observations in the camps, Frankl concluded that, even when faced with the most horrific experiences and suffering, a person can find meaning. He observed that those prisoners who had a reason to live tended to survive. Frankl believed that the search for meaning is a primary motivation in life and is unique for every person. He asserted that a variety of biographical, cultural, and religious factors contributed to such meaning. He also saw meaning to be connected to love, suffering, God, service to others, and a life characterized by giving and self-sacrificing. After the war, Frankl developed a therapy called "logotherapy," which was based on meaning making (Clarke, 2006; Frankl, 1985).

There are cautions with respect to assessing the need for meaning and purpose. When a client asks "Why?" questions (e.g., "Why is this happening to me?" "Why now?"), often the assertion is made in the health care literature that that the client is searching for meaning and purpose. While this may sometimes be the case, Morrison (1992) sees "Why?" questions as being "in reality, a statement of [the clients'] deepest painful feelings. 'Why?' so often means 'I am hurting terribly'" (p. 37). Therefore, before the nurse proceeds to help such a client find meaning in the client's suffering, the nurse may first need to help the client express his or her feelings and also validate his or her feelings. Another caution related to the need for meaning and purpose is with respect to seeing meaning as the primary focus in spirituality. Such a conclusion presupposes an ability of the client to reflect on life and life events. Some people are, by nature, not reflective. Others may have cognitive impairment that can impact their ability to reflect. Thus, nurses need to assess not only the sources of meaning and purpose for clients but also the clients' abilities to engage in contemplation and discussion about meaning and purpose.

THE NEED FOR HOPE AND STRENGTH

Burkhardt and Nagai-Jacobson (2002) describe hope as "desire accompanied by expectation of fulfillment. The expectation of hope goes beyond merely believing or wishing and involves envisioning that the desired circumstances can become reality" (p. 60). They continue with the description of hope, identifying it as "an attitude of the heart, . . . a feeling, a passion for the possible that affects the whole person . . . . Hope helps us deal with fear and uncertainty and enables us to envision positive outcomes [both of which are important factors in dealing with illness and adversity]" (p. 61).

Richardson (2000), who writes about evidence for a biological basis for hope, argues that if hope is present, then life is present. He uses the life of Victor Frankl (referenced earlier) to illustrate that not only meaning and purpose, but also hope, is the key to survival. Frankl hoped for a future where he could share his experiences in the concentration camps with others. Frankl's love for his wife and his work to increase the morale of the other prisoners all provided hope in the midst of a seemingly hopeless situation. Richardson also uses the example of Dietrich Bonhoeffer, a German Christian pastor who was imprisoned and died because of his opposition to the Nazis during the World War II. However, Richardson's example of Bonhoeffer was to illustrate that hope does not always lead to survival. As Bonhoeffer died, his hope remained in the prospect of life after death, or eternal life with God. Thus, hope can have a transcendent aspect and extend beyond this present life.

Hope can be derived from many sources, but it is primarily rooted in relationships of love, security, and mutuality, whether those relationships are with other people or with God/Supreme Being. Hope can motivate people to be open to new ways of coping. If a client is hopeful, the result can be a sense of peace and contentment, a sense of gratitude, courage, and new energy. Hope nurtures the human spirit (Galek et al., 2005; Narayanasamy, 1991; Stoll, 1979).

Hope is intricately connected to meaning and purpose in that meaning and purpose can be derived from hope, and can also be a source of hope (Espeland, 1999). Hope can also be connected to strength, as when hope is present, clients may feel stronger to face situations in life. Hope may be, in itself, a source of strength. Other sources of strength include other people, talking with God through prayer, sacred writings, and so on (Narayanasamy, 2004). Nurses need to inquire about viable sources of hope and strength as part of spiritual assessment.

THE NEED FOR LOVE, BELONGING, AND RELATEDNESS

We are all "wired" for close bonding with other people (Johnson, 2004). The need to give and receive love is a basic human need (Maslow, 1968). Delaney (2005) writes about the scientific basis for a relational aspect to spirituality. Caleb (2003, quoted in Delaney, 2005) sees spirituality as being all about relationships—human to human, human to nature, human to cosmic reality. Aspects related to this spiritual need include not only the need to give and receive love but also the need for unconditional acceptance; and to feel connected not only to other people but also to the world and perhaps to God or a Supreme Being (Galek et al., 2005; Hoshiko, 1994).

When the need for love and relatedness is not met, clients may express feelings of being alone or abandoned by others—or by God (Duff, 1994). In contrast, when the spiritual need for love, belonging, and harmonious relationship is achieved, clients feel valued, secure, joyful, hopeful, and courageous. They also experience a feeling of self-worth and a sense of belonging (Narayanasamy, 2004). Nurses not only need to show unconditional love to clients, but they also need to assess the clients' sources of love and belonging: to whom they are connected and the quality and impact of such connections.

THE NEED FOR FORGIVENESS

Forgiveness is a concept that has been much studied by health care professionals, theologians, therapists, and others. Delineations between cognitive and affective forgiveness have been made. The *choice* to forgive and factors contributing to this choice have been discussed. The emotions connected with forgiveness have been examined, such as benevolence, empathy, and love, plus the replaced emotions of bitterness, anger, and hatred. Approaches to forgiveness therapy as well as instruments to measure forgiveness have also been developed (Hargrave & Sells, 1997; Holeman, Dean, DeShea, & Duba, 2011).

There are many definitions and descriptions of forgiveness spawned by the various people who have studied this concept. For example, Worthington (2009) describes the experience of forgiveness as encompassing two different kinds of forgiveness: decisional, which controls behavioral intentions; and emotional, which replaces negative emotions with positive ones. He points out that forgiveness does not mean reconciliation (others would disagree with this), exoneration, justifying, or condoning. Lawler-Row, Scott, Raines, Edlis-Matityahou, and Moore (2007) found that participants in their study described both intrapersonal forgiveness (focused on self) and interpersonal forgiveness (focused on others). Forgiveness was experienced by them as a behavior, an emotion, and/or a thought.

Forgiveness relates to the need to forgive self, to forgive others, and to be forgiven (Macaskill, 2002; Narayanasamy, 2001) both by others and by God. Spiritual and religious convictions can motivate people to forgive. The need to forgive is identified as a spiritual need in that, when one forgives or receives forgiveness, not only is physical, emotional, and relational health impacted, but spiritual well-being is also experienced (Holeman et al., 2011). Forgiveness is also linked to inner peace, humility, honesty, realism, joy, elation, and renewed self-worth (Espeland, 1999; Macaskill, 2002; Narayanasamy, 2001). Part of the nurse's role is assessing the quality of the client's relationships with others and with God (if applicable) and listening for cues that might indicate the need for forgiveness.

When clients are in spiritual distress, they may feel guilty and may feel that they need to be forgiven by others or by God. Guilt can result if a person feels that he or she is not living up to his or her own personal expectations or to the expectations of others. Guilt can also result from committing or contemplating some action that may be contrary to that person's personal standards of conduct, or, if the person is religious, to the teachings of that person's religion. Therefore, guilt and forgiveness involve an evaluation of one's behavior or transgressions. Guilt can be expressed through feelings of paranoia, hostility, worthlessness, defensiveness, withdrawal, psychosomatic complaints, criticism of self, others, God, and scapegoating (Narayanasamy, 2001). Careful assessment is warranted and the validation of such assessment is crucial as such expressions of guilt can also be indicative of other needs. In such cases, wording a question akin to a hypothesis can be helpful: "I wonder if you are feeling guilty because _____." The client can then verify this or refute it.

THE NEED FOR SPIRITUAL/RELIGIOUS RITUALS AND PRACTICES/EXPRESSIONS OF SPIRITUAL BELIEFS AND VALUES

The need to engage in spiritual or religious practices/rituals and to express spiritual and religious beliefs/values can be connected to organized religion that can involve such practices as prayer, reading sacred writings, participating in sacraments, or worship. This need can also be disconnected from organized religion, such as participation in various forms of private meditation. When engaged in such practices or rituals, a sense of strength and stability can result; and if practiced with other people in a faith community, then a sense of community and belonging can be the outcome (Espeland, 1999; Galek et al. 2005; Stoll, 1979). A client being able to verbally express his or her spiritual beliefs and values can also be insightful and comforting to him or her. For example, a client can believe that God is with him or her through his or her suffering or he or she can believe that everything is under God's control (Keller, 2013). Verbalizing beliefs and values can also be a means of expressing issues and concerns related to these beliefs and values that might result from suffering or being diagnosed with an illness. For example, suffering can shake previously held beliefs and values about God, the world, and so on.

In terms of spiritual assessment, nurses need to assess what spiritual or religious practices and rituals are important to their clients. They must also determine if the need to engage in such practices or rituals should be addressed while the client is hospitalized. It is also important to assess whether such practices and rituals are comforting to the client, and also to assess if changes have occurred in such practices/rituals (or the ability to engage in them) as a result of an illness. For example, a client for whom prayer is a daily practice may experience spiritual distress if that practice is impacted by hospitalization. This may manifest itself both in terms of actually being *able* to pray and perhaps in terms of not feeling the usual comfort or guidance from prayer. The client can also be distressed if he or she is unable to be involved in and with his or her faith community while he or she is in hospital, particularly if the hospitalization is lengthy.

OTHER SPIRITUAL NEEDS

Several additional spiritual needs are identified in the literature, albeit perhaps not as abundantly and thoroughly as those just discussed:

- **The need for trust** is a developmental need for children, but it also relates to adults. Being able to trust is to place confidence in others and to recognize that they are trustworthy. Establishing trusting relationships brings a sense of security (Narayanasamy, 1991, 2001). Nurses who are open and accessible to clients during the assessment process will help meet their clients' need for trust (Narayanasamy, 2004).

- **The need to care for others** takes a person beyond the self to caring for others' well-being. Meeting such a need can provide not only a sense of meaning and purpose, but also result in increased self-esteem, personal empowerment, and spiritual health (Espeland, 1999; Montgomery, 1991). Nurses need to observe clients for cues pertaining to this need and to assess the potential for fulfillment of the need.

- **The need for transcendence** refers to a need to be connected to someone or something beyond the self who will provide guidance and support. This need is often connected to organized religion, and often involves belief in God or a higher power (Espeland, 1999). Transcendence can provide a client with means of dealing with illness and suffering. As Paloutzian, Bufford, and Wildman (2012) maintain, people have a need to "focus on whatever transcends them because it is psychologically functional to do so. That is, by transcending immediate concerns, peoples' minds go beyond themselves and make attributions about the meaning of events in their environment—past, present, and future" (p. 354). Assessing sources of transcendence and the quality of transcendent experiences is important in spiritual assessment.

- **The need for beauty and creativity** is often connected to nature and the arts, such as music, painting, writing, and so on (Narayanasamy, 1991). Assessing where a client finds beauty and how creativity is expressed by the person can provide signposts for interventions that can contribute to the client's spiritual life.

- **The need to prepare for death** includes addressing unmet issues before impending death (including spiritual issues), addressing concerns about life after death, having a deeper understanding of death and dying (which can involve spiritual or religious understandings), forgiving oneself or others, being forgiven by others/God, and reviewing one's life (Galek et al., 2005). Assessment regarding this need is likely to be more prominent in a palliative care context.

Reflection 5.6

- Reflect on each of the spiritual needs discussed. Do you identify such needs within yourself? Appraise each need in terms of whether it is being met in your life, and how.
- Reflect on various clients whom you may have encountered in your practice where there was evidence that one or more spiritual needs of the clients had not been met. How did you respond? What was the impact on the clients? How might you have responded differently to effect a more positive outcome?
- This week, pay attention to cues that clients give indicating that any of the spiritual needs just discussed are being met—or, conversely, are not being met. What are these cues? How did "hearing" the spiritual needs impact on your response to the clients?

As can be seen from the discussion on spiritual needs, merely identifying a client's religious affiliation or determining if the client wants to see a chaplain or pastoral care professional is *not* an adequate spiritual assessment (Taylor, 2002). A dialogue between two nurses recorded in Carson (1989) makes this point:

- Nurse Smith: Were you able to gather any information about the patient's spiritual needs when you did the admission interview?

- Nurse Bramer: Oh sure. Mr. Johns is Catholic, and just recently started going to Mass again.

- Nurse Smith: Does his return to church coincide with the onset of his illness?

- Nurse Bramer: I don't know. I didn't think to ask about that. It seemed too personal.

- Nurse Smith: Any more personal than asking about his bowel habits? I think we need more data about Mr. Johns's spiritual needs. With the surgery facing him, we want to draw on whatever support is available (p. 155).

Spiritual needs cannot be identified from such superficial conversations as that conducted by Nurse Bramer with Mr. Johns. However, the information gained from even a superficial conversation can be "kept on the back burner" for future conversations with Mr. Johns. For example, the nurse can say: "When you were admitted, you mentioned that you were Catholic and had recently started attending Mass again. Where does your faith fit in with the situation that you are facing now?" Carson provides a follow-up conversation between Nurse Bramer and Mr. Johns, giving another example of returning to the earlier conversation:

- Nurse Bramer: Mr. Johns, I was wondering about something you told me earlier. You said you just started going to Mass again. What brought about this change?

- Mr. Johns: To tell you the truth, fear pushed me back to church. When I first discovered I had this heart condition, I was so afraid I would die that I started to pray again.

- Nurse Bramer: You started praying again? What made you stop?

- Mr. Johns: Several years ago, when my wife died, I found myself so angry at God that I didn't want to talk to him. Now I find that I need him again.

- Nurse Bramer: So you returned to church out of fear. Has going to Mass helped you?

- Mr. Johns: Yes, indeed! I went back out of fear, but now I have a sense of peace. Even though the thought of the bypass surgery is frightening, I know that God is with me. (p. 156)

Carson provides three additional conversations between Nurse Bramer and Mr. Johns (pp. 159–160; p. 166). She also gives a summary of the assessment data and a discussion of a nursing care plan for Mr. Johns (pp. 160–163). Reference to Carson is recommended for additional details.

Reflection 5.7

Reflect on clinical situations in which you have inquired about the religious affiliation of a client. What was the response from the client? Might you have conducted a deeper spiritual assessment; and if so, how? What questions might you have asked?

The fact that illness or some other significant life event can precipitate spiritual searching or questions about life and its meaning has already been discussed. As O'Connor (2001) maintains, spiritual needs are often most acutely felt during an illness than at many other times in a person's life. In a sense, spirituality can be "closer to the surface" at such times, thus making it easier for the nurse to access. If a client says, "I don't know what I am going to do or who I am anymore now that I can't return to my work because of this accident," then it should be apparent that such a statement is not only related to an altered sense of meaning and purpose, but also to a sense of self. Both of these are intricately connected to spirituality. If a client says, "I don't know what the man upstairs is thinking about (referring to God)," then such a statement indicates relatedness to meaning and purpose.

It is critical to note that spiritual assessment is not just about identifying spiritual needs or concerns but also about identifying strengths. As has been discussed earlier, spirituality pervades all aspects of life, and the spiritual dimension can be a significant resource for health and well-being for clients. For example, a nurse may observe a client reading religious or spiritual material or saying the rosary. The client may tell the nurse that this activity gives him or her peace and comfort. Or a client may say, "I know that God is helping me through all of this" to which the nurse may inquire: "*How* is your faith helping you?" Such an engagement would draw forth the specifics of this valuable resource. Knowing information about the client's strengths is invaluable not only to support and validate such strengths, but also to provide information that can be helpful in working with other clients who are struggling.

SPIRITUAL NEEDS AND PSYCHOSOCIAL NEEDS

One question that may arise in reading about the various spiritual needs is: Why are some needs characterized as spiritual needs and not as psychosocial needs? Although these two categories of needs are entwined, spiritual needs need to be distinguished so that they are not subsumed under psychological needs and thereby overlooked. Clarke (2006) states:

If nursing wishes to preserve the concept of spirituality there could be an argument for more attempts to articulate the subtle differences between spiritual, and the psychological, and emotional aspects of a person although this should not be at the expense of enforcing artificial or hierarchical separations between the parts of a person and their needs. (p. 918)

Clarke goes on to say that spiritual needs deal with religious discourse (for some), with ultimate explanations and beliefs about the world and with existential aspects of living such as love, hope, and forgiveness.

Greenstreet (1999) sees the psychological dimension of personhood as connected to the person's mind, thereby limiting it to a person's human resources. Piles (1990) maintains that the spiritual dimension seeks to worship something external to human resources and control; therefore, psychological means alone cannot, by that definition, fulfill the spiritual dimension. Piles describes spiritual needs as relating to a person's relationship to a higher power (or God), however that may be defined by the person. She sees psychological needs as being concerned with the person's relationship to himself/herself or to the environment.

It is important to clearly identify a spiritual need. For example, a client may express anxiety and guilt as prime concerns and also complain of insomnia and various physical complaints. All of this may be under investigation by medical professionals with no remarkable findings. If the nurse views the client purely from a psychological perspective, then he or she might speculate that the client's physical complaints are connected to the feelings of anxiety and guilt, and may proceed with various psychological interventions. If, in exploring the guilt further, the nurse discovers that the anxiety and guilt stem from a "wrong" committed against another person, which is in violation of the client's religious or moral code (which the client may term as "sin"), then spiritual interventions may also need to be instituted in order to enable the client to deal with the guilt.

THE NURSE AS ASSESSOR

It is important to recognize that the nurse's own positioning can impact the process of spiritual assessment. For example, Dukes (1999), referenced in Speck (2005), found that if nurses have strong religious belief systems, then they may be more effective in identifying (and also responding to) clients' religious needs. Dukes also found that those nurses who had strong spiritual beliefs (nonreligious) were able to identify and respond to broader spiritual aspects but missed the religious needs of clients (unless the clients raised such issues). Fitchett (1993a) maintains that spiritual assessment makes four demands on the caregiver:

- For modesty in one's treatment of a spiritual assessment model, as the spiritual dimension is complex with complex interrelationships between it and other dimensions of the person

- For playfulness, avoiding rigidity in using the spiritual assessment model and seeing spiritual assessment as a source of delight in one's work

- For continued personal self-awareness inasmuch as no spiritual tool can remove personal bias and distortion

- For cultural self-awareness as any given spiritual assessment tool may have norms against which a person is assessed, which may not be appropriate for all people. Moreover, caregivers, themselves, are influenced by their culture in terms of their personal spiritual beliefs and biases

The manner in which spiritual assessment is conducted is also important. As Burkhart and Hogan (2008) state: "Nurses can create an atmosphere to increase the likelihood that the patient will offer [an invitation to provide spiritual care] by assessing their patients with a spiritual openness of love, hope, and compassionate caring" (p. 931). The competencies discussed in Chapter 4 are also relevant in terms of conducting a spiritual assessment.

Numerous studies of the assessment of the personal spirituality and spiritual well-being of professionals and caregivers have been conducted, in keeping with the truism that professional caregivers' spiritual health and spiritual well-being can impact how they assess and help clients in the provision of spiritual care (Hsiao et al., 2013). Boutell and Bozett (1990) also developed a tool to help nurses determine the extent to which they assess clients' spiritual needs (Boutell's Inventory for Identifying the Nurses' Assessment of Patients' Spiritual Needs). This inventory can be found in Appendix A.

PRINCIPLES OF SPIRITUAL ASSESSMENT

A summary of the principles of spiritual assessment is as follows (Burkhardt & Nagai-Jacobson, 2002; Carson, 2008; Draper, 2012; Ellis & Narayanasamy, 2009; Fitchett, 1993a; 1995; Fitchett & Handzo, 1998; Hodge, 2006; Hungelmann et al., 1996; Labun, 1988; Miner-Williams, 2006; National Health Service [NHS] Education for Scotland, 2009; Stewart, 2014; Stoddard & Burns-Haney, 1990; Stoll, 1979):

- Initiate assessment with a simple, open probe.

- Choose an assessment model/tool appropriate for all people, religious or not.

- Choose an assessment model/tool appropriate to the clinical setting.

- Do not conduct a spiritual assessment if the client acuity level is high.

- Conduct the assessment in a supportive manner, conveying sensitivity and respect.

- Use language appropriate to the client during the assessment.

- Continue to assess after the initial assessment is completed.

- Incorporate spiritual assessment as part of general nursing assessment or as separate assessment.

- Do spiritual assessment only after trust and rapport have been developed.

- Follow a short, brief assessment with more in-depth assessment as needed.

- Complete assessment within a religious, cultural, and developmental context.

- Include categories of spirituality that include religious and nonreligious belief systems.

- Obtain client consent for spiritual assessment.

- Respect client's objection to spiritual assessment or silence regarding spiritual concerns.

- Document spiritual assessment findings.
- Include client as an active partner in the assessment process.
- Avoid stereotyping religious groups and assuming similarity among all adherents.
- Be aware of normative values and beliefs of major world religions.
- Be sensitive to subtle verbal/nonverbal and environmental cues regarding the client's spirituality.
- Be aware that spiritual/religious beliefs and practices can be a source of not only strength but also challenge for the client.
- Explain the rationale for inquiry about spirituality/religion.
- Use effective and appropriate communication skills in assessing, for example, the skills of probing, reflecting content/feeling, and showing empathy.
- Assess for the client's strengths as well as needs, issues, and concerns.
- Remember that intuition can be integral to assessment.
- Respect the client's privacy and adhere to confidentiality boundaries.
- Reflect on your own spiritual/religious beliefs, values, biases, and feelings to avoid imposing your own ideas on the client, proselytizing, or transference/counter-transference.
- Distinguish between spiritual and psychosocial needs but examine the latter to see if any spiritual needs are present.
- Validate assessment data with the client.
- Be aware of bias in assessment tools and adapt if needed.
- Create an internal and external environment conducive to exploring the spiritual dimension.
- Consider any client vision, reading, hearing, or comprehension barriers to assessment.
- Be sensitive to the timing of assessment—time of day, in conversation, in nurse–client relationship.
- Use open-ended questions if possible in the assessment.
- Be ethical in the assessment process.
- Do not rely on spiritual assessment tools and ignore the nurse–client relationship.
- If time is an issue, complete spiritual assessment simultaneously with routine physical care.
- Focus on the spiritual needs of the client's family as well as the client.
- If you cannot address a spiritual need for a variety of reasons, refer to a pastoral care professional.

SUMMARIZATION OF SPIRITUAL ASSESSMENT FINDINGS

A common approach to the summarization of spiritual assessment information/data in nursing is to make a nursing diagnosis. Spiritual needs can be diagnosed using the need statement itself, for example, "loss of meaning and purpose in life related to job loss due to an injury." Another way is to select a nursing diagnosis from already formulated diagnoses, for example, diagnoses developed by the North American Nursing Diagnosis Association (NANDA; Carpenito, 2017). Fitchett (1993a) has provided a critique of this model that is well-worth reading (pp. 123–127). Fitchett describes it as a useful model for clinical practice and identifies its major strengths as the list of defining characteristics of the diagnoses as well as the practicality of the model. It is important to note that nursing diagnoses can focus on strengths as well as problems or concerns. Moreover, nursing diagnoses can refer not only to individual clients, but also to families and groups (Carpenito, 2013).

Examples of diagnoses related to spirituality and religion are identified by NANDA and given in Box 5.3 (Carpenito, 2017). As is common within an NANDA framework, the defining characteristics and related factors for each diagnosis are described by Carpenito, and reference to this resource for further elaboration is recommended.

A nursing diagnosis approach to spiritual assessment is not without its issues. Generally, diagnosing is a nurse-centered activity where the nurse as "expert" makes a diagnosis. Yet, as has been mentioned several times in this chapter, the recommended approach for spiritual assessment is to be a partnership approach between the nurse and the client. The *client* is the "expert" on his or her life, not the nurse! Another issue with respect to a nursing diagnosis approach is that each client's situation is unique, and may not "fit" within a given diagnosis. Nevertheless, a nursing diagnosis approach *can* still be a helpful framework if care is taken to include the client as a partner throughout the diagnostic process.

Closely akin to the diagnosis of spiritual distress is spiritual crisis, a concept described by Agrimson and Taft (2009) as follows:

> A unique form of grieving or sense of loss, marked by a profound questioning of or lack of meaning in life, in which an individual reaches a turning point or juncture, leading to a significant alteration in the way oneself and life is viewed. (p. 457)

Box 5.3 *Nursing Diagnoses Related to Spirituality and Religion*

Spiritual distress, defined as "a state of suffering related to impaired ability to experience meaning in life through connection with self, others, the world, or a superior being" (p. 766).

Impaired religiosity, defined as "impaired ability to exercise reliance on beliefs and/or participate in rituals of a particular faith tradition" (p. 778).

Source: Carpenito (2017).

From this description, it can be seen that the person is changed by the crisis. This change can be a negative one (e.g., depression and discontinuation of a relationship) or a positive one (e.g., spiritual insight and spiritual growth). Agrimson and Taft (2008) provide attributes of spiritual crisis as well as give a "model" case of spiritual crisis. A reference to this article for further elaboration is recommended.

Spiritual pain is a concept that is found in the health care literature. Morrison (1992) describes spiritual pain as a "shattering of a view of life" (p. 37)—in essence, a relationship to life as one has experienced and known it is catastrophically shattered. This type of pain can be particularly agonizing. Morrison describes indicators of spiritual pain to be found in such phrases as "'nothing makes sense anymore,' 'nothing adds up any more,' 'my world is in pieces,' 'I can't see any meaning in anything.' Their picture of life has been smashed" (p. 37). At the center of such pain, then, is loss of meaning and purpose. A referral to Morrison for further elaboration of spiritual pain, including the management of such pain, plus the implications for nursing practice, is recommended.

Others have identified "diagnoses" related to spirituality and religion. For example, O'Brien (1982), quoted and discussed in O'Brien 2011 (pp. 76–77), also identifies and describes spiritual pain but adds six other "diagnoses" related to spiritual concerns:

- Spiritual pain: . . . evidenced by expressions of discomfort or suffering relative to one's relationship with God; verbalization of feelings of having a void or lack of spiritual fulfillment, and/or a lack of peace in terms of one's relationship to one's creator (O'Brien, 1982, p. 106)

- Spiritual alienation: . . . evidenced by expressions of loneliness, or the feeling that God seems very far away and remote from one's everyday life; verbalization that one has to depend upon oneself in times of trial or need; and/or a negative attitude toward receiving any comfort or help from God (O'Brien, 1982, p. 106)

- Spiritual anxiety: . . . evidenced by an expression of fear of God's wrath and punishment; fear that God might not take care of one, either immediately or in the future; and/or worry that God is displeased with one's behavior (O'Brien, 1982, p. 106)

- Spiritual guilt: . . . evidenced by expressions suggesting that one has failed to do the things which he or she should have done in life, and/or done things which were not pleasing to God; articulation of concerns about the "kind of life one has lived" (O'Brien, 1982, p. 106)

- Spiritual anger: . . . evidenced by expressions of frustration, anguish or outrage at God for having allowed illness or other trials; comments about the "unfairness" of God; and/or negative remarks about institutionalized religion and its ministers or spiritual caregivers (O'Brien, 1982, p. 107)

- Spiritual loss: . . . evidenced by expression of feelings of having temporarily lost or terminated the love of God; fear that one's relationship with God has been threatened; and/or a feeling of emptiness with regard to spiritual things (O'Brien, 1982, p. 107)

- Spiritual despair: . . . evidenced by expressions suggesting that there is no hope of ever having a relationship with God, or of pleasing Him; and/or a feeling that God no longer can or does care for one (O'Brien, 1982, p. 107)

These six diagnostic terms arose out of O'Brien's research on spirituality in life-threatening illness. As can be seen from the descriptions, these diagnoses are rooted in a Judeo-Christian worldview. Aspects of some of the descriptions may, however, be applicable to those who do not ascribe to that particular worldview. Hay (1989) also provides four diagnoses related to spirituality and religion, along with discussion about their defining characteristics, the assessment, goals/outcomes, and interventions for each diagnosis (pp. 26–29). He labeled these diagnoses as "spiritual suffering," "inner resource deficiency," "belief system inquiry," and "religious needs" (p. 27). Again, a referral to these resources for further review is recommended.

Pesut (2008) makes an important point when she asserts that a nursing diagnosis of spiritual distress (or even of spiritual crisis, pain, etc.) implies that something needs to be "solved," rather than acknowledging that a person can suffer with all of the resulting emotions, and yet be spiritually well. For example, a person can experience hurt, pain, discouragement, or other emotions, but his or her connectedness to God or a higher power may be so strong that he or she perceives himself or herself to be spiritually well. Again, this calls for careful assessment and interpretation of the assessment.

Once spiritual needs/concerns and strengths have been identified by the nurse, together with the client, a plan can be cocreated to address the needs and concerns. There are no "standardized" nursing care plans when it comes to spiritual care, as each plan needs to be individualized for each client. Careful and accurate assessment with the client as an active partner is invaluable to this process. While there are challenges and barriers to spiritual assessment—such as biases in assessment tools, the elusiveness of spiritual needs, time constraints, and many notions of spirituality—the positive outcomes of spiritual assessment can far outweigh the barriers.

The Bottom Line

- Spiritual assessment is crucial to effective, ethical, and comprehensive client care.

- Be aware of various spiritual assessment tools and choose those that best fit your context of practice.

- Assessment should focus on both spirituality and religion and be tailored to the client's worldview.

- Assessment should include the client as an active partner.

- Tailor the processes of assessment to your particular clinical setting and context.

- Be aware of context when conducting spiritual assessment—culture, developmental stage, and so forth.

- Know fundamental spiritual needs and how to assess if they are met.

- Be able to distinguish between spiritual and psychosocial needs.

- Remember that spiritual assessment can identify strengths as well as problems/concerns.

- Be aware of how your own spiritual positioning may impact the process of spiritual assessment.

- Follow the principles of spiritual assessment.

- Know how to make a diagnosis related to spiritual and/or religious concerns.

Taking It Further

1. Research the spiritual assessment tools in Tables 5.2 and 5.3:
   a. Complete each tool to assess your own spirituality while reflecting on a current or past illness or some other adversity in your life. What insights, if any, have you gained about your own spirituality, spiritual/religious biases, and so forth?
   b. Are there questions missing from the tool that you would deem important in assessing your spirituality? If so, what are those questions?
   c. What questions might you reword in the tool; and why?
   d. Examine each tool for its possible applicability in your own clinical practice, adapting them as warranted for your particular client population or clinical setting. Pilot one or two tools in your clinical practice and evaluate the impact, with ongoing adaption of the tools as warranted.

2. Using the guidelines given in this chapter for evaluating spiritual assessment tools, choose one or two tools that might be most applicable to your clinical setting; and evaluate the tool(s). What changes might you need to make in the tool(s) in order for them to fit the criteria for suitability to your practice?

3. Consult a number of reviews found in the literature on spiritual assessment tools. How do the reviews inform your appraisal of the various assessment tools?

4. For each spiritual need identified in this chapter, write a few questions that could be asked of clients to assess whether this need is being met or not. Pilot the questions with clients, appraising the impact and changing the tool as warranted. How has this exercise sensitized you to the importance of assessing spiritual needs?

5. Review Carpenito's nursing diagnoses related to spirituality/religion (Carpenito, 2017). Have you witnessed any defining characteristics associated with each diagnosis in your clinical practice and if so, had you considered whether they might indicate a spiritual need? In your clinical practice, heighten your awareness of such defining characteristics as they are presented by clients, and seek to

further assess whether they are indicative of a spiritual need. Evaluate the impact of this exercise on client outcomes, and also on your competence in assessing for spiritual distress.

6. Research O'Brien's "diagnoses" (O'Brien, 1982) related to spirituality (O'Brien, 2011, pp. 76–77). Have you witnessed such diagnoses in clients whom you have encountered? How might O'Brien's work in this area inform your clinical practice, in particular, in identifying spiritual issues and concerns?

7. Write a guide for nurses in terms of initiating conversations with clients about spirituality for the purpose of spiritual assessment. What would you include in this guide, and why? Pilot the guide with a number of nurses and evaluate its effectiveness and usefulness in clinical practice.

8. Interview a number of people who have experienced adversity in their lives, for example, illness, suffering, and/or loss. Inquire about how the experience may have impacted their sense of meaning and purpose; and also how the experience may have developed new meanings for them. How can their stories of this journey be useful in your clinical practice?

9. Review the literature on studies that focus on clients' perceptions of their spiritual needs. How do the clients' perspectives compare with what is found in the health care literature?

10. If you deem it appropriate to advocate for more inclusion of spiritual assessment in your clinical setting, then prepare a brief to be presented to senior management staff in your clinical setting. Include in the brief an outline of the importance of nurses' spiritual assessment to comprehensive care. Anticipate the barriers that they will raise and be prepared to discuss how each barrier might be addressed in the brief. Present the brief and evaluate the outcome. What is your next step?

11. Interview spiritual care professionals about how they conduct a spiritual assessment. How is their role similar in this regard to the nurse's role in spiritual assessment? How is the context of their practice different? How might they be of assistance to nurses in terms of spiritual assessment of clients?

12. Review the T.R.U.S.T. Model for Spiritual Assessment and Care (Barss, 2012). Reflect on the following questions in relation to this model:

    a. What is your appraisal of the underlying assumptions of this model?

    b. Use the model to conduct a spiritual reflection on your own person/life using the sample reflection questions in Table 2 in Barss's article. What insights, if any, did you gain from this exercise in terms of your own spiritual positioning?

    c. Use some or all of the spiritual reflection questions in Table 2 in the article in your conversations with clients. What was the outcome, and what are the implications for your clinical practice?

    d. What potential does this model have for nursing practice in your own setting? How can the model be piloted and evaluated in your clinical setting?

13. Review Boutell's Inventory for Identifying the Nurses' Assessment of Patients' Spiritual Needs in Appendix A. Complete this inventory. What is your appraisal of your practice with respect to the inclusion of assessment of spiritual needs? What areas do you need to develop further and how can this be done?

14. Research the impact of human development and developmental stages on the process of spiritual assessment. How can the findings from your research inform your clinical practice?

15. Reflect on the spiritual need for forgiveness. Think of a person who has hurt or offended you in some way. Write a brief description of this event.

    a. Rate the degree of hurt you experienced on a scale of 1 to 10, with 1 being "very little hurt" and 10 being "great degree of hurt."

    b. How did this event impact you emotionally, cognitively, socially, and spiritually?

    c. Do you feel that something "sacred" was taken from you as a result of this event? If so, how?

    d. Where are you with respect to forgiving this person?

    e. If you have not forgiven this person, what needs to happen in order for you to do so? What do you envision the impact of forgiving this person may be on you?

    f. If you have forgiven this person, how did you replace negative emotions and thoughts about the person (e.g., no longer feeling upset when thinking about the person) with positive emotions and thoughts (e.g., empathy)? How did forgiving this person impact you?

    (Adapted from Holeman et al., 2011)

16. Write a one-sentence epitaph as you would like to see your life described in your obituary. What do you identify as your purpose in life from this exercise?

    (Adapted from Espeland, 1999)

17. Review a number of current movies or television shows that have themes that touch upon one or more spiritual needs. From the movie or show, what are the defining characteristics of such needs? How are the characters meeting their needs or seeking to meet their needs?

18. Review the literature for discussion about the differences between spiritual needs and psychosocial needs. Compare and contrast the two based on your review.

19. With respect to the spiritual need for love and belonging, review the literature for information about various forms of love: "agape" love and "eros" love. How does the information gained assist you in assessing this spiritual need in clients?

20. Review the literature for information on spiritual needs that consider or present a continuum from spiritual well-being to spiritual distress. What characteristics are typical of each of these extremes? Where would you rate yourself on such a continuum? How is mapping a client on a continuum helpful in terms of planning and providing spiritual care?

21. Reflect on clinical situations where one or more of the clients' spiritual needs were not being met, for example, when the clients were hopeless, felt alone, or felt the need for forgiveness. Critically analyze your assessment of such clients as well as develop a plan to address such needs. What recommendations do you have for future assessment of such clients (Greenstreet, 1999)?

22. Some professionals and clients may see spirituality/religion as a "private" topic, and therefore for a nurse to address it with a client is an invasion activity. Do you agree with this stance? If "Yes," then what factors contributed to this stance? What opportunities might be missed in your practice because of this stance? What other "private" areas do nurses assess in clients? How is assessing spirituality or religion different from these other areas? Or *is* it different (Groer, O'Connor, & Droppleman, 1996)?

23. Consult the model developed by Hawley and Taylor (2003, p. 207) and reflect on the following questions:

    a. What are the relationships between the various components of the model?

    b. Develop a list of questions to ask clients to obtain information about each of the model's components.

    c. Compare your questions with those developed by Hawley and Taylor (p. 208).

    d. Ask these questions of yourself. What insights, if any, have you gained about your spirituality?

    e. Use your questions or those of Howley and Taylor (or a mixture of both) in the spiritual assessment of clients in your clinical practice. What was the outcome for the clients and for your relationship with these clients?

    f. How can this model be used to understand your own spirituality and that of clients?

24. Reflect on any barriers/challenges to spiritual assessment: those personally internal to yourself, those in your particular nursing care setting, those within the profession of nursing, and those within in the health care system. How can you address each barrier/challenge?

25. Reflect on a situation where you were able to satisfactorily assess a client's spirituality/religion and the impact on his or her care. What factors contributed to this sense of satisfaction?

26. Have you ever asked "Why?" questions in dealing with particular events in your own life? Were your questions indicative of your pain? Were you searching for meaning in the event? Did you express your questioning to another person? If such interactions with others were helpful to you, then what characteristics or actions on their part contributed to this helpfulness? If they were not helpful, then what factors contributed to this lack of helpfulness? How can this reflection be of assistance to you in further exploring "Why?" questions with clients?

27. Reflect on a current/past illness or other adverse life event in your life. If a clinician were to explore spiritual aspects related to such an event, what qualities, attitudes, and characteristics would you prefer to be present within this clinician? Write a list of questions that would facilitate an exploration between you and the clinician of the spiritual aspects of this event.

28. Fenske (2011) makes the following statement in her article about creating "soul" to make meaning of her severely disabled son's life and death: "The human condition requires we 'make meaning' out of our experiences. Before we understand or comprehend, we must make meaning. We perceive, recognize and attribute meaning to our experiences before responding or reacting" (p. 230).

    a. Do you agree with Fenske's statement? Why or why not?

    b. Can you relate Fenske's statement to experiences in your own life? And if so, how?

    c. What might be the implications of Fenske's statement for nursing spiritual assessment?

29. In considering the concept of "story" as an appropriate method for clients to explore their experiences with illness, reflect on the stories your clients have related to you:

    a. Have any of these stories had explicit or implicit content related to faith/spirituality/religion?

    b. How have the stories enabled you to see the impact of faith/spirituality/religion on illness experiences, including making meaning of such experiences?

    c. Do these stories show a connection between the client's faith and others, including God or a higher power?

    d. What nonverbal or emotional overtones accompanied the stories?

    e. What role did you play (or might you have played) in using the story to assess the client's spirituality?

30. What is your comfort level in assessing aspects of a client's religion, as well as his or her spirituality? What factors contribute to your comfort or lack of comfort? If the latter, how can you become more comfortable in assessing aspects of religion when it is pertinent to clients?

31. Respond to the following idea about why you might not record spiritual/religious information about a client. Use a Likert scale, where 1 denotes "strongly disagree" and 5 denotes "strongly agree":

    I do not always ask about or record religious or spiritual information about a client because:

    a. I think that it is unnecessary to record this information for some clients.

    b. I sometimes feel embarrassed to ask clients about religion/spirituality.

    c. I think that asking about spirituality/religion is intrusive.

d. Clinical factors make it impossible for me to record such information.

e. Religion does not mean much to me.

f. I feel that asking clients about spirituality/religion is related mostly to death.

g. Collecting such information will not impact the care that might/should be given.

h. Sometimes, I do not understand clients' responses to such inquiries.

i. It is something that I can skip as there are more important things to record.

j. The clinical agency is not concerned about whether I record such information.

k. Sometimes, I do not have time to ask or record such information.

l. I do not feel confident asking about or recording such information.

m. I do not know why such information is collected.

n. The information is already recorded before I have contact with the client.

(Adapted from Swift, Calcutawalla, & Elliot, 2007)

What do your responses suggest about your recording of spiritual/religious information? Which factors are intrinsic to you and which are connected to the agency in which you practice? How can you improve your recording of this information?

32. Reflect on a time when you told someone a story, which had spiritual or religious overtones, either your own story or that of another person:

a. What personal beliefs and values were operant in the story?

b. What meaning and purpose overtones were present in the story?

c. How did/does the story help you to understand yourself or the other person?

d. How easy was it to relate the story; and why?

e. What communication skills did you use to facilitate the telling of the story?

f. Did your story have a beginning, a middle, and an end so as to encourage making sense of the story?

g. Could the story connect to future goals/aspirations; and how?

h. Was your worldview similar to or different from the person hearing the story? What was the impact of these worldview(s) in the telling of the story? (Adapted from National Health Service [NHS] Education for Scotland, 2009)

What insights, if any, have you gained from this reflection that might impact the use of story to encourage clients to talk about their spirituality or in terms of you listening to clients' stories that have spiritual/religious overtones?

33. Identify times in your life when you have personally felt spiritually content, or spiritually distressed. What caused this feeling? What did you think and feel? How was this different from other types of contentment or distress?

34. With respect to the spiritual need for forgiveness:

    a. What are your feelings and beliefs about forgiveness?

    b. How have you experienced forgiveness in your life—both in terms of giving and receiving it?

    c. Consider a time when you experienced healing through forgiveness. What helped you in this process? Have you experienced hurts or are you holding grudges that you cannot seem to release? Consider how holding on to these feelings is affecting your life, your health, and your relationships with others and, if appropriate, with God. What would help you begin to release these feelings?

REFERENCES

Agostino, J. N. (1988). Religiosity and religious participation in the later years: A reflection of the spiritual needs of the elderly. *Journal of Religion & Aging, 4*(2), 75–82. doi:10.1300/J491v04n02_06

Agrimson, L. B., & Taft, L. B. (2009). Spiritual crisis: A concept analysis. *Journal of Advanced Nursing, 65*(2), 454–461. doi:10.1111/j.1365-2648.2008.04869.x

Anandarajah, G., & Hight, E. (2001). Spirituality and medical practice: Using the HOPE questions as a practical tool for spiritual assessment. *American Family Physician, 63*(1), 81–89.

Barss, K. S. (2012). T.R.U.S.T.: An affirming model for inclusive spiritual care. *Journal of Holistic Nursing, 30*(1), 24–34. doi:10.1177/0898010111418118

Battey, B. W. (2012). Perspectives of spiritual care for nurse managers. *Journal of Nursing Management, 20*(8), 1012–1020. doi:10.1111/j.1365-2834.2012.01360.x

Boutell, K. A., & Bozett, F. W. (1990). Nurses' assessment of patients' spirituality: Continuing education implications. *Journal of Continuing Education, 21*(4), 172–176. doi:10.3928/0022-0124-19900701-10

Browning, D. (2008). Internists of the mind or physicians of the soul: Does psychiatry need a public philosophy? *Zygon: Journal of Religion and Science, 43*(2), 371–383. doi:10.1111/j.1467-9744.2008.00922.x

Burkhardt, M. A., & Nagai-Jacobson, M. G. (2002). *Spirituality: Living our connectedness.* Albany, NY: Delmar.

Burkhart, L., & Hogan, N. (2008). An experiential theory of spiritual care in nursing practice. *Qualitative Health Research, 18*(7), 928–938. doi:10.1177/1049732308318027

Carpenito, L. J. (2013). *Handbook of nursing diagnosis* (14th ed.). Philadelphia, PA: Lippincott Williams & Wilkins.

Carpenito, L. J. (2017). *Nursing diagnosis: Application to clinical practice* (15th ed.). Philadelphia, PA: Wolters Kluwer.

Carpenito-Moyet, L. J. (2004). *Nursing diagnosis: Application to clinical practice* (10th ed.). Philadelphia, PA: F. A. Davis.

Carroll, B. (2001). A phenomenological exploration of the nature of spirituality and spiritual care. *Mortality, 6*(1), 81–98. doi:10.1080/13576270020028656

Carson, V. B. (1989). *Spiritual dimensions of nursing practice.* Philadelphia, PA: Saunders.

Carson, V. B. (2008). Spirituality: Identifying and meeting spiritual needs. In V. B. Carson & H. G. Koenig (Eds.), *Spiritual dimensions of nursing practice* (Rev. ed., pp. 125–153). West Conshohocken, PA: Templeton Foundation.

Chan, C. L. W., Ng, S. M., Ho, R. T. H., & Chow, A. Y. M. (2006). East meets West: Applying Eastern spirituality in clinical practice. *Journal of Clinical Nursing, 15*(7), 822–832. doi:10.1111/j.1365-2702.2006.01649.x

Chrash, M., Mulich, B., & Patton, C. M. (2011). The APN role in holistic assessment and integration of spiritual assessment for advance care planning. *Journal of the American Academy of Nurse Practitioners, 23*(10), 530–536. doi:10.1111/j.1745-7599.2011.00644.x

Clarke, J. (2006). A discussion paper about "meaning" in the nursing literature on spirituality: An interpretation of meaning as "ultimate concern" using the work of Paul Tillich. *International Journal of Nursing Studies, 43*(7), 915–921. doi:10.1016/j.ijnurstu.2006.05.005

Darden, R. A. (2005). Spiritual assessment and treatment strategies. *The Remuda Review: The Christian Journal of Eating Disorders, 4*, 14–16.

Davidhizar, R., Bechtel, G. A., & Juratovac, A. L. (2000). Responding to the cultural and spiritual needs of clients. *The Journal of Practical Nursing, 50*(4), 20–23.

Delaney, C. (2005). The Spirituality Scale: Development and psychometric testing of a holistic instrument to assess the human spiritual dimension. *Journal of Holistic Nursing, 23*(2), 145–167. doi:10.1177/0898010105276180

de Jager Meezenbroek, E., Garssen, B., van den Berg, M., Tuytel, G., van Dierendonck, D., Visser, A., & Schaufeli, W. (2012). Measuring spirituality as a universal human experience: Development of the spiritual attitude and involvement list (SAIL). *Journal of Psychosocial Oncology, 30*(2), 141–167. doi:10.1080/07347332.2011.651258

Draper, P. (2012). An integrative review of spiritual assessment: Implications for nursing management. *Journal of Nursing Management, 20*(8), 970–980. doi:10.1111/jonm.12005

Duff, V. (1994). Spiritual distress: Deciding to care. *Journal of Christian Nursing, 11*(1), 29–31.

Dukes, C. (1999). *Nurses' assessment of spiritual need* (Unpublished bachelor's thesis). University of Southampton, Southampton, England.

Dunn, K. S. (2008). Development and psychometric testing of a new geriatric spiritual well-being scale. *International Journal of Older People Nursing, 3*(3), 161–169. doi:10.1111/j.1748-3743.2007 .00107.x

Eliopoulos, C. (2005). *Gerontological nursing* (6th ed.). Philadelphia, PA: Lippincott Williams & Wilkins.

Ellis, H. K., & Narayanasamy, A. (2009). An investigation into the role of spirituality in nursing. *British Journal of Nursing, 18*(14), 886–890. doi:10.12968/bjon.2009.18.14.43358

Ellison, C. W. (1983). Spiritual well-being: Conceptualization and measurement. *Journal of Psychology & Theology, 11*(4), 330–338.

Emblen, J., & Pesut, B. (2001). Strengthening transcendent meaning: A model for the spiritual care of patients experiencing suffering. *Journal of Holistic Nursing, 19*(1), 42–56. doi:10.1177/08980 1010101900105

Espeland, K. (1999). Achieving spiritual wellness: Using reflective questions. *Journal of Psychosocial Nursing, 37*(7), 36–40. doi:10.3928/0279-3695-19990701-22

Fenske, J. M. (2011). Soul mate: Exploring the concept of soul. *Journal of Holistic Nursing, 29*(3), 229–232. doi:10.1177/0898010111398661

Fetzer Institute. (1999). *Multidimensional measurement of religiousness/spirituality for use in health care research: A report of the Fetzer Institute/National Institute on Aging Working Group.* Retrieved from http://fetzer.org/sites/default/files/images/resources/attachment/[current-date:tiny]/Multidi mensional_Measurement_of_Religousness_Spirituality.pdf

Fish, S., & Shelly, J. (1988). *Spiritual care: The nurse's role* (3rd ed.). Downers Grove, IL: Intervarsity Press.

Fisher, J. (2010). Development and application of a spiritual well-being questionnaire called SHA-LOM. *Religions, 1*(1), 105–121. doi:10.3390/rel1010105

Fitchett, G. (1993a). *Assessing spiritual needs: A guide for caregivers.* Minneapolis, MN: Augsburg.

Fitchett, G. (1993b). *Spiritual assessment in pastoral care: A guide to selected resources.* Decatur, GA: Journal of Pastoral Care Publications.

Fitchett, G. (1995). Linda Krauss and the lap of God: A spiritual assessment case study. *Second Opinion, 20*(4), 41–49.

Fitchett, G., & Handzo, G. F. (1998). Spiritual assessment, screening, and intervention. In J. C. Holland, W. Breitbart, P. B. Jacobsen, M. S. Lederberg, M. Loscalzo, M. J. Massie, & R. McCorkle (Eds.), *Psycho-Oncology* (pp. 790–808). New York, NY: Oxford University Press.

Flannelly, K. J., Galek, K., & Flannelly, L. T. (2006). A test of the factor structure of the patient spiritual needs assessment scale. *Holistic Nursing Practice, 20*(4), 187–190.

Frankl, V. E. (1985). *Man's search for meaning.* New York, NY: Simon & Schuster.

Fulton, R. A. B., & Carson, V. (1995). The spiritual variable: Essential to the client system. In B. Neuman (Ed.), *The Neuman systems model* (3rd ed., pp. 77–91). East Norwalk, CT: Appleton & Lange.

Galek, K., Flannelly, K. J., Vane, A., & Galek, R. M. (2005). Assessing a patient's spiritual needs: A comprehensive instrument. *Holistic Nursing Practice, 19*(2), 62–69.

Gow, A. J., Watson, R., Whiteman, M., & Deary, I. J. (2011). A stairway to heaven? Structure of the religious involvement scale and spiritual well-being scale. *Journal of Religion & Health, 50*(1), 5–19.

Greenstreet, W. M. (1999). Teaching spirituality in nursing: A literature review. *Nurse Education Today, 19*(8), 649–658. doi:10.1054/nedt.1999.0355

Groer, M. W., O'Connor, B., & Droppleman, P. G. (1996). A course in health care spirituality. *Journal of Nursing Education, 35*(8), 375–377.

Hargrave, T. D., & Sells, J. N. (1997). The development of a forgiveness scale. *Journal of Marital and Family Therapy, 23*(1), 41–62. doi:10.1111/j.1752-0606.1997.tb00230.x

Harris, G. M., Allen, R. S., Dunn, L., & Parmelee, P. (2013). "Trouble won't last always": Religious coping and meaning in the stress process. *Qualitative Health Research, 23*(6), 773–781. doi:10.1177/1049732313482590

Hatch, R. L., Burg, M. A., Naberhaus, D. S., & Hellmich, L. K. (1998). The spiritual involvement and beliefs scale: Development and testing of a new instrument. *The Journal of Family Practice, 46*, 476–486.

Hawley, G., & Taylor, P. C. (2003). Using research skills to inform the teaching of spirituality. *Nurse Education in Practice, 3*(4), 204–211. doi:10.1016/S1471-5953(03)00003-9

Hay, M. W. (1989). Principles in building spiritual assessment tools. *The American Journal of Hospice and Palliative Care, 6*(5), 25–31. doi:10.1177/104990918900600514

Hermann, C. P. (2007). The degree to which spiritual needs of patients near the end of life are met. *Oncology Nursing Forum, 34*(1), 70–78. doi:10.1188/07.ONF.70-78

Hilty, D. M., & Morgan, R. L. (1985). Construct validation for the religious involvement inventory: Replication. *Journal for the Scientific Study of Religion, 24*, 75–86.

Hodge, D. R. (2006). Template for spiritual assessment: A review of the JCAHO requirements and guidelines for implementation. *Social Work, 51*(4), 317–326. doi:10.1093/sw/51.4.317

Hoge, R. (1972). A validated intrinsic religious motivation scale. *Journal of the Scientific Study of Religion, 11*(4), 369–376. doi:10.2307/1384677

Holeman, V. T., Dean, J. B., DeShea, L., & Duba, J. D. (2011). The multidimensional nature of the quest construct forgiveness, spiritual perception, and differentiation of self. *Journal of Psychology & Theology, 39*, 31–43.

Hoshiko, B. R. (1994). *Worldview: A practical model of spirituality*. Lecture given at Kent State University, Spring, 1994.

Howden, J. (1992). *Development and psychometric characteristics of the spirituality assessment scale* (Doctoral dissertation). Retrieved from http://poar.twu.edu/handle/11274/187

Hsiao, Y. C., Chiang, Y. C., Lee, H. C., & Han, C. Y. (2013). Psychometric testing of the properties of the spiritual health scale short form. *Journal of Clinical Nursing, 22*(21–22), 2981–2990. doi:10.1111/jocn.12410

Hungelmann, J., Kenkel-Rossi, E., Klassen, L., & Stollenwerk, R. (1996). Focus on spiritual well-being: Harmonious interconnectedness of mind–body–spirit-use of the JAREL Spiritual Well-Being Scale. *Geriatric Nursing, 17*(6), 262–266.

Jackson, J. (2004). The challenge of providing spiritual care. *Professional Nurse, 20*(3), 24–26.

Johnson, S. M. (2004). *The practice of emotionally focused couple therapy: Creating connection.* New York, NY: Brunner-Routledge.

Joint Commission on the Accreditation of Health Care Organizations. (2016). Spiritual assessment: Standards FAQ details. Retrieved from www.jointcommission.org/standards_information/jcfaq details.aspx?StandardsFaqId=290&ProgramId=47

Katerberg, R. (1997, January). *And then I got this pain . . . Spiritual assessment using the narrative approach*. Paper presented at the Canadian Association of Pastoral Professional Education (CAPPE), St. John's, NL, Canada.

Kearns, M. L. (2002). Managing the spiritual needs of patients: Simple steps to enhance well-being. *Advance for Nurse Practitioners, 10*(3), 101–104.

Keller, T. (2013). *Walking with God through pain and suffering.* New York, NY: Dutton.

Kerrigan, R., & Harkulich, J. T. (1993). A spiritual tool. *Health Progress, 74*(4), 46–49.

Kilpatrick, S. D., Weaver, A. J., McCullough, M. E., Puchalski, C., Larson, D. B., Hays, J. C., . . . Flannelly, K. J. (2005). A review of spiritual and religious measures in nursing research journals: 1995–1999. *Journal of Religion & Health, 44*(1), 55–66.

Kumar, K. (2004). Spiritual care: What's worldview got to do with it? *Journal of Christian Nursing, 21*(1), 24–28. doi:10.1097/01.CNJ.0000262275.10582.66

Labun, E. (1988). Spiritual care: An element in nursing care planning. *Journal of Advanced Nursing, 13*(3), 314–320. doi:10.1111/j.1365-2648.1988.tb01424.x

Larson, K. (2003). The importance of spiritual assessment: One clinician's journey. *Geriatric Nursing, 24*(6), 370–371. doi:10.1016/j.gerinurse.2003.10.020

Lawler-Row, K. A., Scott, C. A., Raines, R. L., Edlis-Matityahou, M., & Moore, E. W. (2007). The varieties of forgiveness experience: Working toward a comprehensive definition of forgiveness. *Journal of Religion & Health, 46*(2), 233–248.

Leetun, M. C. (1996). Wellness spirituality in the older adult: Assessment and intervention protocol. *Nurse Practitioner, 21*(8), 60–70.

Lemmer, C. M. (2010). Reflections on teaching spirituality in the healthcare environment. *Journal of Holistic Nursing, 28*(2), 145–149. doi:10.1177/08980109350770

Life Advance. (2009). Spiritual Well-Being Scale: FAQS. Retrieved from http://ww.lifeadvance.com/spiritual-well-being-scale/6-faqs.html

Macaskill, A. (2002). *Heal the hurt: How to forgive and move on.* London, England: Sheldon Press.

Maslow, A. H. (1968). *Toward a psychology of being.* New York, NY: Van Nostrand.

Massey, K., Fitchett, G., & Roberts, P. A. (2004). Assessment and diagnosis in spiritual care. In K. L. Mauk & N. A. Schmidt (Eds.), *Spiritual care in nursing practice* (pp. 209–242). Philadelphia, PA: Lippincott Williams & Wilkins.

Maugens, T. A. (1996). The SPIRITual history. *Archives of Family Medicine, 5*(1), 11–16.

McSherry, W., & Watson, R. (2002). Spirituality in nursing care: Evidence of a gap between theory and practice. *Journal of Clinical Nursing, 11*(6), 843–844. doi:10.1046/j.1365-2702.2002.00656.x

Miner-Williams, D. (2006). Putting a puzzle together: Making spirituality meaningful for nursing using an evolving theoretical framework. *Journal of Clinical Nursing, 15*(7), 811–821. doi:10.1111/j.1365-2702.2006.01351.x

Monod, S., Brennan, M., Rochat, E., Martin, E., Rochat, S., & Büla, C. J. (2011). Instruments measuring spirituality in clinical research: A systematic review. *Journal of General Internal Medicine, 26*(11), 1345–1357. doi:10.1007/s11606-011-1769-7

Montgomery, C. (1991). The care-giving relationship: Paradoxical and transcendent aspects. *The Journal of Transpersonal Psychology, 23*(2), 91–104.

Morrison, R. (1992). Diagnosing spiritual pain in patients. *Nursing Standard, 6*(25), 36–38.

Musa, A. S., & Pevalin, D. J (2012). An Arabic version of the spiritual well-being scale. *The International Journal for the Psychology of Religion, 22*(2), 119–134. doi:10.1080/10508619.2011.638592

Narayanasamy, A. (1991). *Spiritual care: A resource guide.* Lancaster, England: Quay Books.

Narayanasamy, A. (1999). ASSET: A model for auctioning spirituality and spiritual care education and training in nursing. *Nurse Education Today, 19*(4), 274–285. doi:10.1054/nedt.1999.0637

Narayanasamy, A. (2001). *Spiritual care: A practical guide for nurses and health care practitioners* (2nd ed.). Dinton, England: Quay Books.

Narayanasamy, A. (2002). Spiritual coping mechanisms in chronically ill patients. *British Journal of Nursing, 11*(22), 1461–1470. doi:10.12968/bjon.2002.11.22.10957

Narayanasamy, A. (2004). The puzzle of spirituality for nursing: A guide to practical assessment. *British Journal of Nursing, 13*(19), 1140–1144. doi:10.12968/bjon.2004.13.19.16322

National Health Service (NHS) Education for Scotland. (2009). Spiritual care matters: An introductory resource for all NHS Scotland staff. Retrieved from http://www.nes.scot.nhs.uk/media/3723/spiritualcaremattersfinal.pdf

O'Brien, M. E. (1982). The need for spiritual integrity. In H. Yura & M. Walsh (Eds.), *Human needs and the nursing process* (Vol. 2, pp. 82–115). Norwalk, CT: Appleton Century Crofts.

O'Brien, M. E. (2011). *Spirituality in Nursing: Standing on holy ground* (4th ed.). Sudbury, MA: Jones & Bartlett.

O'Connor, C. I. (2001). Characteristics of spirituality, assessment, and prayer in holistic nursing. *Holistic Nursing Care, 36*(1), 33–45.

Paloutzian, R. F., Bufford, R. K., & Wildman, A. J. (2012). Spiritual Well-Being Scale: Mental and physical health relationships. In M. Cobb, C. M. Puchalski, & B. Rumbold (Eds.), *Oxford textbook of spirituality in healthcare* (pp. 353–358). New York, NY: Oxford University Press.

Pargament, K. I., Smith, B. W., Koenig, H. G., & Perez, L. (1998). Patterns of positive and negative religious coping with major life stressors. *Journal for the Scientific Study of Religion, 37*(4), 710–724. doi:10.2307/1388152

Pesut, B. (2008). Spirituality and spiritual care in nursing fundamentals textbooks. *Journal of Nursing Education, 47*(4), 167–173. doi:10.3928/01484834-20080401-05

Pesut, B., Fowler, M., Reimer-Kirkham, S., Taylor, E. J., & Sawatzky, R. (2009). Particularizing spirituality in points of tension: Enriching the discourse. *Nursing Inquiry, 16*(4), 337–346. doi:10.1111/j.1440-1800.2009.00462.x

Piedmont, R. L. (1999). Does spirituality represent the sixth factor of personality? Spiritual transcendence and the five-factor model. *Journal of Personality, 67*(6), 985–1013. doi:10.1111/1467-6494.00080

Piles, C. (1990). Providing spiritual care. *Nurse Educator, 15*(1), 36–41.

Puchalski, C., & Romer, A. L. (2000). Taking a spiritual history allows clinicians to understand patients more fully. *Journal of Palliative Medicine, 3*(1), 129–137. doi:10.1089/jpm.2000.3.129

Reed, P. G. (1991). Self-transcendence and mental health in oldest-old adults. *Nursing Research, 40*(1), 5–11.

Richardson, R. L. (2000). Where there is hope, there is life: Toward a biology of hope. *Journal of Pastoral Care & Counseling, 54*(1), 75–83. doi:10.1177/002234090005400109

Roberts, K., & Aspy, C. (1993). Development of the serenity scale. *Journal of Nursing Measurement, 1*(2), 145–164.

Sessanna, L., Finnell, D. S., Underhill, M., Chang, Y., & Peng, H. (2011). Measures assessing spirituality as more than religiosity: A methodological review of nursing and health-related literature. *Journal of Advanced Nursing, 67*(8), 1677–1694. doi:10.1111/j.1365-2648.2010.05596.x

Stewart, M. (2014). Spiritual assessment: A patient-centered approach to oncology social work practice. *Social Work in Health Care, 53*(1), 59–73. doi:10.1080/00981389.2013.834033

Stoddard, G., & Burns-Haney, J. (1990). Developing an integrated approach to spiritual assessment: One department's experience. *The Caregiver Journal, 7*(1), 63–86. doi:10.1080/1077842X.1990.10781565

Stoll, R. I. (1979). Guidelines for spiritual assessment. *American Journal of Nursing, 79*(9), 1574–1577. doi:10.1097/00000446-197909000-00041

Sumner, C. H. (1998). CE Credit: Recognizing and responding to spiritual distress. *American Journal of Nursing, 98*(1), 26–30. doi:10.2307/3471826

Swift, C., Calcutawalla, S., & Elliot, R. (2007). Nursing attitudes towards recording of religious and spiritual data. *British Journal of Nursing, 16*(20), 1279–1282. doi:10.12968/bjon.2007.16.20.27575

Swinton, J., & Narayanasamy, A. (2002). Response to "A critical view of spirituality and spiritual assessment" by P. Draper & W. McSherry (2002) Journal of Advanced Nursing 39, 1–2. *Journal of Advanced Nursing, 40*(2), 1–2. doi:10.1046/j.1365-2648.2002.02401.x

Taylor, E. J. (2001). Spiritual assessment. In B. Ferrell & N. Coyle (Eds.), *Textbook of palliative nursing* (pp. 397–406). New York, NY: Oxford University Press.

Taylor, E. J. (2002). *Spiritual care: Nursing theory, research and practice.* Upper Saddle River, NJ: Pearson Education.

Taylor, E. J. (2011). Spiritual care: Evangelism at the bedside? *Journal of Christian Nursing, 28*(4), 194–202. doi:10.1097/CNJ.0b013e31822b494d

The Free Library. (2014). What is healthy spirituality? Remuda Ranch provides health professionals with a spiritual assessment questionnaire. Retrieved from http://www.thefreelibrary.com/What +is+Healthy+Spirituality%3f+Remuda=Ranch=Provides=health . . . -a0100546679

Timmins, F., & Kelly, J. (2008). Spiritual assessment in intensive and cardiac care nursing. *Nursing in Critical Care, 13*(3), 124–131. doi:10.1111/j.1478-5153.2008.00276.x

Travelbee, J. (1971). *Interpersonal aspects of nursing* (2nd ed.). Philadelphia, PA: F. A. Davis.

Treloar, L. L. (2001). Spiritual care: Safe, appropriate, ethical. *Journal of Christian Nursing, 18*(2), 16–20.

Underwood, L. G., & Teresi, J. A. (2002). The daily experience scale: Development, theoretical description, reliability, exploratory factor analysis, and preliminary construct validity using health-related data. *Annals of Behavioral Medicine, 24*(1), 22–33. doi:10.1207/S15324796ABM2401_04

Vella-Brodrick, D. A., & Allen, F. C. L. (1995). Development and psychometric validation of the mental, physical, and spiritual well-being scale. *Psychological Reports, 77*(2), 659–674. doi:10.2466/pr0.1995.77.2.659

Walter, T. (2002). Spirituality in palliative care: Opportunity or burden? *Palliative Medicine, 16*(2), 138–139. doi:10.1191/0269216302pm516oa

Willard, D. (1998). *The divine conspiracy: Rediscovering our hidden life in God.* New York, NY: Harper-Collins.

World Health Organization Quality of Life-Spirituality, Religiousness and Personal Beliefs Group. (2006). A cross-cultural study of spirituality, religion, and personal beliefs as components of quality of life. *Social Science & Medicine, 62*(6), 1486–1497. doi:10.1016/j.socscimed.2005.08.001

Worthington, E. L. Jr. (2009). *A just forgiveness: Responsible healing without excusing injustice.* Downers Grove, IL: Intervarsity.

Wright, K. B. (1998). Professional, ethical and legal implications for spiritual care in nursing. *Journal of Nursing Scholarship, 30*(1), 81–83. doi:10.1111/j.1547-5069.1998.tb01241.x

6

Spiritual Care

The rationale in favor of inclusion of spiritual care into nursing practice has already been addressed in Chapter 2, in which some of the points regarding spiritual care were considered, such as spiritual care is an ethical care; it results in better client health outcomes; it is consistent with providing holistic care; and it is consistent with the nature of nursing. The challenges to incorporating spiritual care in nursing practice were also addressed, for example, lack of time, a sense of incompetence on the part of the nurse, and issues within the health care environment. A review of Chapter 2 in conjunction with Chapter 6 is recommended.

There is much discussion in the nursing literature with respect to the assertion that the provision of spiritual care in nursing is often overlooked and neglected (Battey, 2012; Ellis & Narayanasamy, 2009; & Piotrowski, 2013). Concurrently, there is recognition that spiritual care is integral to nursing practice. For example, Giske (2012) says that spiritual care is "part of the art of nursing" (p. 1054). The International Council of Nurses (ICN, 2007) in *Vision for the Future of Nursing* states, "We are determined that science and technology remain the servant of compassionate and ethical caring that includes meeting spiritual and emotional needs" (para 3). And Reimer-Kirkham, Pesut, Sawatzky, Cochrane, and Redman (2012) predict that spiritual care is certain to become prominent in nursing care as "Global migration has brought unprecedented plurality to modern societies and spirituality and religion into the purview of nurse leaders" (p. 1029).

How do nurses perceive spiritual care? Although not all nurses perceive spiritual care as integral to their practice, there have been encouraging findings in several studies that have explored nurses and spiritual care. For example, McSherry and Jamieson (2013) found in their research that nurses consider spirituality and spiritual care to be fundamental (i.e., core, essential) to nursing practice and to providing holistic care. The nurses also recognized the expansive breadth and understanding of spirituality and spiritual beliefs, and observed that attending to spiritual needs enhanced overall quality of care. Cavendish, Konecny, Luise, and Lanza (2004) found that nurses accept spirituality as promoting health and supportive of their practice. Milligan (2004) concluded that current research shows nurses to be favorable toward spiritual care. Grant (2004) found that almost all nurses in his study thought that spiritual care resources should be made available to clients, especially when clients request for these resources; face serious and emotionally difficult situations such as death and grieving; struggle with meaning in life; face surgery; are depressed or subject to abuse; and/or exhibit religious behavior such as praying.

Several tools have been developed to assess nurses' perceptions and deliverance of spiritual care, for example, the Spirituality and Spiritual Care Rating Scale (SSCRS; McSherry, Draper, & Kendrick, 2002); the Spiritual Care Perspective Scale (SCPS— developed for an Iranian context; Iranmanesh, Tirgari, & Cheraghi, 2011); the Spiritual Care Perspectives Survey (Taylor, Highfield, & Amenta, 1999); the Spiritual Care Competency Scale (van Leeuwen, 2008; van Leeuwen, Tiesinga, Middel, Post, & Jochemsen, 2009); and the Spiritual Care-Giving Scale (SCGS; Tiew & Creedy, 2012). An exploration of these and other similar tools should serve to increase awareness of your own perceptions and execution of spiritual care.

DEFINING SPIRITUAL CARE

In Chapter 1 (see section on Defining Spirituality), examples of the multiple definitions of spirituality were presented, illustrating a wide range of perceptions about spirituality. How spirituality is defined will impact not only the focus for spiritual assessment but also how spiritual care is defined and described. A few definitions are presented in this chapter.

The National Health Service (NHS) Education for Scotland (2009) describes spiritual care as

> that care which recognizes and responds to the needs of the human spirit when faced with trauma, ill health or sadness and can include the need for meaning, for self worth, to express oneself, for faith support, perhaps for rites or prayer or sacrament, or simply for a sensitive listener. (p. 6)

MacLaren (2004) describes spiritual nursing [care] as "a way for nurses to enquire into that which is fundamental about the human condition and to give truly whole person care in a multi-faith society" (p. 461). Van Leeuwen, Tiesinga, Middel, Post, and Jochemsen (2008) describe spiritual care as "the care nurses provide to meet the spiritual needs and/or problems of patients" (p. 2769). Drawing on the interdisciplinary literature, Barss (2012) defines inclusive spiritual care as "relevant, nonintrusive care which tends to the spiritual dimension of health by addressing universal spiritual needs, honouring unique spiritual worldviews and helping individuals explore and mobilize factors that can help them gain/regain a sense of trust to promote optimum healing (Capsi, 2007; Lemner, 2010; Puchalski & Ferrell, 2010)" (p. 25). Creel (2007) describes spiritual care as "a multifaceted phenomenon that cannot be separated from other aspects of nursing care but is directed at caring for the unique spiritual needs of each person" (p. 15). Ruder (2013) identifies spiritual care as care that "includes building intuitive, caring, interpersonal relationships with patients that reflect patients' spiritual/religious reality" (p. 357). Carr (2008) concluded that participants in her study (nurses, clients, families, and others) perceived spiritual care to be " . . . at its most basic level (. . .) developing caring relationships through fostering connections to promote spiritual comfort and well-being" (p. 690). Sawatzky and Pesut (2005) describe spiritual care as "an intuitive, interpersonal, altruistic, and integrative experience that rests on the nurse's awareness of the transcendent dimension, yet reflects the patient's reality" (p. 30). Burkhart and Schmidt (2012) provide a definition of spiritual care that arises out of a theory used as a framework for their study, namely the Burkhart/Hogan Spiritual Care in Nursing Practice Framework (Burkhart & Hogan, 2008). The definition adds another dimension to the description of spiritual care:

> [S]piritual care is an interactive process between patient(s) and nurse designed to promote patient spirituality, but it can also affect nurse spirituality. It is not a list of assessment questions and prescribed interventions, but rather a purposeful monitoring and compassionate responding to patients' spiritual needs toward greater meaning and/or hope. (p. 316)

Burkhart and Schmidt continue with their description: "Spiritual care begins when the nurse recognizes the patient's spiritual need (verbally or non-verbally) at the moment it is expressed, consciously decides to intervene, and provides the appropriate intervention" (p. 316).

As can be surmised from these multiple descriptions, spiritual care is care that is seen as relational, integral to all nursing care, and focused on the spiritual dimension of persons. It is also focused not only on needs, but also on exploring, affirming, and supporting clients' strengths. Other authors describe spiritual care from explicit worldviews. For example, Shelly (2000) presents spiritual care from the Christian worldview; Meyer (2000) from an Eastern worldview; and Pesut (2006) describes spiritual care from three perspectives: a humanistic worldview, a theistic worldview, and a monastic worldview.

Reflection 6.1

- Reflect on each of the aforementioned descriptions of spiritual care. Which most closely fits your personal view of spirituality and why?
- Write your own definition of spiritual care. What worldview is represented in your definition? What are the implications of your definition for your nursing practice?

THE NATURE OF SPIRITUAL CARE

Generally speaking, the nature of spiritual care flows from spiritual assessment. For example, in the assessment process, if a client identifies with a particular religion, then religious care may be part of spiritual care. Conversely, if the client is assessed to not be connected to a religious perspective but still self-identifies as "very spiritual," then the nature of how spirituality is addressed should be consistent with the client's worldview.

The attributes and competencies described in Chapter 4 (see sections on Competencies for Spiritual Assessment and Care and Attributes for Spiritual Assessment and Caregiving) are applicable to the provision of spiritual care and spiritual assessment. For example, the professional relationship between the nurse and the client provides the context within which spiritual care is provided, and, therefore, nurses need to strive to develop therapeutic, trusting relationships with clients. As the National Health Service (NHS) Education for Scotland (2009) states, "Spiritual care begins with encouraging human contact in compassionate relationship, and moves in whatever direction need requires" (p. 6). Being friendly, gentle, honest, sensitive, present, open, nonjudgmental, compassionate, and empathetic is conducive to effective spiritual care. Being a good listener and using the effective/appropriate communication skills are also critical. Contextual factors of the client, such as gender, age, hearing ability, culture, and so on are also important to consider.

What level of spiritual care is appropriate and who should provide spiritual care? Although all nurses need to be able to assess the spirituality of clients and nurses must respect clients' spiritual/religious beliefs and practices, Barss (2012) stresses the need for nurses to clarify with the client who it is that the client wishes to attend to his or her spiritual needs. This is in keeping with client-centered, nonintrusive, and respectful care. Barss also points out the necessity for nurses to discern whether the nature and context of their relationship with clients is conducive to and/or appropriate to in-depth exploration of spiritual concerns. For example, in acute care settings, short-term episodic relationships may be the norm such that in-depth exploration of the client's spirituality is not feasible. However, nurses in long-term care facilities will generally have ample opportunity to explore the client's spiritual needs. The expertise and competence of the nurse can also impact the nature and level of spiritual care provided. Not all nurses can be expected to provide the same level of spiritual care in all situations of the client. However, in some instances, it must be remembered that the nurse is the health care professional whom the client trusts the most, or who is present when the client's spiritual needs are most acutely felt. Because of all of these factors, there is no "standardized" spiritual care.

Some descriptions of spiritual care involve active listening, presence, compassion, and other aspects that are generally noted to be basic to good nursing care (Barss, 2012; Battey, 2012; McSherry, 2006; Molzahn & Sheilds, 2008; Murphy & Walker, 2013). Thus, *all* nurses can provide such spiritual care. Narayanasamy (1999a) captures the importance of good nursing care as constituting spiritual care when he states:

> [G]iving a bath to a patient too weak to bathe himself certainly meets physical needs of comfort and hygiene. However, if during the bath the nurse is gentle in her approach, is aware of the patient's feelings and mental state, and responds appropriately, then a bath becomes a way of serving the patient and touching the very core of his spirit. (p. 387)

Spiritual care, then, can be contained in expressions of empathy, in listening to clients' hopes, fears, and stories, in responding to their feelings, and/or in the nurse recognizing and accepting their beliefs, faith, or culture. All of these are related to and indicative of the human spirit (Molzahn & Sheilds, 2008; National Health Service [NHS] Education for Scotland, 2009). In such a manner, spiritual care is caring for the *person* of the client and can easily be incorporated into daily nursing practice—an assertion made by many who research and write about spiritual care in nursing, for example, MacLaren (2004) and Miner-Williams (2006). As Johnson (2001) states, "All good nursing care is . . . considered to be 'spiritual', conveying to the patient that they have value and are cared for regardless of their illness, colour or creed" (p. 180). Laukhuf and Werner (1998) also summarize this perspective well:

Spiritual care involves the caring practices we exhibit as nurses. It takes the guise of those practices we do daily that affects our patients in profound ways. Spiritual care is more than realizing a patient's spiritual beliefs and incorporating these into our interventions. Spiritual care is anything that touches the spirit of another. It can be shared laughter, tears, keeping vigil with a family as a loved one struggles to recover. It can be crying with that family when the patient dies. It can be soothing a chronically ill individual . . . sitting there . . . . It can be the 3 a.m. conversation prior to surgery. It can be shared prayer or religious reading from the Bible, Koran or other religious book that has special meaning to the patient. (p. 67)

Reflection 6.2

Reflect on the notion of good nursing care as constituting spiritual care. What aspects of good nursing care are integral to your own practice? Where do you need to improve and how can you do this?

Although it is right and proper to conceptualize good generic nursing care as providing spiritual care, it should not preclude specific spiritual-oriented interventions or the religious aspect of spiritual care (Reimer-Kirkham, 2009), as such may be important to clients. Neither should spiritual care be perceived *only* as religious care. In instances where religious care is important because of a client's view of his or her spirituality, not all nurses may feel comfortable or have the expertise to address the explicit religious needs of such clients in the fullest sense. This is particularly the case if the client has issues and concerns directly related to his or her religion. Although all nurses should have a basic understanding of the beliefs and practices of major world religions (at least those beliefs and practices that have possible health implications), it cannot be expected that nurses will be expert in all aspects related to such religions. If the nurse is not possessed with a sufficient understanding or expertise with respect to the religion of the client, then a consultation with or referral to a religious leader or spiritual care professional may be in order, depending on the client's wishes. In instances where the nurse shares the same religion as the client, more in-depth spiritual care may be provided by adapting such care to the manner in which the client practices his or her religion. Paramount in such instances is that the nurse respects the client's beliefs, and has an approach that is centered on the client (Matthew, 2000).

Kumar (2004) addresses spiritual care provision at different levels depending on the spiritual/religious worldviews of nurses and clients. She acknowledges that nurses who share a client's worldview can provide spiritual care interventions different from those of the nurses whose worldview may be different from the client's. In the case of disparate worldviews, Kumar advocates for nurses to try and understand clients, be sensitive to them and their beliefs, and be nonjudgmental. Kumar also points out that, even in disparate worldviews between nurses and clients, there may still be common beliefs and agreement. Again, understanding and respect are the norms. Pesut (2013) also addresses the worldviews of nurses and clients, the impact on spiritual care, and commonality across disparate worldviews. Her comment regarding the latter is particularly insightful when, as writing from her own perspective as a nurse from an evangelical Christian worldview, she states, "I learned how often these differences [with clients' worldviews] melted away in the presence of authentic human engagement. In our research . . . we heard how healthcare providers found human connection even across seemingly chasms of differing beliefs" (p. 6).

What is the nature of spiritual care relative to psychosocial care? The World Health Organization Quality of Life-Spirituality, Religion and Personal Beliefs (WHOQOL-SRPB) Group, (2006) identifies eight factors distinguishing spiritual care from psychosocial care when it states that spiritual care is connected to a spiritual being or force; the meaning of life; awe, wholeness, and integration; spiritual strength; inner peace/serenity/harmony; hope; and optimism and faith. One can see from this list of factors a correlation with the focus of several spiritual needs as discussed in Chapter 5 (see section on Spiritual Needs).

SPIRITUAL CARE INTERVENTIONS

Pesut (2008) points out that codes of ethics stipulate a mandate to respect and support clients' spiritual and religious beliefs, values, and practices. She suggests that the nursing literature goes beyond that ethical provision of respect and support to the actual intervention. The importance of good nursing care cannot be overemphasized when it comes to any discussion about spiritual care. In this regard, caution needs to be exercised in using the term "spiritual interventions." If one thinks of interventions, then it can all too easily become nurse-centered; and also assumes a stance of "doing to" as opposed to "being with." However, consistent with a nursing process framework and terminology, the word "interventions" continues to be used.

There are specific spiritual care nursing interventions that have been noted as appropriate not only for individual clients but also for groups of clients. For example, Tuck (2012) developed and tested a spiritual intervention group for clients with chronic health problems.

Much has been written about spiritual coping strategies, both from clients' perspectives as well as nurses' perspectives. For example, Baldacchino and Draper (2001) reviewed studies in the nursing literature to determine the coping strategies used by clients during times of illness. Their list included: meditation; contemplation or the connection to one's inner self and one's strengths; relationships with others such as family, friends, and a faith community; relationship with a Supreme Being; developing hope for a better future; helping others as well as receiving love from others; appreciating nature, art, music; religious beliefs and practices; and participation in worship. Baldacchino and Draper (2001) conclude that illness stimulates a person's spirituality and that using spiritual coping strategies is a way for people to meet their spiritual needs. Obviously, their literature review implies that nurses need to assess the client's usual spiritual coping strategies and then facilitate the use of the same strategies during times of illness.

FACILITATIVE INTERVENTIONS

When nurses enter the experience of clients, accompanying them on their journey through illness and suffering, nurses can encourage and facilitate clients in exploring their values, goals, and spiritual beliefs, and practices. Changes within clients can be facilitated and decisions encouraged that may positively impact on their spiritual health (Narayanasamy, 1999a). Personal spiritual coping strategies can be enhanced as spirituality is explored as a resource for clients. The nurse can also support the facilitation of spiritual or religious rituals or practices in which clients want to engage. For example, some religions have specific rituals that need to be performed before prayer; or clients may need to face in a particular direction or assume a certain posture while praying. Nurses can do as much as possible to ensure that these requirements are met. Also, clients may wish to partake of various sacraments that may be associated with their faith, which require the presence of a religious leader. Again, the nurse can facilitate this process.

Facilitative interventions take their direction from clients, so such interventions need to be client centered. In a facilitative role, the nurse *works with* clients to ensure that any interventions are according to the wishes and goals of the clients (Stanhope, Lancaster, Jessup-Falcioni, & Viverais-Dresler, 2011). This does not mean that the nurse has no input in the process for he or she may have knowledge or expertise that clients can access. Ideally, in a partnership stance, decisions are made with respect to how to best meet clients' spiritual needs. Then nurses can facilitate the chosen interventions, using any resources that may be available to them. A facilitative role is critical to the provision of quality spiritual care.

Spiritual Need Interventions

Various spiritual needs were identified in Chapter 5 (see section on Spiritual Needs). It may be determined through the process of assessment that the client may require help in meeting one or more of these spiritual needs, perhaps due to illness or suffering. The following suggestions for interventions aimed at some select spiritual needs are by no means an exhaustive list. There are further resources available when one deals with clients who require interventions directed at specific spiritual needs.

The Need for Meaning and Purpose

As discussed earlier, the need for meaning and purpose is a predominant need for clients during illness and loss experiences, and this need is often the target of nursing interventions. For example, 81% of the nurses in a study by Grant (2004) said that they provided spiritual care when clients questioned the meaning of life and life events. There are many theorists who have written the articles that specifically focus on the struggle for meaning and how nurses can respond, for example, Meyerhoff, van Hofwegen, Harwood, Drury, and Emblen (2002).

Nurses cannot provide meaning for clients because developing meaning is a process that must be driven by the client. Nurses can, however, be present and supportive with clients who are trying to develop meaning. Nurses can facilitate the process by asking questions, making empathetic responses, and employing other facilitative communication skills (Miner-Williams, 2006). Specific strategies for meaning making can be employed. Discussing the importance of finding meaning in and during illness/suffering is among such strategies (Carpenito, 2013). Normalizing the client's questions that often accompany the search for meaning is another strategy. Exploring meaning and purpose through activities that promote the client's self-knowledge and self-awareness (e.g., journaling, reflection, and meditation) is yet another strategy (Delaney, 2005). Finally, listening to clients' stories and facilitating the expression of such stories is important in making meaning (Browning, 2008; National Health Service [NHS] Education for Scotland, 2009). As Liehr and Smith (2008) state:

> The human story is a health story in the broadest sense. It is a recounting of one's current life situation to clarify present meaning in relation to the past with an eye toward the future, all in the present moment (p. 207) . . . . Through story . . . Patterns surface as individuals shed a momentary light on the meaning of important experiences. (p. 212)

The following example of a spiritual story illustrates the point that spiritual stories can hold many meanings for clients and that meaning can be found in the stories:

> A woman had been admitted to a hospital following a miscarriage, her third in three successive pregnancies. Her great sorrow, expressed to me as the visiting chaplain, was that she was left with nothing, that is, there were no human remains with which she could have a funeral, or remember and mark the lives which had been there. At the same time, she indicated a vase of daffodils on the bedside cabinet. These had been given to her by her mother, but in the heat of the ward, they had all withered on their stems and not one of them had opened. She said it seemed to be a visual reminder to her of her losses, "The buds that never came to flower." I then suggested that we might do something symbolic with these buds, since we had no human remains with which to conduct a funeral. She found the idea a helpful one, and we ended up cocreating a rite involving us digging a hole in her garden, laying three of the buds at the bottom of it along with some poems she had written about her experiences and a form of words appropriate to what we were doing, and planting a rose bush on top, which comes to full flower each year. (National Health Service [NHS] Education for Scotland, 2009, p. 36)

The actual activity conducted in this story to help the client with making meaning of her experiences may not be carried out by a nurse per se. However, the nurse discussing such activities with clients as possibilities for them to carry out, perhaps with significant others, may be in order.

Thompson and Janigian (1988) developed a conceptual framework for understanding "finding meaning." They focused on what they call the "life scheme" of a person. A life scheme is defined by Thompson and Janigian as "a cognitive representation of one's life, much like a story, which organizes one's perspectives of the world and oneself, goals one wishes to attain, and events that are relevant to those goals" (p. 260). Therefore, a life scheme provides a sense of purpose and order to one's life. Illness can often disrupt a person's life scheme and correspondingly his or her sense of order and purpose. Thompson and Janigian propose changing the life scheme of a person as a means of finding meaning in the midst of illness.

Scales can be used not only as a means of measuring aspects of meaning and purpose in life, but can also aid in discussion about finding meaning and purpose. For example, Ryff's Purpose-in-Life Scale (Ryff & Keyes, 1995) can be a valuable tool to assist the nurse in this regard. Moreover, giving information to clients about strategies known to be helpful in meaning making can be an effective way to facilitate clients moving through this process. For example, Taylor (2002) identifies various cognitive and behavioral approaches as well as relationship approaches (pp. 163–168) and she illustrates each in client scenarios. Reference to Taylor for an in-depth discussion of such approaches is recommended.

Clarke (2006) identifies that helping clients find significance in their health situation and helping clients clarify their spiritual beliefs are important in assisting them to develop meaning. Helping clients recognize the variety of ways that meaning can be found is also important, for example, through spiritual or religious beliefs, through relationships, and through drawing on past experiences. Nurses can "hypothesize" about possible and potential sources of meaning for clients to consider and then affirm sources that clients may find useful in developing meaning (Burkhart, Schmidt, & Hogan, 2011; Como, 2007; Wright, 2005).

Narayanasamy (2004) points out that it is important for nurses to recognize that often, when people are searching for meaning and purpose, they may be looking primarily for an opportunity to talk about their feelings. This point was discussed in Chapter 5 (see section on The Need for Meaning and Purpose). In such an instance, the nurse can respond by facilitating the expression of such feelings, which can then bring clarity and a renewed sense of meaning, purpose, and hope to the client.

Reflection 6.3

- Reflect on a situation in your own life where you were engaged in the process of "meaning making." What was that experience like for you? Did you eventually come to make sense of the situation, that is, develop some sense of meaning and purpose in it? If so, what was helpful in the process and how was it helpful?
- Think of a past or present situation in which clients with whom you worked were/are in the process of making meaning of life in general or of some life event in particular. How were you aware that this process was/is occurring? How did/can you facilitate the process for the client?

The Need for Hope

Nurses can assist clients to develop and maintain hope by such activities as reflecting on the past memories where joy and happiness were present; identifying and hypothesizing about sources of hope; encouraging expressions of hope; encouraging hope inherent in spiritual or religious beliefs and practices; and helping clients find forgiveness from self, God, or other people (Espeland, 1999; Fitchett & Handzo, 1998; Piotrowski, 2013).

The Need for Forgiveness

Nurses can help clients meet the need for forgiveness by initially facilitating discussion about any "wrong doing" in which clients feel they have engaged or even thought about. Clients can then be encouraged to forgive themselves, or to seek forgiveness from others and God (or a Supreme Being) if relevant for them. Clients may also want to forgive others who they feel have wronged them in some way. Nurses can then assist clients with a plan to forgive. Referral to a religious leader or spiritual care provider may be in order if clients so wish.

The Need for Love, Belonging, and Relatedness

Interventions directed at connecting clients with other people, God, or a Supreme Being can help to meet the clients' need for love, belonging, and relatedness. The provision of support, love, security, belonging, and strength can be provided through such relationships, all of which can facilitate spiritual and general well-being (Delgado, 2007; Meyerhoff et al., 2002). During the assessment process, the nurse may be able to identify people and processes in which the client has engaged in the past to address this need. Where possible, support and encouragement of these can occur, but accommodations due to the client's health status may be required. For example, a client may have been part of a faith community, but, due to ill health, may now not be able to be involved with that community. The nurse can then contact representatives of the faith community to visit the client and involve him or her in the life of the community in a different way. For example, a certain woman may be unable to regularly attend her faith community due to her precarious health status. She can feel part of this community when she is made responsible for making sure that greeting cards get completed and sent to people who are having birthdays, who are celebrating anniversaries, or who are grieving. Another person who is in a similar situation could accomplish the same connectivity by developing the roster for greeters at his or her faith community and by telephoning them on a weekly basis to remind others of their upcoming duties.

Spiritual Distress Interventions

Carpenito (2013, 2017) outlines spiritual care interventions directed toward the various nursing diagnoses related to spirituality and religion as identified by the North American Nursing Diagnosis Association-International (NANDA-I). Some examples of interventions given for the nursing diagnosis of "spiritual distress" include the following (Carpenito, 2017):

- Use questions about past beliefs and spiritual experiences to assist the person in putting this life event into wider perspective (p. 775).

- Inform individuals and families about the importance of finding meaning in illness and suffering (p. 774).

- Be available and willing to listen when person expresses self-doubt, guilt, or other negative feelings (p. 775).

- Give "permission" to discuss spiritual matters with the nurse by bringing up the subject of spiritual welfare, if necessary (p. 774).

Examples of interventions to address the diagnosis of "impaired religiosity" include (Carpenito, 2017, pp. 779–781):

- Provide privacy and quiet as needed for daily prayer, visit by a spiritual leader, and spiritual reading and contemplation (p. 780).

- Express the willingness of the health care team to help the person meet spiritual needs (p. 781).

- Communicate acceptance of various beliefs and practices (p. 780).

- Explore whether the person desires to engage in an allowable religious or spiritual practice or ritual; if so, provide opportunities to do so (p. 779).

For a complete list of spiritual care associated with the NANDA-I nursing diagnoses, refer to Carpenito (2013, 2017).

RELIGIOUS INTERVENTIONS

Reference to various religious interventions has already been made. When a client is connected to a particular religion, then there may be specific interventions that are focused on various aspects of that religion. Before any interventions are considered, it must be remembered that nurses are to respect clients' religious beliefs and practices. They may facilitate and encourage religious beliefs and practices that provide comfort, strength, and security for clients. Faith communities can be invaluable resources to the physical, emotional, and spiritual care of clients and families (Carr, 2008; Casarez & Engebretson, 2012; Lemmer, 2005; Stoll, 1979). Nurses may encourage clients to actively participate in their faith community as a means of support, both social and spiritual. In instances where a client is unable to participate in a faith community due to the client's health status, the nurse can facilitate bringing members of the faith community to the client—or refer the client to a religious leader or spiritual care professional, if it is desired. Some faith communities have parish nurses to whom the nurse can refer the client for follow-up after the client is discharged from the health care institution. If clients are not connected to a religion, then they may still seek to engage in spiritual rituals and practices that provide strength and comfort for them. In such a context, nurses can facilitate the clients' engagement in such activities.

If clients desire such activities, then religious beliefs and practices may be integrated into the general treatment or nursing care plan. For example, if a client's normal routine is to have daily readings from a book sacred to his or her religion (e.g., the Bible or the Quran) and cannot do this due to illness, the nurse can incorporate such a reading into the nursing care plan, perhaps recruiting the assistance of family members to carry out the plan. Participation of the client in a religious ritual that is important to him or her can also be facilitated by ensuring privacy for same, or by arranging for such rituals to be carried out by an appropriate person. The nurse being present during these times may be important for relationship building and also for support (Carson, 2008; Delany, 2005; Koenig, 1997; Taylor, 2002).

Sometimes, nurses can deem clients' religious beliefs, values, and practices to be harmful to the clients' spiritual or overall well-being. For example, a client may believe that only God can heal him or her and may refuse any medical intervention even when that intervention is known to be effective in addressing whatever health issue the client is experiencing. Depending on the context, the age of the client, and the relationship with the client, the nurse can challenge the client to think about such beliefs, values, and practices. It is wise to consult with a religious leader or spiritual care professional in such instances (Koenig, 1997; Taylor, 2002; Unruh, 2007).

Besides facilitating rituals, nurses can also assist clients to create their own rituals that are meaningful to them and that facilitate their spiritual well-being (Taylor, 2002). For example, in a situation where a client is experiencing a profound grief reaction to the death of a loved one, the client may be encouraged to go to the ocean or some body of water, place a bouquet of flowers in the water, and watch them recede from the shore.

This can be helpful to the client in terms of "letting go." As with any other intervention, the ritual needs to be client centered and may be a cocreation between the nurse and the client. Imposing a ritual on a client simply will not work. Taylor (2002) gives helpful guidelines when planning a ritual with clients (pp. 212–214), illustrating such in a case scenario. Reference to Taylor for more information on these guidelines is recommended.

Prayer as Intervention

Prayer is a practice that is common to all major world religions, albeit the form and nature of prayer vary among and within various religions. Prayer is defined by Sciarra (2013) as the speaking through the mind or voice to a power that the person believes is higher than himself/herself" (p. 28). Thus, it is a means of connecting with God, a higher power, or something or someone beyond the self. Prayer has perhaps been the most researched of all spiritual interventions. It has been noted to be used as a resource by clients and families during times of illness or other adversity (Koenig, King, & Carson, 2012; McCaffrey, Eisenberg, Legedza, Davis, & Phillips, 2004; O'Connor, Pronk, Tan, & Whitebird, 2005). For example, prayer has been used by clients dealing with breast and other types of cancer (Lengacher et al., 2002; Taylor & Outlaw, 2002), chronic illness (Narayanasamy, 2002), and kidney disease (Lindqvist, Carlsson, & Sjöden, 2004). Clients can gain strength and hope from prayer and it can be helpful in developing or restoring meaning (Meyerhoff et al., 2002). Other benefits of prayer include promoting calm feelings, rest, and well-being; engendering a sense of peace; promoting healing and recovery; providing a means to overcome negative feelings that often accompany illness such as anger and sadness; improving quality of life; and increasing the ability to cope (Hubbartt, Corey, & Kautz, 2012; Oliver, 2013; Sciarra, 2013). The ethical issues surrounding the use of prayer have been discussed (French & Narayanasamy, 2011; Taylor, 2003). In general, the research indicates that prayer can contribute positively to physical and emotional health, as well as contribute positively to the client's coping ability (Taylor, 2002). Furthermore, there is indication that clients want nurses to pray with them (Narayanasamy, 2011; Reig, Mason, & Preston, 2006; Taylor, 2003).

Although prayer is traditionally associated with a religion, people who do not claim to be religious report praying. In such instances, I have heard people describe prayer as "a quiet moment of reflection," "petitioning the universe about _____," and "positive thoughts and petitions directed at a person who is suffering or in need." Thus, prayer does not have to be connected to religion. As Rossiter-Thornton (2002) maintains, making a distinction between the two will "permit the use [by clients] of techniques of prayer without having to subscribe to a particular set of religious beliefs. It will also permit the study of the technique being used by practitioners with and without religious beliefs" (p. 23).

In nursing codes of ethics, there are directives for nurses to respect the spiritual beliefs of clients (see section on Nursing Codes of Ethics in Chapter 3). The implication of these directives is that if clients believe in the benefits of prayer, then to respect such a belief, it may be incumbent upon nurses to utilize prayer as part of the health care of such clients. Nursing diagnostic bodies also specifically include prayer as part of meeting spiritual needs (Hubbartt et al., 2012). Nurses can use prayer as an intervention in a number of ways. For example, they can pray silently for clients or they can pray aloud with and for clients (Carson, 2008). Research has indicated that nurses also pray for themselves, their own spiritual well-being, and their work demands and issues (Cavendish et al., 2004; Holt-Ashley, 2000).

Some of the challenges to the use of prayer by nurses as an intervention include not knowing what to say when praying with clients; fear of offending clients; lack of confidence in the use of prayer; cultural issues connected to prayer; time pressures; and uncertainty regarding praying for someone from a different religion (Hubbartt et al., 2012). With respect to the last challenge, Hubbartt and colleagues suggest asking clients to pray or referring them to someone from their faith tradition who can pray with them. Moreover, there are generic prayers available for different faith traditions (e.g., see www.worldprayer.org). Some of the challenges to the use of prayer can be addressed by following specific guidelines regarding the use of prayer with clients. On the basis of a number of sources from the literature, Kim-Godwin (2013) and Hubbartt and colleagues (2012) provide examples of useful guidelines:

- Carefully assess the client's spiritual beliefs and wishes regarding prayer.

- Obtain permission from the client to pray for the client.

- Ensure that the client is not made to feel uncomfortable or is coerced in any way.

- Do not proselytize or evangelize.

- Ensure that optimal practices for use of prayer are followed.

- Respect and accommodate the client's choices regarding prayer.

- Use prayer that has more general and universal overtones in certain contexts.

- Offer privacy and spiritual space if possible.

- Be present with the client if he or she wishes to pray and desires the nurse to be present.

- Assist the client to find prayers that can be helpful, for example, from books or YouTube.

- Ensure that the focus is on the client, that is, the prayer is client centered and not nurse centered.

- Refer the client to a religious leader/spiritual care professional if the situation warrants it.

- Use silent prayer in situations where praying with the client is problematic.

Reflection 6.5

- Reflect on prayer as a ritual. Is prayer part of your life? If so, how does it function in your life, for example, in your coping with various life events?

(continued)

Reflection 6.5 **(continued)**

- How might you conduct an assessment of the place of prayer in a client's life? Write two or three questions that you might ask. Pilot these in an interaction with a couple of clients, noting not only how their responses facilitated your understanding of the role and impact of prayer in their lives, but also how it impacted your spiritual care of these clients.

STORIES AND INTERVENTION

The connection between stories and the spiritual need for meaning and purpose has already been addressed. Clients often relate stories of their illness experiences and their lives to nurses. As O'Connor (2001) states:

> We are people of the story. Every patient has a story, and the caregiver has his or her story. [The role of the nurse] is to hear the patient into speech, to be a midwife of the spirit . . . . Sometimes [nurses] are the interpreter of the person to himself to herself, or at times [they] may be the interpreter of meaning-making, hope, suffering, fear, anxiety, or joy . . . . [Nurses need to] . . . receive their story through the eyes of compassion and gentleness. (p. 38)

As can be seen from this quote, a vital intervention for nurses with respect to stories is to listen carefully to them. Listening is a powerful intervention, one that is often minimized in terms of its impact on clients. Nurses can also play a role in the interpretation of the story to the client. However, this interpretation needs to be conducted in a "hypothesis-generating" manner rather than an authoritative manner. For example, the nurse can think of various possible interpretations inherent in the story, and begin with the phrase, "I wonder if _____," continuing on with a possible interpretation for the client to consider.

Taylor (1998) identifies some practical suggestions for nurses as they listen to and encourage clients' stories (p. 253). Although these suggestions were specifically focused for use by oncology nurses, they are also relevant for other contexts of care:

- Encourage storytelling as the resultant connectedness and meaningfulness are components of spiritual health.

- Listen attentively and accept stories that are repetitive, as such may be part of the client processing the story. Recognize the client's need to be heard.

- Facilitate linkages between clients' stories and their present situation.

- Facilitate the client's self-understanding from stories by asking such questions and making comments such as: "How is the story you've just told me a metaphor/lesson for your life?" "The stories you've been telling me about your life seem to have a theme or focus about . . . ; can you tell me more about that?" "I learned from your story that you believe or value . . . ; how does that help you now?" (p. 253)

- Analyze clients' stories to facilitate understanding of the clients. Taylor gives a number of questions that nurses can ask themselves to aid in this analysis (p. 253).

- Place clients' stories into a purposeful context, perhaps by reframing stories to provide meaning. Taylor suggests asking questions such as the following can be helpful in facilitating this process: "This is your life so far, now how would you like the story to end?" "Although you've had a lot of tough times in your life, what are the good things that have come out of them?" . . . "How has this (what happened in the story) helped you to become the person you are meant to be—or the person you think you were meant to be?" (p. 253)

- Consider stories to be more than mere recall of what is remembered. They also reflect what is chosen to be remembered. It is important for the nurse to consider how clients want nurses to see them, how they see themselves, and how accepting they are of themselves.

- Recognize that clients' stories can evoke aspects of a nurse's own stories and use this self-awareness for the benefit of the client.

Stories that nurses tell clients can also be therapeutic spiritually in that they can provide connection, meaning, comfort, and hope. They can also normalize feelings and experiences and provide a more positive aspect to the clients' situations. Sometimes, these stories can come from a biography or an autobiography that has been written about someone's life experiences. Other clients' stories can also be helpful but permission to share that story with other people must be obtained. Clients can also be referred to appropriate client groups where the sharing of stories can be part of the therapeutic value of the group.

The concept of "holding the story" (p. 37) described by the National Health Service (NHS) Education for Scotland (2009) is an interesting one. This involves the professional "holding the story" for the client in the form in which it is told. This is especially crucial if the story's content is at variance with what the nurse might think or believe. For example, a client may talk about a time in his or her illness experience when the presence of God was felt in a powerful way. The nurse, however, may not believe that there is a God. Holding the story for the client enables the client to find his or her own meaning in the stories told. Partial stories can also be "held" so that clients can determine how they will end. Such a practice is empowering for clients, acknowledging their right to autonomy as they tell their stories, own them, and participate in their completion. It is truly a client-centered approach!

Nouwen, quoted and affirmed in Taylor (2002, p. 254), is worth repeating here to end the discussion about interventions pertaining to stories:

As healers, we have to receive the story of our fellow human beings with a compassionate heart, a heart that does not judge or condemn but recognizes how the stranger's story connects with our own. We have to offer safe boundaries within which the often painful past can be revealed and the search for a new life can find a start. Our most important question as healers is not, "What to say or do?", but, "How to develop enough inner space where the story can be received?" Healing is the humble but also the very demanding task of creating and offering a friendly empty space where strangers can reflect on their pain and suffering without fear, and find the confidence that makes them look for new ways right in the center of their confusion. (Nouwen, 1975, p. 90)

Reflection 6.6

- Write a significant story of your own life, focusing on an adverse event in your life such as illness or loss. What meaning can you find in your story? Would reframing aspects of the story provide opportunities for you to grow personally and spiritually? What possible interpretations might you make in reflecting on your story?
- Pay particular attention to client stories this week using Taylor's guidelines for listening to and encouraging clients' stories. What was the outcome of your endeavors for both the client and yourself?

CONSULTATION AND REFERRAL INTERVENTIONS

Sometimes, the help of other health care professionals is needed. Such professionals can be religious leaders, parish nurses, or spiritual care professionals. These professionals have advanced training and education that is focused on spirituality/religion. Their role is to assist clients in facing difficult questions about life and death, in searching for meaning in life or in illness and suffering, to encourage clients to express feelings regarding the emotions that often accompany illness and suffering, to engage in religious rituals with clients, and to support people at difficult times in their lives in a variety of ways. They also support other health care professionals by providing information and education about various faith groups, other resources, and about spiritual care. Moreover, support can be provided to health care professionals when they, themselves, may be impacted by the client's situations (Abu-Ras & Laird, 2001; National Health Service [NHS] Education for Scotland, 2009; Pesut, Reimer-Kirkham, Sawatzky, Woodland, & Peverall, 2012). Reciprocally, nurses can be helpful to spiritual care professionals in terms of gathering information about clients and then sharing that information with the spiritual care professionals. This bilateral process enables both nurses and spiritual care providers to be more effective in carrying out their roles as part of the health care team. A partnership between nurses and spiritual care professionals can ensure that the spiritual needs of clients and their families are better met.

It is incumbent upon the nurse to be familiar with the religious leaders within the main faith groupings in the community at large. Often, in institutions, an up-to-date list may be kept of such leaders. Consulting with religious leaders may help nurses broaden their knowledge about various religious groups and their beliefs and practices relative to health and illness. However, such leaders are not considered to be a formal part of the health care team as is the case for spiritual care professionals who are employed by the institution or the regional health authority, usually in pastoral care departments within the institution. The point is that nurses need to be aware of confidentiality issues when consulting religious leaders.

When does the nurse consult with a religious leader or a spiritual care professional? There are a number of instances when such a consultation may be in the best interest of the client. For example, if the client has a good relationship with the nurse and wishes to discuss spiritual issues with only him or her, then consultation may be best to better equip the nurse to deal with the client. Moreover, the nurse may have a question about a particular aspect of a religion that might impact health. In that case, consultation may provide the information that the nurse requires to attend to the client's needs. With respect to referral, it is paramount that the wishes of the client are considered before referring him or her. Referral may be the best intervention when the client's spiritual or religious issues are complex and beyond the competency level of the nurse, when time pressures prevent the nurse from addressing the client's spiritual or religious issues, and/or when the client expresses an explicit desire to talk with a religious leader or spiritual care professional.

Sometimes, consultation or referral can be directed at another nurse on the health care team who may be more particularly interested, knowledgeable, experienced, and/or comfortable with the spiritual dimension of care. Although such persons may not have formal training and education in the spiritual dimension of care, they may have studied this aspect of care because of their own interest in it, or they may have been mentored by others with more formal training and education. For example, early in my nursing career, I worked on a multidisciplinary care team in an emergency department of a general hospital. The focus of this team was to do short-term crisis counseling for clients who presented in the emergency department with nonphysical health problems. I indicated to the team that I was particularly interested in spirituality and would like to work with clients who were presenting with issues related to spirituality or religion. Several times, other team members would refer a client to me for specific interventions related to spirituality or religion. At other times, team members would consult with me about a particular client with whom they were working. This model worked well, and it emphasizes the fact that nurses bring a diversity of strengths to the health care team. A team approach to spiritual care can be an effective means of providing comprehensive care.

An important point to keep in mind is that the nurse is often the only person available to the client at a particular time that spiritual concerns come to the forefront (e.g., in the middle of the night). In such cases, nurses need to provide spiritual care at the level of their personal competence and also employ the generic spiritual care that is so important for clients. Consultation and/or referral can be made at a later time.

Reflection 6.7

- What has been your experience in working with spiritual care professionals or religious leaders? Do you have a partnership with such people, or do you merely refer clients to them?
- How can the relationship between pastoral care professionals and nurses be strengthened?

OTHER INTERVENTIONS

There are other interventions identified in the health care literature as spiritual care interventions. Although many are not interventions that are *only and specifically* directed at the spiritual needs of clients, they can also be helpful in nurturing spirituality and also as a means of spiritual coping. One example is *imagery*, which uses mental pictures or images, figurative speech representing objects, actions or ideas, images pertaining to the arts, and representative images such as icons or statues (Green & Harkness, 1997). Imagery can facilitate the expression of feelings or provide comfort and meaning to clients. For example, the imagery of climbing a mountain can be used to capture both the "danger" and "treachery" that can accompany illness and suffering, as well as the possibilities of joy as one completes each leg of the journey. A statue of a person being encircled by a large hand may evoke feelings of being protected, sheltered, loved by God, and so on. Imagery that is more closely related to the client's background will be most effective. For example, if a client is familiar with the sea, guided imagery using images that are related to the sea may be more useful in discussing spiritual issues. Clients will sometimes use imagery themselves to describe their experiences and feelings. In such cases, nurses can expand the use of the imagery so as to maximize spiritual growth.

The use of *humor* is another identified spiritual care intervention (Creel, 2007). Caution must be exercised in that humor can be used inappropriately—for example, as an expression of the nurse's own anxiety and discomfort, or in a forced manner. Clinical judgment regarding the use of humor is crucial. Effective use of humor can occur when the lead is taken from the client. If humor is used by the client as a normal way of experiencing life, then he or she may be also more likely to accept its use to deal with an illness experience. In such cases, the nurse can "match" the style of the client, encouraging the use of humor as a coping strategy. For example, I know of a man with Parkinson's disease (PD) who makes humorous videos chronicling various aspects of his experience with the disease and he posts these videos on YouTube. He does this as a means not only to chronicle his journey and make sense of it, but also to encourage and help others who are experiencing the disease. This activity provides great meaning for him.

Meditation is another spiritual care intervention (Barnum, 2011; Murphy & Walker, 2013; Taylor, 2002). Meditation involves reflection on and contemplation of some phenomenon, especially that of a spiritual nature (Green & Harkness, 1997). There are many forms of meditation, such as Christian meditation, mindfulness meditation, and transcendental meditation, each with roots in various worldviews. Critical to the use of any meditation as a spiritual intervention is to ensure its compatibility with the client's worldview.

Advocacy for clients with respect to spiritual care is an identified spiritual care intervention. Such advocacy can be for a single client or for a group of clients, as when spiritual care is advocated within institutions, in the health care system generally, and in governance policies such as advocating for spiritual care to be part of the quality assurance process (Lemmer, 2005; Sumner, 1998). Advocating for spiritual care professionals to be present in institutions is also important (Reimer-Kirkham et al., 2012; Sherwood, 2000). Advocacy for spirituality to be part of the health care workplace is also becoming a topic of interest as recognition of the benefits of such grows. For example, environments that consider and foster spirituality in their workers contribute to the spiritual growth of the workers, the development of meaning and purpose in their work, their ability to be creative and empathetic, and their ability to cope with stressful situations (Hensel, 2011; Jurkiewicz & Giacalone, 2004; Kazemipour & Amin, 2012; Krishnakumar & Neck, 2002; National Health Service [NHS] Education for Scotland, 2009). Benefits have also been noted at the organizational level: an increase in organizational success and performance, an increase in organizational citizenship behavior, better provision of holistic care, a healthier work environment, and a culture of service to clients (Batcheller, Davis, & Yoder-Wise, 2013; Kazemipour, Amin, & Pourseidi, 2012; Swinton & McSherry, 2006). There is much discussion in the literature about how nurse managers can facilitate the provision of spiritual care in their work settings, for example, Battey (2012), Biro (2012), and Kevern (2012).

Connecting clients to *support groups* that have spiritual support and growth as part of their mandate can be helpful for clients spiritually. Groups such as Alcoholics Anonymous, Al-Anon, and Narcotics Anonymous, for example, are known for their inclusion of spirituality as part of the recovery process. Other examples include Christian Recovery International and Survivors of Sexual Abuse (Darden, 2005).

Lane (2005) describes the potential for *spiritual-body-healing practices*, such as music, drawing, dance, and writing to be effective spiritual care interventions. Nurses can include such practices into the client's care plan or work with creative arts professionals to bring such activities to client care. Some institutions have such professionals who regularly provide these practices for clients, often in a group context.

Bibliotherapy, or the use of books and other reading materials, can promote spiritual healing as well as provide hope and strength to clients (Meyerhoff et al., 2002). When clients identify with characters and their situations in books or other reading materials, it can help them recognize and express feelings, as well as to reframe their situations in a more positive light. Reading materials that more closely approximate the experience of the client will be most effective. Finding appropriate reading materials can be quite a challenge, but amassing such a list for a variety of client contexts can be invaluable. An example from my own nursing experience illustrates the power of bibliotherapy. A couple's young adult son died in a car accident. Knowing that they both were avid readers and of a Christian faith perspective, I recommended a book entitled *Lament for a Son*. Several weeks later, the couple commented on how helpful the book was in dealing with their grief, including the spiritual aspects of this grief. The father read the book several times. This example also illustrates the importance of careful assessment as to the relevance of this type of intervention for clients. For example, if a client does not enjoy or engage in reading, then bibliotherapy will likely not be the best choice.

The use of *nature or horticulture* has been identified as useful spiritual interventions (Emblen & Pesut, 2001). I was reminded of the power of this intervention when I conducted a workshop on spirituality in nursing practice in a province in Canada for which agriculture is a primary industry. Nurses there told me about taking long-term care residents with agricultural backgrounds to a farm during harvest time. They described the residents' spirits as being rejuvenated as they reexperienced something that was meaningful to them in terms of their connection to the land. Some institutions now incorporate small gardens within their grounds or try to bring nature inside the institution in the form of fish tanks or pictures. It is worthwhile to explore this further in Taylor (2002, pp. 267–268) who summarizes the spiritual benefits of a connection to nature that were identified by Cumes (1998).

Other interventions connected to spiritual care in the literature include: massage; therapeutic touch; the "laying on of hands"; aromatherapy; journaling, blogging, or some other literary expression; and biofeedback (Grant, 2004). Offering commendations can also be related to spiritual care where the nurse identifies something positive in the client's patterns of behavior and intentionally verbalizes observations of strengths to the client as a means of reframing a situation in a more positive light—and perhaps deriving meaning from it (Hoglund, 2013; Wright & Leahey, 2009).

Although all of the interventions described in this section are legitimate and effective in the right contexts and situations, it is important to emphasize several factors in determining which interventions might be most therapeutic for a client. The need to tailor the intervention to each client based on his or her personal and spiritual beliefs has been stressed, that is, to provide client-centered spiritual care. The necessity of the client (and the family in some contexts) being a full partner in the decision making about spiritual care interventions cannot be overemphasized. The importance of seeing spiritual care interventions from a stance of educating clients about a resource as opposed to prescribing such interventions is important (Shelly, 2001). The age and gender of the client needs to be taken into account. For example, nurses need to adjust interventions when working with children. The acuity level of clients is also important, as physical needs can take priority over other types of needs when acuity levels are high. In cases where a client is comatose or in an acute psychotic state, generic spiritual care can be the norm until the client is well enough to focus on other needs. The spiritual needs of the client's family should also be addressed in order to provide family-centered care; and at times, the spiritual needs of the family will take precedence over that of the client. Cultural factors are important to consider given the diversity of culture in today's society. Being aware of one's own cultural and spiritual positioning and one's own attitudes and biases in terms of spirituality/religion is also important for nurses to consider. In addition to cultural factors that affect the individual/family, the culture of nursing itself, as well as the culture of health care organizations, should be considered (Carr, 2010).

Upadhaya and Kautz (2012) discuss instances where clients' spiritual beliefs may actually interfere with treatment goals; for example, when they believe that God is punishing them by inflicting some adverse health event upon them, or when they believe that sinful actions have caused an illness. Such beliefs can prevent clients from fully engaging in the therapeutic process. Upadhaya and Kautz suggest strategies that nurses can use to deal with such instances: active listening while helping clients express not only surface feelings but also underlying feelings; reframing; and providing an environment conducive to spiritual healing.

Proper documentation of spiritual care is important to avoid discontinuity of care and to identify and convey the outcomes of spiritual interventions. Some institutions have developed specific forms to assist health care professionals in this regard. For example, Kerrigan and Harkulich (1993) prepared a form for use in a nursing home so that staff could quickly document spiritual interventions, including the frequency of such interventions (refer to Kerrigan & Harkulich [p. 47] for a copy of this form). Tools have also been developed to ensure that spiritual care is addressed, which can be helpful in documentation. For example, Mitchell, Bennett, and Manfrin-Ledet (2006) developed spiritual care maps, which are plans of care depicted in the schematic form of the client's total response to illness—physical, emotional, social, and spiritual. Refer to Mitchell and colleagues (2006) for an example of such a map.

Reflection 6.8

Reflect on all of the interventions discussed in this chapter (see section on Spiritual Care Interventions). Which do you regularly include in your own nursing practice? Which might you like to include, but are unsure about how to do this? How might you develop competence in such interventions?

EVALUATION OF SPIRITUAL CARE

Outcomes of spiritual care have been determined for each of the spiritual interventions discussed, but it is beyond the scope of this work to identify these. A worthwhile exercise would be to explore each intervention more thoroughly, including outcomes of the interventions noted in the literature. Considering spiritual care generally, examples of outcomes include the following:

- Spiritual integrity, demonstrated through a sense of tranquility and peace that is reality based, through developing meaningful and purposeful behavior, and through a sense of integrity that has been restored (Narayanasamy, 2004)

- Positive impact on psychological, social, physical, and spiritual health (Culliford, 2002; Tyler & Raynor, 2006)

- Promotion of a sense of wholeness and well-being (Taylor, 2002)

- Enhancement of coping (Baldacchino & Draper, 2001)

- Ability to transcend the illness experience (Taylor, Amenta, & Highfield, 1995)

- Development of meaning and purpose (Taylor et al., 1995)

- Verbalization by clients that spiritual needs have been met or that they have enhanced spiritual well-being

- Enhanced and rapid recovery (Culliford, 2002)

- Maximization of the quality of health care and health care organizations (Pesut, 2009; Timmins & McSherry, 2012)

With respect to the documented outcomes of spiritual care, Sawatzky and Pesut (2005) point out that such outcomes should reflect the client's reality. The outcomes may or may not be observable. The outcomes of spiritual care can also be perceived by some to be negative as they may include experiences of suffering and pain. However, such experiences may lead to profound spiritual growth. As Sawatzky and Pesut maintain, "Inherent in [times of spiritual] growth are times of suffering and pain. Who are we as nurses to view emotions often associated with suffering as negative spiritual outcomes?" (p. 29). Sawatzky and Pesut also point to the fact that the spiritual journey is unique to clients and "may not be readily understood by those standing on the outside" (Sawatzky & Pesut, p. 30). It is important to realize that outcomes of spiritual care not only are experienced by clients, but, incidentally, may also be experienced by nurses. For example, nurses have reported that *they* benefit from spiritual care encounters in terms of their own personal spiritual growth, finding personal and professional depth, experiencing increased job satisfaction, and feeling less "burned out" (Price, Stevens, & LaBarre, 1995).

MODELS OF SPIRITUAL CARE

As discussed previously, nurse theorists have included spirituality either as an embedded concept or as a major concept in their nursing theories and frameworks. There are a number of dedicated spiritual caregiving models/theories that can be quite helpful in guiding nursing practice in spiritual care. An overview is presented in Table 6.1. Further exploration of these models is recommended by consulting the references given.

Table 6.1 **Models/Theories of Spiritual Care**

Models	Focus
Trinity Model (Wright, 2005)	Meaning; interactions between spirituality, suffering, and beliefs
Synergy Model (Smith, 2006)	Critical care
ASSET Model (adapted from Ellis & Narayanasamy, 2009)	Nurses' reflection on own spiritual care
Spiritual Care in Nursing Practice Theory (Burkhart & Hogan, 2008)	Interaction between nurses and clients in spiritual encounter
Mid-Range Theory of Spiritual Empathy (Chism, 2007)	Spiritual empathy as a form of spiritual care
Connecting Spiritually Theory (Hood, Olson, & Allen, 2007)	Connection as a means to meet spiritual needs
Emblen & Pesut's Model for Spiritual Assessment/Care in Suffering (Emblen & Pesut, 2001)	Assessment and intervention focused on transcendent meaning
Model for Spiritual Care (Delgado, 2007)	Spiritual environment (assessment, communication, and support)

(continued)

Table 6.1 **Models/Theories of Spiritual Care (*continued*)**

Models	Focus
T.R.U.S.T. Model for Spiritual Assessment (Barss, 2012)	Five domains; for clients and clinicians
Careful Nursing Spiritual Values Model (Meehan, 2012)	Human dignity; spiritual values
Body-Mind-Spirit Framework (Chan, Ng, Ho, & Chow, 2006)	Eastern spirituality
Gadow's Ethical Framework (Gadow, 1999; Pesut, 2009)	Three-level ethical tool: immediacy, universalism, relational narrative
Principal Components Model (McSherry, 2006)	Six components of spiritual care
Health Services Framework of Spiritual Care (Daaleman, 2012)	Nursing management
Model of Spirituality (Miner-Williams, 2006)	Aspects of spirituality-guiding spiritual care

ETHICAL CONSIDERATIONS

Many ethical aspects of care have already been discussed earlier, for example, the issue of nurses sharing their spiritual or religious beliefs with clients. A brief summary of ethical considerations regarding spiritual care is as follows:

- Codes of ethics for nursing require nurses to respect a client's beliefs and practices and to provide care that is sensitive to the client's spiritual beliefs and values.

- It is an ethical responsibility for nurses to address spiritual needs if holistic care is to be provided.

- Client-centered caregiving precedence to clients' choices is an ethical responsibility of the nurse.

- Nurses are to provide spiritual care following the general ethical principles of beneficence, nonmaleficence, autonomy, justice and fairness, and advocacy.

- Nursing codes of ethics protect nurses when faced with the need for nursing care that is in conflict with their moral/religious beliefs and values.

- Ethical spiritual care recognizes the vulnerability of clients, respects their autonomy, and ensures that nurses are not proselytizing or being coercive.

- Competency to provide spiritual care needs to be ensured by adequate nursing education in the spiritual dimension.

- Nurses are to refer clients to spiritual care professionals or religious leaders when they are not competent to deal with a client's spiritual or religious needs.

- Confidentiality is an ethical standard for spiritual care as for other aspects of client care.

Reflection 6.9

What ethical issues have you encountered with respect to spiritual or religious care? How did you deal with these issues and what was the outcome? If an ethical issue presented itself now, would you deal with it differently? If so, why, and how?

This chapter has presented an introduction to providing spiritual care in nursing practice. There are a myriad of interventions that can be considered as fitting under the umbrella of spiritual care. Generic spiritual care is critical for all clients. Other interventions more specific to the spiritual and religious concerns of clients can be implemented as they are warranted and must be based on the client's worldview and preferences.

The Bottom Line

- Nurses need to be competent in providing spiritual care and providing care spiritually.

- Nurses need to refer clients if they cannot meet their spiritual needs for a variety of reasons.

- Nurses are to follow ethical principles and guidelines in providing spiritual care.

- Nurses need to be aware of and comfortable with their own spirituality in order to provide appropriate and ethical spiritual care.

- Nurses need to be aware of the various spiritual care interventions and tailor them to meet each client's spiritual needs.

- Nurses need to remember that spiritual care flows from careful spiritual assessment.

- Models and frameworks of spiritual care can assist the nurse in providing spiritual care.

- Evaluation of spiritual care is important to ensure that spiritual needs are met.

Taking It Further

1. Interview a spiritual care professional (pastoral care) and gather information about the scope and nature of his or her practice in terms of the spiritual care of clients and staff. How can this information inform your nursing practice? How can the relationship between nursing and pastoral care be strengthened?

2. Consult Taylor (2002) and read the guidelines for nurses in terms of dealing with "harmful religiosity" (pp. 258–259). On a scale of 1 to 10, with 1 being "not at all" and 10 being "very much so," how many of these guidelines have you followed with respect to clients whose religious beliefs may have a harmful impact on them? What do you need to do in order to follow guidelines that you wish to incorporate more fully into your practice?

3. Use the nursing process to document spiritual assessment and spiritual care given to a client who exhibits one or more spiritual/religious needs. What benefits and challenges did you encounter in your use of the nursing process to focus on spiritual needs? What was the outcome in terms of documenting your assessment and intervention and in terms of continuity of care from other members of the health care team?

4. Complete a nursing care plan using an NANDA-I nursing diagnosis related to spirituality or religion for a client who has one or more spiritual or religious needs. Discuss this care plan with a colleague, including interventions carried out from the plan (Lovanio & Kazer, 2006).

5. Review the models/frameworks of spiritual care presented in Table 6.1. Which of these models/frameworks might be helpful in your nursing practice? Pilot the use of this model/framework in your work with clients, noting the outcome(s) in terms of spiritual care provided. If appropriate, prepare a proposal to include this model as a guide to the provision of spiritual care to clients in the setting in which you work.

6. Interview a number of people who have experienced, or who are experiencing, health issues similar to clients in your area of practice. Focus the discussion on the following topics: (a) What qualities/attributes do the interviewees think should be inherent in nurses who provide spiritual care or care spiritually? (b) What care would be deemed by them to be "spiritual care?" (c) What guidelines might be helpful for nurses in terms of providing spiritual care? Work with these people to develop an education module on spiritual care for nursing staff in your setting. Pilot this module and evaluate its effectiveness in terms of preparing nurses to provide spiritual care.

7. Review the Marie Curie model of reflective practice and competency (Gordon & Mitchell, 2004). Assess the potential of this model (or an adaptation thereof) for educating nurses in your clinical setting about spiritual care.

8. Review the nursing literature for studies that use various nursing theories or models focusing on aspects of spiritual care. How can these studies inform your nursing practice?

9. Review the Careful Nursing spiritual values model described in Meehan (2012). Reflect on and discuss the following:

   a. Does the philosophy underlying the model fit with your view of nursing? Why or why not?

   b. How can this philosophy/model contribute to the development of a therapeutic milieu that facilitates healing, effective interpersonal relationships, and cooperation?

   c. How do the spiritual values of the Careful Nursing philosophy/model compare with analogous generic values of nursing, which can be used in your particular setting or context of practice?

   d. How can the Careful Nursing philosophy/model facilitate nurses' care for themselves and one another? How might attainment of this care impact the setting in which you work?

   e. How can the spiritual values of the Careful Nursing philosophy/model be taught? How can you obtain organizational support and commitment for such learning?

   f. What action statements can be developed in order to incorporate the spiritual values of the Careful Nursing philosophy/model into practice?

   g. Might this model be appropriate to provide a spiritual approach to nursing in your area of nursing practice? Why or why not?

10. In this chapter, stories have been identified as a method for clients to explore meaning and as a way to cope with illness (see section on Stories and Intervention). Conduct a discussion with your peers/colleagues about the stories that they hear from clients. What insights do you gather from the discussion with respect to the potential of stories as a spiritual intervention methodology?

11. Timmins and McSherry (2012) make the following statement about the organizational structure of an institution with respect to spirituality:

    > [The concept of spirituality has the potential] . . . to transform organizational cultures, values and attitudes; all of which influence the patient and staff experience. Organizational structures and values are created and communicated through management structure systems. Nursing managers and nurses are the custodians of caring—this caring must be person-centered and incorporate the spiritual dimension. (p. 955)

a. Do you agree with this statement? Why or why not?

b. How can spirituality transform organizational cultures, values, and attitudes?

c. What role can nurses/nurse managers play in shaping organizational culture, values, and attitudes so as to incorporate spirituality?

12. Identify an adverse event in your life that impacted you, or someone close to you. Write a description of the circumstances of this event. Identify the physical, emotional, social, and spiritual difficulties that you/someone close to you had to deal with in terms of this event. Review the nursing literature with respect to the event and the known difficulties surrounding it. Write a theoretical nursing care plan to address the spiritual needs that arise (or could arise) from the event (Glick, 2012, p. 76–77).

13. Interview a number of spiritual care professionals (pastoral care) with respect to their role in spiritual care. Inquire about the way that they promote their role within health care contexts, how they view themselves as members of the health care team, how they respond to the diversity of spiritual/religious traditions in clients and challenges that they may perceive in their role or in working in the health care team/system (Pesut et al., 2012).

14. When you encounter clients who self-identify as having no religious affiliation, ask them the following questions:

a. What is the meaning of spiritual care for you?

b. Can you describe an experience that you had when you received what you consider to be spiritual care?

c. If you feel that you have not experienced spiritual nursing care, what would this type of care look like for you?

Record themes that are present in the interview(s). How will the clients' responses impact your future care of clients with no religious affiliation (Creel, 2007)? Now ask the same questions to clients who self-identify with a particular religion. Compare the responses and themes inherent in their answers with those of the clients who do not self-identify with a religion. How can this analysis be of use to you in your nursing practice?

15. Review a number of group approaches to spiritual care, such as those described by Lechner and colleagues (2003), Levine and Targ (2002), Phillips, Lakin, and Pargament (2002), and Tuck (2012). Reflect on or discuss the following:

a. Appraise each of these approaches in terms of the study design used to identify outcomes of the group intervention.

b. Might any of these approaches be relevant in your clinical context? Why or why not?

16. Complete Ruder's Perceptions of Spiritual Care Assessment Scale (Ruder, 2013, pp. 366–367). What observations and insights do you have as a result of completing the scale? What items in the scale require your further attention in terms of improving your spiritual care of clients? How can this be accomplished?

17. Conduct a literature review on the place and efficacy of prayer as a spiritual care intervention in nursing practice. Use the following questions as a guide to analyze the literature:

    a. What rationale is provided for the use of prayer in the context of illness?

    b. What rationale is provided for the use of prayer by nurses?

    c. What are the potential ethical issues associated with the use of prayer?

    d. What is your response to the information on the use of prayer in the literature? What issues does it raise for you personally relative to your own beliefs about prayer?

    e. Form a list of guidelines for appropriate use of prayer in nursing practice.

18. Kevern (2012) presents a discussion of a model, which has the potential to assist nurse managers in helping manage nurses' provision of spiritual care. This model is drawn from the social psychology of religion. What is your reaction to the usefulness of this model for nurse managers? Can this model be useful to you in your nursing practice? Why/why not?

19. Visit the World Prayers Project site (www.worldprayers.org) to examine the prayers there. How can this resource be of assistance to you in your clinical practice? Which prayers do you feel comfortable/uncomfortable with in terms of praying them with clients and why? How might you modify some of these prayers for use in your own practice?

20. Cockell and McSherry (2012) conducted an overview of international research on spiritual care in nursing to enable nurse managers to use evidence so as to improve quality of care and implement best practices in their settings. Thinking of nursing management, reflect on or discuss the following questions:

    a. What are the current understandings of spiritual care in your setting of practice?

    b. What spiritual care is offered there?

    c. What training/education is given to nurses on spiritual care? Is this ongoing?

    d. What support is offered to nurses themselves?

    e. How can you promote an organizational culture that supports spiritual care/nurses' provision of spiritual care?

    f. What insights regarding spiritual care can you gain from this article that might be applied to your nursing context?

    g. How can you ensure that your own education/support in the area of spiritual care is current so that you can demonstrate not only what to expect from others but also model good practice?

    h. How can you use pastoral care resources to assist you in implementing spiritual care in your nursing setting? (Adapted from Cockell & McSherry, 2012, p. 966)

21. Cockell and McSherry (2012) identify possible activities for nurse managers who wish to respond to the evidence-based rationale for the inclusion of spiritual care in client care. Review these activities, assessing the extent and level of each activity for the setting in which you work. Identify ways to enhance activities that would encourage the incorporation of spiritual care into the setting in which you work.

22. Review the 18 items of the Spiritual Care Inventory (SCI) designed by Burkhart, Schmidt, and Hogan (2011):

    a. Complete this inventory reflecting on your own practice. Based on your score (a higher score denotes a greater tendency to provide spiritual care), how well do you fare in your beliefs about providing spiritual care?

    b. Review the Spiritual Care in Practice (SCIP) instrument, also developed by Burkhart and Schmidt (2012). Reflecting on your own nursing practice, complete the 12 items on this scale. How do you rate in recognizing patient cues regarding spiritual needs and providing spiritual care interventions?

    c. Compare your SCI score (beliefs) with your SCIP score (actions). Is there a discrepancy in the two scores? If so, what do you need to do to translate your beliefs into actions?

23. Review the hope-fostering strategies presented by Narayanasamy (1999b, p. 282). Discuss these strategies for fostering hope as a spiritual need. Which might you be able to include in your nursing practice?

24. Read and reflect on Virginia Henderson's poem "To Make Complete" (Fulton, 1987). How does this poem illustrate the desired outcomes of optimal nursing care? What qualities does the nurse need to achieve such outcomes? How are these qualities related to the spirituality of the nurse (Hermann, 2003)? How do these qualities relate to you personally?

25. Read the proposal by Haase, Britt, Coward, Leidy, and Penn (1992) that nursing focuses on a person's "spiritual perspective" rather than a person's spirituality (as the latter is a universal quality of all people, whereas the former is highly individualized). Does this distinction provide clarity for you in terms of spiritual care, and if so, how?

26. Reflect on ethical issues identified by Caserez and Engebretson (2012):

    a. Do you omit spiritual/religious care in your practice? What does this reflect about your own spiritual/religious positioning or view of spiritual/religious care?

    b. Have you ever been guilty of inappropriate application of spiritual care (e.g., coercion of the client or overstepping your competence in spiritual care)? Have you witnessed such in your clinical setting? What was the impact on the client?

    c. What conditions do you identify in your own clinical setting, your clinical practice, or within yourself that are especially conducive to offering spiritual care?

d. Are you guilty of prescriptive spiritual care where *you* identify spiritual goals for clients? What are the outcomes of such an approach versus approaching spiritual care from the *client's* perspective?

27. Reflect on or discuss a time when you gave spiritual care to a client:

a. What were the health problems or concerns of the client?

b. How long and how well did you know the client?

c. How did the episode of spiritual caregiving begin?

d. What prompted you to provide spiritual care in this situation?

e. What particular actions did you take in this incident? What did the client do?

f. What was the outcome of the provision of spiritual care for the client and for you? (Adapted from van Dover & Bacon, 2001, p. 19)

REFERENCES

Abu-Ras, W., & Laird, L. D. (2011). How Muslim and non-Muslim chaplains serve Muslim patients? Does the interfaith chaplaincy model have room for Muslims' experiences? *Journal of Religion & Health, 50*(1), 46–61. doi:10.1007/s10943-010-9357-4

Baldacchino, D., & Draper, P. (2001). Spiritual coping strategies: A review of the nursing research literature. *Journal of Advanced Nursing, 34*(6), 833–841. doi:10.1046/j.1365-2648.2001.01814.x

Barnum, B. S. (2011). *Spirituality in nursing: The challenges of complexity* (3rd ed.). New York, NY: Springer Publishing Company.

Barss, K. S. (2012). T.R.U.S.T.: An affirming model for inclusive spiritual care. *Journal of Holistic Nursing, 30*(1), 24–34. doi:10.1177/0898010111418118

Batcheller, J., Davis, J., & Yoder-Wise, P. S. (2013). Hope for the future: Intensifying spirituality in the workplace. *Nursing Administration Quarterly, 37*(4), 309–316. doi:10.1097/NAQ.0b013e3182a2f9ae

Battey, B. W. (2012). Perspectives of spiritual care for nurse managers. *Journal of Nursing Management, 20*(8), 1012–1020. doi:10.1111/j.1365-2834.2012.01360.x

Biro, A. (2012). Creating conditions for good nursing care by attending to the spiritual. *Journal of Nursing Management, 20*(8), 1002–1011. doi:10.1111/j.1365-2834.2012.01444.x

Browning, D. (2008). Internists of the mind or physicians of the soul: Does psychiatry need a public philosophy? *Zygon: Journal of Religion and Science, 43*(2), 371–383. doi:10.1111/j.1467-9744.2008.00922.x

Burkhart, L., & Hogan, N. (2008). An experiential theory of spiritual care in nursing practice. *Qualitative Health Research, 18*(7), 928–938. doi:10.1177/1049732308318027

Burkhart, L., & Schmidt, W. (2012). Measuring effectiveness of a spiritual care pedagogy in nursing education. *Journal of Professional Nursing, 28*(5), 315–321. doi:10.1016/j.profnurs.2012.03.003

Burkhart, L., Schmidt, L., & Hogan, N. (2011). Development and psychometric testing of the Spiritual Care Inventory instrument. *Journal of Advanced Nursing, 67*(11), 2463–2472. doi:10.1111/j.1365-2648.2011.05654.x

Carpenito, L. J. (2013). *Handbook of nursing diagnosis* (14th ed.). Philadelphia, PA: Lippincott Williams & Wilkins.

Carpenito, L. J. (2017). *Handbook of Nursing Diagnosis* (15th ed.). Philadelphia, PA: Lippincott Williams & Wilkins.

Carr, T. (2008). Mapping the processes and qualities of spiritual nursing care. *Qualitative Health Research, 18*(5), 686–700. doi:10.1177/1049732307308979

Carr, T. J. (2010). Facing existential realities: Exploring barriers and challenges to spiritual nursing care. *Qualitative Health Research, 20*(10), 1379–1392. doi:10.1177/1049732310372377

Carson, V. B. (2008). Spirituality: Identifying and meeting spiritual needs. In V. B. Carson & H. G. Koenig (Eds.), *Spiritual dimensions of nursing practice* (Rev. ed., pp. 125–153). West Conshohocken, PA: Templeton Foundation Press.

Casarez, R. L. P., & Engebretson, J. C. (2012). Ethical issues of incorporating spiritual care into clinical practice. *Journal of Clinical Nursing, 21*(15–16), 2099–2107. doi:10.1111/j.1365-2702 .2012.04168.x

Cavendish, R., Konecny, L., Luise, B. K., & Lanza, M. (2004). Nurses enhance performance through prayer. *Holistic Nursing Practice, 18*(1), 26–31. doi:10.1097/00004650-200401000-00005

Chan, C. L. W., Ng, S. M., Ho, R. T. H., & Chow, A. Y. M. (2006). East meets West: applying Eastern spirituality in clinical practice. *Journal of Clinical Nursing, 15*(7), 822–832. doi:10.1111/ j.1365-2702.2006.01649.x

Chism, L. (2007). *Spiritual empathy: A model for spiritual well-being* (Unpublished doctoral dissertation). Oakland University, Rochester, MI.

Clarke, J. (2006). A discussion paper about "meaning" in the nursing literature on spirituality: An interpretation of meaning as "ultimate concern" using the work of Paul Tillich. *International Journal of Nursing Studies, 43*(7), 915–921. doi:10.1016/j.ijnurstu.2006.05.005

Cockell, N., & McSherry, W. (2012). Spiritual care in nursing: An overview of published international research. *Journal of Nursing Management, 20*(8), 958–969. doi:10.1111/j.1365-2834.2012.01450.x

Como, J. M. (2007). Spiritual practice: A literature review relative to spiritual health and health outcomes. *Holistic Nursing Practice, 21*(5), 224–236. doi:10.1097/01.HNP.0000287986.17344.02

Creel, E. (2007). The meaning of spiritual nursing care for the ill individual with no religious affiliation. *International Journal for Human Caring, 11*(3), 14–21.

Culliford, L. (2002). Spirituality and clinical care. *British Medical Journal, 325*, 1434–1435. doi:10.1136/ bmj.325.7378.1434

Cumes, D. (1998). Nature as medicine: The healing power of the wilderness. *Alternative Therapies in Health and Medicine, 4*(2), 79–85.

Daaleman, T. P. (2012). A health services framework of spiritual care. *Journal of Nursing Management, 20*(8), 1021–1028. doi:10.1111/j.1365-2834.2012.01482.x

Darden, R. A. (2005). Spiritual assessment and treatment strategies. *The Remuda Review: The Christian Journal of Eating Disorders, 4*, 14–16.

Delaney, C. (2005). The Spirituality Scale: Development and psychometric testing of a holistic instrument to assess the human spiritual dimension. *Journal of Holistic Nursing, 23*(2), 145–167. doi:10.1177/0898010105276180

Delgado, C. (2007). Meeting clients' spiritual needs. *Nursing Clinics of North America, 42*(2), 279–293. doi:10.1016/j.cnur.2007.03.002

Ellis, H. K., & Narayanasamy, A. (2009). An investigation into the role of spirituality in nursing. *British Journal of Nursing, 18*(14), 886–890. doi:10.12968/bjon.2009.18.14.43358

Emblen, J., & Pesut, B. (2001). Strengthening transcendent meaning: A model for the spiritual care of patients experiencing suffering. *Journal of Holistic Nursing, 19*(1), 42–56. doi:10.1177/08980 1010101900105

Espeland, K. (1999). Achieving spiritual wellness: Using reflective questions. *Journal of Psychosocial Nursing, 37*(7), 36–40. doi:10.3928/0279-3695-19990701-22

Fitchett, G., & Handzo, G. F. (1998). Spiritual assessment, screening, and intervention. In J. C. Holland, W. Breitbart, P. B. Jacobsen, M. S. Lederberg, M. Loscalzo, M. J. Massie, & R. McCorkle (Eds.), *Psycho-Oncology* (pp. 790–808). New York, NY: Oxford University Press.

French, C., & Narayanasamy, A. (2011). To pray or not to pray: A question of ethics. *British Journal of Nursing, 20*(18), 1198–1204. doi:10.12968/bjon.2011.20.18.1198

Fulton, J. (1987). Virginia Henderson: Theorist, prophet, poet. *Advances in Nursing Science, 10*(1), 1–9.

Gadow, S. (1999). Relational narrative: The postmodern turn in nursing ethics. *Scholarly Inquiry for Nursing Practice, 13*(1), 57–70.

Giske, T. (2012). How undergraduate nursing students learn to care for patients spiritually in clinical studies: A review of literature. *Journal of Nursing Management, 20*(8), 1049–1057. doi:10.1111/jonm.12019

Glick, L. H. (2012). Nurturing nursing students' sensitivity to spiritual care in a Jewish Israeli nursing program. *Holistic Nursing Practice, 26*(2), 74–78. doi:10.1097/HNP.0b013e31824621e6

Gordon, T., & Mitchell, D. (2004). A competency model for the assessment and delivery of spiritual care. *Palliative Medicine, 18*(7), 646–651. doi:10.1191/0269216304pm936oa

Grant, D. (2004). Spiritual interventions: How, when, and why nurses use them. *Holistic Nursing Practice, 18*(1), 36–41.

Green, S., & Harkness, J. (1997). *ITP Nelson Canadian Dictionary of the English Language: An Encyclopedic Reference.* Scarborough, ON, Canada: Thomson.

Haase, J. E., Britt, T., Coward, D. D., Leidy, N. K., & Penn, P. E. (1992). Simultaneous concept analysis of spiritual perspective, hope, acceptance and self-transcendence. *Journal of Nursing Scholarship, 24*(2) 141–147.

Hensel, D. (2011). Relationships among nurses' professional self-concept, health, and lifestyles. *Western Journal of Nursing Research, 33*(1), 45–62. doi:10.1177/0193945910373754

Hermann, M. L. S. (2003). Keeping the magic alive in nursing care: Advice from the Dalai Lama. *Nurse Educator, 28*(6), 245–246.

Hoglund, B. A. (2013). Practicing the code of ethics, finding the image of God. *Journal of Christian Nursing, 30*(4), 228–233. doi:10.1097/CNJ.0b013e3182a18d40

Holt-Ashley, M. (2000). Nurses pray: Use of prayer and spirituality as a complementary therapy in the intensive care setting. *AACN Clinical Issues Advanced Practice in Acute and Critical Care, 11*(1), 60–67. doi:10.1097/00044067-200002000-00008

Hood, L. E., Olson, J. K., & Allen, M. (2007). Learning to care for spiritual needs: Connecting spiritually. *Qualitative Health Research, 17*(9), 1198–1206. doi:10.1177/1049732307306921

Hubbartt, B., Corey, D., & Kautz, D. D. (2012). Prayer at the bedside. *International Journal for Human Caring, 16*(1), 42–46.

International Council of Nurses. (2007). Vision for the future of nursing. Retrieved from http://www.icn.ch/who-we-are/icns-vision-for-the-future-of-nursing

Iranmanesh, S., Tirgari, B., & Cheraghi, M. A. (2011). Developing and testing a spiritual care questionnaire in the Iranian context. *Journal of Religion & Health, 51*(4), 1104–1116. doi:10.1007/s10943-011-9458-8

Johnson, C. P. (2001). Assessment tools: Are they an effective approach to implementing spiritual health care within the NHS? *Accident and Emergency Nursing, 9*(3), 177–186. doi:10.1054/aaen2001.0259

Jurkiewicz, C. L., & Giacalone, R. A. (2004). A values framework for measuring the impact of workplace spirituality on organizational performance. *Journal of Business Ethics, 49*(2), 129–142. doi:10.1023/B:BUSI.0000015843.22195.b9

Kazemipour, F., & Amin, S. M. (2012). The impact of workplace spirituality dimensions on organizational citizenship behaviour among nurses with the mediating effect of affective organizational commitment. *Journal of Nursing Management, 20*(8), 1039–1048. doi:10.1111/jonm.12025

Kazemipour, F., Amin, S. M., & Pourseidi, B. (2012). Relationship between workplace spirituality and organizational citizenship behavior among nurses through mediation of affective organizational commitment. *Journal of Nursing Scholarship, 44*(3), 302–310. doi:10.1111/j.1547-5069.2012.01456.x

Kerrigan, R., & Harkulich, J. T. (1993). A spiritual tool. *Health Progress, 74*(4), 46–49.

Kevern, P. (2012). Who can give "spiritual care?" The management of spiritually sensitive interactions between nurses and patients. *Journal of Nursing Management, 20*(8), 981–989. doi:10.1111/j.1365-2834.2012.01428.x

Kim-Godwin, Y. (2013). Prayer in clinical practice: What does evidence support? *Journal of Christian Nursing, 30*(4), 208–215. doi:10.1097/cnj.0b013e31826c2219

Koenig, H. G. (1997). *Is religion good for your health? The effects of religion on physical and mental health.* London, England: Routledge.

Koenig, H. G., King, D. E., & Carson, V. B. (2012). *Handbook of religion and health* (2nd ed.). New York, NY: Oxford University Press.

Krishnakumar, S., & Neck, C. P. (2002). The "what," "why" and "how" of spirituality in the workplace. *Journal of Managerial Psychology, 17*(3), 153–164. doi:10.1108/02683940210423060

Kumar, K. (2004). Spiritual care: What's worldview got to do with it? *Journal of Christian Nursing, 21*(1), 24–28. doi:10.1097/01.CNJ.0000262275.10582.66

Lane, M. R. (2005). Creativity and spirituality in nursing: Implementing art in healing. *Holistic Nursing Practice, 19*(3), 122–125. doi:10.1097/00004650-200505000-00008

Laukhuf, G., & Werner, H. (1998). Spirituality: The missing link. *Journal of Neuroscience Nursing, 30*(1), 60–67. doi:10.1097/01376517-199802000-00007

Lechner, S. C., Antoni, M. H., Lydston, D., LaPerriere, A., Ishii, M., Devieux, J., . . . Weiss, S. (2003). Cognitive-behavioural interventions improve quality of life in women with AIDS. *Journal of Psychosomatic Research, 54*(3), 253–261. doi:10.1016/S0022-3999(02)00480-4

Lemmer, C. (2005). Recognizing and caring for spiritual needs of clients. *Journal of Holistic Nursing, 23*(3), 310–322. doi:10.1177/0898010105277652

Lengacher, C. A., Bennett, M. P., Kip, K. E., Keller, R., LaVance, M. S., Smith, L. S., & Cox, C. E. (2002). Frequency of use of complementary and alternative medicine in women with breast cancer. *Oncology Nursing Forum, 29*(10), 1445–1452. doi:10.1188/02.ONF.1445-1452

Levine, E., & Targ, E. (2002). Spiritual correlates of functional well-being in women with breast cancer. *Integrative Cancer Therapies, 1*(2), 166–174. doi:10.1177/1534735402001002008

Liehr, P. R., & Smith, M. J. (2008). Story theory. In M. J. Smith & P. R. Liehr (Eds.), *Middle range theory for nursing* (2nd ed., pp. 205–224). New York, NY: Springer Publishing Company.

Lindqvist, R., Carlsson, M., & Sjödén, P. (2004). Coping strategies of people with kidney transplants. *Journal of Advanced Nursing, 45*(1), 47–52. doi:10.1046/j.1365-2648.2003.02859.x

Lovanio, K., & Kazer, M. W. (2006). Promoting spiritual knowledge and attitudes. *Holistic Nursing Practice, 21*(1), 42–47. doi:10.1097/00004650-200701000-00008

MacLaren, J. (2004). A kaleidoscope of understandings: Spiritual nursing in a multi-faith society. *Journal of Advanced Nursing, 45*(5), 457–464. doi:10.1111/j.1365-2648.2004.2929_1.x

Matthew, D. (2000). Can every nurse give spiritual care? *Kansas Nurse, 75*(10), 4–5.

McCaffrey, A. M., Eisenberg, D. M., Legedza, A. T. R., Davis, R. B., & Phillips, R. S. (2004). Prayer for health concerns: Results of a national survey on prevalence and patterns of use. *Archives of Internal Medicine, 164*(8), 858–862. doi:10.1001/archinte.164.8.858

McSherry, W. (2006). The principal components model: A model for advancing spirituality and spiritual care within nursing and health care practice. *Journal of Clinical Nursing, 15*(7), 905–917. doi:10.1111/j.1365-2702.2006.01648.x

McSherry, W., Draper, P., & Kendrick, D. (2002). The construct validity of a rating scale designed to assess spirituality and spiritual care. *International Journal of Nursing Studies, 39*(7), 723–734. doi:10.1016/S0020-7489(02)00014-7

McSherry, W., & Jamieson, S. (2013). The qualitative findings from an online survey investigating nurses' perceptions of spirituality and spiritual care. *Journal of Clinical Nursing, 22*(21–22), 3170–3182. doi:10.1111/jocn.12411

Meehan, T. C. (2012). Spirituality and spiritual care from a careful nursing perspective. *Journal of Nursing Management, 20*(8), 990–1001. doi:10.1111/j.1365-2834.2012.01462.x

Meyer, C. (2000). Providing spiritual care: Mutual journey of discovery. *Kansas Nurse, 75*(10), 1–3.

Meyerhoff, M., van Hofwegen, L., Harwood, C. H., Drury, M., & Emblen, J. (2002). Spiritual nursing interventions. *Canadian Nurse, 98*(3), 21–24.

Milligan, S. (2004). Perceptions of spiritual care among nurses undertaking postregistration education. *International Journal of Palliative Nursing, 10*(4), 162–171. doi:10.12968/ijpn.2004.10.4.12792

Miner-Williams, D. (2006). Putting a puzzle together: Making spirituality meaningful for nursing using an evolving theoretical framework. *Journal of Clinical Nursing, 15*(7), 811–821. doi:10.1111/j.1365-2702.2006.01351.x

Mitchell, D. l., Bennett, M. J., & Manfrin-Ledet, L. (2006). Spiritual development of nursing students: Developing competency to provide spiritual care to patients at the end of life. *Journal of Nursing Education, 45*(9), 365–370.

Molzahn, A. E., & Sheilds, L. (2008). Why is it so hard to talk about spirituality? *Canadian Nurse*, *104*(1), 25–29.

Murphy, L. S., & Walker, M. (2013). Spirit-guided care: Christian nursing for the whole person. *Journal of Christian Nursing*, *30*(3), 144–152. doi:10.1097/CNJ.0b013e318294c289

Narayanasamy, A. (1999a). Learning spiritual dimensions of care from a historical perspective. *Nurse Education Today*, *19*(5), 386–395. doi:10.1054/nedt.1999.0325

Narayanasamy, A. (1999b). ASSET: A model for actioning spirituality and spiritual care training in nursing. *Nurse Education Today*, *19*(4), 274–285. doi: 10.1054/nedt.1999.0637

Narayanasamy, A. (2002). Spiritual coping mechanisms in chronically ill patients. *British Journal of Nursing*, *11*(22), 1461–1470. doi:10.12968/bjon.2002.11.22.10957

Narayanasamy, A. (2004). The puzzle of spirituality for nursing: A guide to practical assessment. *British Journal of Nursing*, *13*(19), 1140–1144. doi:10.12968/bjon.2004.13.19.16322

Narayanasamy, A. (2011). Commentary on Chan MF (2009): Factors affecting nursing staff in practicing spiritual care. Journal of Clinical Nursing, 19 2128–2136. *Journal of Clinical Nursing*, *20*(5–6), 915–916. doi:10.1111/j.1365-2702.2010.03653.x

National Health Service (NHS) Education for Scotland. (2009). Spiritual care matters: An introductory resource for all NHS Scotland staff. Retrieved from http://www.nes.scot.nhs.uk/media/3723/spiritualcaremattersfinal.pdf

O'Connor, C. I. (2001). Characteristics of spirituality, assessment, and prayer in holistic nursing. *Holistic Nursing*, *36*(1), 33–46.

O'Connor, P. J., Pronk, N. P., Tan, A., & Whitebird, R. R. (2005). Characteristics of adults who use prayer as an alternative therapy. *American Journal of Health Promotion*, *19*(5), 369–375. doi:10.4278/0890-1171-19.5.369

Oliver, I. (2013). *Investigating prayer: Impact on health and quality of life*. New York, NY: Springer.

Pesut, B. (2006). Fundamental or foundational obligation? Problematizing the ethical call to spiritual care in nursing. *Advances in Nursing Science*, *29*(2), 125–133. doi:10.1097/00012272-200604000-00006

Pesut, B. (2008). Spirituality and spiritual care in nursing fundamentals textbooks. *Journal of Nursing Education*, *47*(4), 167–173. doi:10.3928/01484834-20080401-05

Pesut, B. (2009). Incorporating patients' spirituality into care using Gadow's ethical framework. *Nursing Ethics*, *16*(4), 418–428. doi:10.1177/0969733009104606

Pesut, B. (2013). Nursings' need for the idea of spirituality. *Nursing Inquiry*, *20*(1), 5–10. doi:10.1111/j.1440-1800.2012.00608.x

Pesut, B., Reimer-Kirkham, S., Sawatzky, R., Woodland, G., & Peverall, P. (2012). Hospitable hospitals in a diverse society: From chaplains to spiritual care providers. *Journal of Religion & Health*, *51*(3), 825–836. doi:10.1007/s10943-010-9392-1

Phillips, R. E., Lakin, R., & Pargament, K. I. (2002). Development and implementation of a spiritual issues psychoeducational group for those with serious mental illness. *Community Mental Health Journal*, *38*(6), 487–495.

Piotrowski, L. F. (2013). Advocating and educating for spiritual screening assessment and referrals to chaplains. *Omega Journal of Death and Dying*, *67*(1–2), 185–192. doi:10.2190/OM.67.1-2.v

Price, J. L., Stevens, H. O., & LaBarre, M. C. (1995). Spiritual caregiving in nursing practice. *Journal of Psychosocial Nursing*, *33*(12), 5–9. doi:10.3928/0279-3695-19951201-04

Reig, L., Mason, C., & Preston, K. (2006). Spiritual care: Practice guidelines for rehabilitation nurses. *Rehabilitation Nursing*, *31*(6), 249–256. doi:10.1002/j.2048-7940.2006.tb0021.x

Reimer-Kirkham, S. (2009). Lived religion: Implications for nursing ethics. *Nursing Ethics*, *16*(4), 406–417. doi:10.1177/0969733009104605

Reimer-Kirkham, S., Pesut, B., Sawatzky, R., Cochrane, M., & Redmond, A. (2012). Discourses of spirituality and leadership in nursing: A mixed methods analysis. *Journal of Nursing Management*, *20*(8), 1029–1038. doi:10.1111/j.1365-2834.2012.01480.x

Rossiter-Thornton, J. (2002). Prayer in your practice. *Complementary Therapies in Nursing and Midwifery*, *8*(1), 21–28. doi:10.1054/ctnm.2001.0594

Ruder, S. (2013). Spirituality in nursing: Nurses' perceptions about providing spiritual care. *Home Healthcare Now*, *31*(7), 356–367. doi:10.1097/NHH.0b013e3182976135

Ryff, C. D., & Keyes, C. L. M. (1995). The structure of psychological well-being revisited. *Journal of Personality and Social Psychology, 69*(4), 719–727. doi:10.1037/0022-3514.69.4.719

Sawatzky, R., & Pesut, B. (2005). Attributes of spiritual care in nursing practice. *Journal of Holistic Nursing, 23*(1), 19–33. doi:10.1177/0898010104272010

Sciarra, E. (2013). Should prayer be used in medicine? *Dimensions of Critical Care Nursing, 32*(1), 28–29. doi:10.1097/DCC.0b013e31826bc635

Shelly, J. A. (2000). *Spiritual care: A guide for caregivers.* Downers Grove, IL: IVP Books.

Shelly, J. A. (2001). Is spiritual care ethical? *Journal of Christian Nursing, 18*(2), 3.

Sherwood, G. D. (2000). The power of nurse-client encounters: Interpreting spiritual themes. *Journal of Holistic Nursing, 18*(2), 159–175. doi:10.1177/089801010001800207

Smith, A. R. (2006). Using the synergy model to provide spiritual care in critical care settings. *Critical Care Nurse, 26*(4), 41–47.

Stanhope, M., Lancaster, J., Jessup-Falcioni, H., & Viverais-Dresler, G. A. (2011). *Community health nursing in Canada* (2nd ed.). Toronto, ON, Canada: Elsevier.

Stoll, R. I. (1979). Guidelines for spiritual assessment. *American Journal of Nursing, 79*(9), 1574–1577. doi:10.1097/00000446-197909000-00041

Sumner, C. H. (1998). CE Credit: Recognizing and responding to spiritual distress. *American Journal of Nursing, 98*(1), 26–30. doi:10.2307/3471826

Swinton, J., & McSherry, W. (2006). Editorial: Critical reflections on the current state of spirituality-in-nursing. *Journal of Clinical Nursing, 15*(7), 801–802. doi:10.1111/j.1365-2702.2006.01687.x

Taylor, E. J. (1998). The story behind the story: The use of storytelling in spiritual caregiving. *Seminars in Oncology Nursing, 13*(4), 252–254. doi:10.1016/S0749-2081(97)80020-4

Taylor, E. J. (2002). *Spiritual care: Nursing theory, research, and practice.* Upper Saddle River, NJ: Prentice-Hall.

Taylor, E. J. (2003). Prayer's clinical issues and implications. *Holistic Nursing Practice, 17*(4), 179–188.

Taylor, E. J., Amenta, M., & Highfield, M. (1995). Spiritual care practices of oncology nurses. *Oncology Nursing Forum, 22*(1), 31–39.

Taylor, E. J., Highfield, M. F., & Amenta, M. (1999). Predictors of oncology and hospice nurses' spiritual care perspectives and practices. *Applied Nursing Research, 12*(1), 30–37. doi:10.1061S0897-1897(99)80156-6

Taylor, E. J., & Outlaw, F. H. (2002). Use of prayer among persons with cancer. *Holistic Nursing Practice, 16*(3), 46–60. doi:10.1097/00004650-200204000-00010

Thompson, S. C., & Janigian, A. S. (1988). Life Schemes: A framework for understanding the search for meaning. *Journal of Social and Clinical Psychology, 7*(2–3), 260–280. doi:10.1521/jscp.1988.7.2-3.260

Tiew, L. H., & Creedy, D. K. (2012). Development and preliminary validation of a composite spiritual care-giving scale. *International Journal of Nursing Studies, 49*(6), 682–690. doi:10.1016/j.ijnurstu.2011.11.014

Timmins, F., & McSherry, W. (2012). Spirituality: The Holy Grail of contemporary nursing practice. *Journal of Nursing Management, 20*(8), 951–957. doi:10.1111/jonm.12038

Tuck, I. (2012). A critical review of a spirituality intervention. *Western Journal of Nursing, 34*(6), 712–735. doi:10.1177/0193945911433891

Tyler, I. D., & Raynor, J. E. (2006). Spirituality in the natural sciences and nursing: An interdisciplinary perspective. *The Association of Black Nurses' Faculty Journal, 17*(2), 63–66.

Unruh, A. M. (2007). Spirituality, religion, and pain. *Canadian Journal of Nursing Research, 39*(2), 66–86.

Upadhaya, R. C., & Kautz, D. D. (2012). God doesn't treat his children that way: How to care when faith interferes. *International Journal for Human Caring, 16*(4), 71–72.

Van Dover, L. J., & Bacon, J. M. (2001). Spiritual care in practice: A close-up view. *Nursing Forum, 36*(3), 18–28. doi:10.1111/j.1744-6198.2001.tb00245.x

van Leeuwen, R. R. (2008). *Towards nursing competencies in spiritual care* (Doctoral dissertation, University of Groningen). Retrieved from http://www.rug.nl/research/portal/publications/towards-nursing-competencies-in-spiritual-care(4e556c37-6639-4b36-9065-f37a63dbeb87).html van Leeuwen, R., Tiesinga, L. J., Middel, B., Post, D., & Jochemsen, H. (2008). The effectiveness of an educational programme for nursing students on developing competence in the provision of spiritual care. *Journal of Clinical Nursing, 17*(20), 2768–2781. doi:10.1111/j.1365-2702.2008.02366.x

van Leeuwen, R., Tiesinga, L. J., Middel, B., Post, D., & Jochemsen, H. (2009). The validity and reliability of an instrument to assess nursing competencies in spiritual care. *Journal of Clinical Nursing, 18*(20), 2857–2869. doi:10.1111/j.1365-2702.2008.02594.x

World Health Organization Quality of Life-Spirituality, Religiousness and Personal Beliefs Group. (2006). A cross-cultural study of spirituality, religion, and personal beliefs as components of quality of life. *Social Science & Medicine, 62*(6), 1486–1497. doi:10.1016/j.socscimed.2005.08.001

Wright, L. M. (2005). *Spirituality, suffering and illness: Ideas for healing.* Philadelphia, PA: F. A. Davis.

Wright, L. M., & Leahey, M. (2009). *Nurses and families: A guide to family assessment and intervention* (5th ed.). Philadelphia, PA: F. A. Davis.

Spiritual Assessment and Care in Various Clinical Contexts

7

Spirituality in Serious, Life-Threatening, and Chronic Illness

The general connections and associations between spirituality, religion, and illness were addressed in Chapter 2 (see section on Religion/Spirituality in Health and Illness). However, in this chapter, the focus is on a more specific examination of spirituality and religion in the context of serious or life-threatening illness, as well as chronic illness. Because they are common illnesses, several specific illnesses have been chosen for this discussion.

SERIOUS, LIFE-THREATENING ILLNESS AND SPIRITUALITY

Serious illness (an illness that can limit one's life and cause significant risk of death) can usually cause great emotional distress as well as reflection on existential questions pertaining to life and death (Molzahn et al., 2012). When faced with critical illness, a person can feel frightened, powerless, vulnerable, isolated, and alienated, and be in a state of panic as his or her world seems to crumble (Nussbaum, 2003). Serious illness can cause significant stress because personal roles can change, pain is experienced, symptoms can be severe, and death can potentially be hastened. Spiritual distress can be the result (Deal & Grassley, 2012). Stoll's comment, although somewhat dated, is still relevant today (Stoll, 1979):

> Crisis situations, whether they be loss, illness, or hospitalization, bring one
> face-to-face with the ultimate issues of life—the limitations of one's humanness,
> the loss of personal and environmental control, and the meaning of pain and
> suffering in the overall purpose of life. (p. 1575)

In a qualitative study focused on the stories of spirituality in people with serious illness, Molzahn and colleagues (2012) found that several themes emerged from their stories:

- Clients reflected on spirituality, religion, and personal beliefs during this time.
- Clients used spiritual and religious practices to cope with the situation.
- Finding meaning and purpose in the midst of illness was important to them.
- Clients were aware of transcendence.

Molzahn and colleagues conclude that people with serious illness can discuss, and are often willing to discuss, spirituality. This has important implications for nurses.

Johnson and colleagues (2011) examined the connection between two domains of spirituality/religion, which research confirmed to be important to the experience of some people with serious illness: past spiritual experiences (spiritual history) and current spiritual well-being (which includes beliefs about the role of faith in illness and meaning, purpose, and peace in life). In their study of clients with serious illness, they found that an increase in negative past religious experiences was associated with more symptoms of anxiety and depression. Moreover, greater spiritual well-being was associated with fewer such symptoms. Johnson and colleagues suggest that the search for meaning in the context of serious illness can bring to the surface struggles related to the past religious life, even if the clients do not presently consider themselves to be overtly religious. Johnson and colleagues conclude from their study that "the search for meaning, peace, and purpose in life and the role of faith in illness are important to the spiritual experience of many patients facing serious illness regardless of their specific diagnosis" (p. 755). This conclusion has been noted by others, namely deWit and Kumagai (2013), Dzul-Church, Cimino, Adler, Wong, and Anderson (2010), Hilbers, Haynes, and Kivikko (2010), Neuman (2011), and O'Brien (2011).

The search for meaning and purpose in serious illness, and the pain/suffering inherent in such illnesses, can cause people to reexamine and even challenge previously held spiritual and religious beliefs (O'Brien, 2011; Stoll, 1979; Vachon, 2008). Although such an introspective examination *can* lead to spiritual growth, it can also cause spiritual distress because clients may feel that their previously held beliefs no longer "fit" for them. For example, a client may believe that God will not give him or her more than he or she can bear. Yet, when faced with serious illness, the client may now feel overwhelmed by the illness at hand. Such confusion and uncertainty can be quite distressing and he or she may need assistance to work through the situation. Spiritual or religious beliefs can also come into play and cause distress in terms of the client's perspective concerning his or her illness. For example, if a client perceives the illness to be a consequence of sin or some wrongdoing and it is God's way of punishing him or her, then the client may feel guilty, which can lead to a spiritual crisis (Stoll, 1979).

Interviewing clients with serious illness, Frybeck and Reinert (1999) found that spirituality was perceived to be essential to their health and well-being. The participants in this study "viewed spirituality as a bridge between hopelessness and meaningfulness in life. Those who found meaning in their disease thought they had better quality of life now than they had before the diagnosis" (p. 13). This observation points to the spiritual growth that can occur in the midst of serious illness, as previously commented. Dombeck

(1996) writes about the intense uncertainty that can accompany serious illness, which can inspire people to reformulate their lives. Dombeck also comments on the resulting potential for change: " . . . spiritual disequilibrium sets into motion turbulent fluctuations that have the potential of altering the whole system . . . . Even small changes in the spiritual aspects of life seem to catalyze significant changes" (p. 45). O'Brien (2011) takes it a step further in stating: "Even though an acutely ill person may be facing a potentially life-threatening situation, the concept of spiritual health is not only possible, but may be the key factor in his or her coping successfully" (p. 172). She goes on to say: "An acutely ill person who is spiritually healthy can find comfort and strength in his or her spiritual or religious philosophy of life" (p. 173).

One factor that can lead to spiritual growth in the midst of serious illness is the power inherent within spiritual and religious coping strategies. Baldacchino, Borg, Muscat, and Sturgeon (2012) found in a sample of individuals with life-threatening illness that the individuals used both existential and religious coping strategies. Existential coping strategies included fostering relationships with others and also finding meaning and purpose. Religious coping strategies included prayer and having a relationship with God. Interestingly, Baldacchino and colleagues (2012) also found that if individuals positively appraised their illness, then outcomes included reevaluating their lives, searching for meaning, seeking God's help, and prioritizing relationships with others. If illness was negatively appraised, then uncertainty, insecurity, difficulty searching for meaning, and spiritual distress resulted.

Spiritual and religious beliefs can be otherwise helpful to clients. O'Brien (2011) maintains: "Religious or spiritual beliefs may . . . provide the person in pain with a vehicle for finding meaning in suffering, or for 'offering' the pain experience to God, in expiation for one's failings or the failings of others" (p. 188). Both spiritual beliefs and spiritual coping strategies have been found to not only assist in the development of meaning and purpose in serious illness, but also encourage, strengthen, provide hope, and enhance connection to others and God (McCord et al., 2004; Molzahn & Sheilds, 2008; Taylor, 2012).

Weiland (2010) supports the notion of spiritual care being relational in the context of critical illness and asserts that ignoring the spiritual dimension may be robbing clients of a powerful source of strength and hope. This is especially important when considering the vulnerability of the critically ill client. Like other authors discussed, Weiland sees spirituality not only as fostering a sense of hope and strength in clients, but also as contributing to clients' coping abilities, enabling them to transcend suffering and pain. Weiland also brings up an important point with respect to nursing practice when she discusses the fact that the suffering inherent in serious illness impacts not only clients but also their families and caregivers. Consequently, spiritual coping extends beyond clients to their families and caregivers. Other authors and researchers similarly point to the need to include family and caregivers in the spiritual care of seriously ill clients (e.g., Puchalski, 2004).

Various models have been utilized as a means of incorporating spirituality into the care of clients who have life-threatening illness. For example, Moorman (2010) writes about the use of Betty Neuman's (Neuman, 1995) theory to address spiritual and other needs in a young woman who experienced necrotizing fasciitis. Weiland (2010) discusses the use of Roy Adaptation Model (Roy & Andrews, 2009) to integrate spiritual care into the critical care unit, using a case study to illustrate the process (pp. 287–289). This model is highlighted by Weiland to be suitable because several of the model's major concepts are consistent with a focus on spirituality, for example, that life has meaning and purpose, and that the care of clients and families should be holistic and multidimensional. Smith (2006) advocates for the use of the American Association of Critical-Care Nurses Synergy Model for Patient Care (Kaplow, 2003) in nursing critically ill clients. In contrast to the first two models just described, the Synergy Model was developed as a framework specifically for acute care and critical care nursing. Reference to these resources for an in-depth discussion of each model and its applicability to clients with serious illnesses is recommended.

From this brief discussion, it can be seen that the nature of serious or life-threatening illness can be disruptive and distressing, with resulting spiritual issues and concerns. However, it can also be a time of spiritual growth.

Reflection 7.1

Reflect on the characteristics of acute illness and any connection to spirituality and religion. Do these connections correlate with your clinical experience in working with clients with serious illness? How can the aforementioned discussion and your reflection contribute to your nursing care of seriously ill clients and their families?

SPIRITUALITY AND EMERGENCY NURSING

The emergency room (ER) is one setting in which nurses can provide spiritual care for clients experiencing serious or life-threatening illness. In this setting, clients and their families can be quite vulnerable and anxious due to the urgency of medical issues experienced. In fact, O'Brien (2011) points out that spiritual care and spiritual support might be especially important in the ER setting when the admitting diagnosis is a life-threatening situation. However, the ER poses some interesting challenges with respect to incorporating spirituality into the care of clients. For example, the fast pace in an ER can create issues related to the available time required to focus on spirituality. The level of acuity of some clients can also be a factor, with the priority focus on medical management. The ER environment itself can be challenging in terms of providing any privacy to discuss spiritual issues or concerns.

McBrien, a nurse with considerable experience in ER nursing, has focused on spirituality in the ER setting. In fact, he credits his experience in the ER with stimulating his interest in spiritual care. McBrien observed that spiritual care *is* given in the ER context, in particular the generic spiritual care that is part of "good nursing care." He cites, as examples, active listening, use of touch, good interpersonal skills, and presence (McBrien, 2008, 2009). On the basis of this observation, McBrien conducted an exploratory study focusing on how Irish ER nurses provide spiritual care (McBrien, 2009). The study revealed that spiritual care was seen by these nurses as integral to their role. These nurses considered interpersonal communication skills to be important in providing spiritual care, as well as therapeutic touch, presence, and the use of intuition. The nurse–client relationship was seen as foundational to such care. Concerns expressed by the nurses included the limited time in the ER for connections, as well as feelings of fear, apprehension, and a sense of incompetence with respect to providing spiritual care. Religious care was deemed to be important for some clients, especially the need for clients to engage in religious practices such as prayer. Due to the time constraints and the chaotic environment that is often characteristic of the ER, the nurses felt that a spiritual care professional or chaplain was better placed to focus on the spiritual needs of clients and families (note that spiritual assessment would have to be completed for such a referral to occur). Providing comfort, being honest, listening to concerns, and providing reassurance were deemed to be important in fostering hope. In spite of the constraints of the ER setting to provide spiritual care, the nurses felt that their words and body language compensated for these constraints. The use of touch was also consistently highlighted as a means of responding to the whole person and as a means of conveying spiritual care. Furthermore, these nurses indicated that they derive positive personal outcomes from providing spiritual care, such as self-satisfaction and a sense of well-being. McBrien also conducted a literature review (1989–2006) of the provision of spiritual care by ER nurses (McBrien, 2010a). From this review, the following conclusions were made:

- The spiritual dimension intensifies when clients are faced with critical illness.

- The main priority in the ER is physical care, even with the recognition that holistic care is important. Given the discussion about the prevalence and importance of spiritual needs in acute illness, this finding is somewhat disconcerting.

- Nurses report a communication pattern of "popping in and out" instead of spending time connecting with clients and families. This finding is also disconcerting, considering the importance of the nurse–client relationship and communication skills in the provision of spiritual care.

- Barriers to spiritual care in the ER include problems in communicating with clients, fragmented care, and a focus on tasks and documentation.

McBrien (2010b) acknowledges that there are difficulties and barriers to identifying and addressing spiritual needs in the ER. Nevertheless, he believes that ER nurses have a role to play in health crisis situations in promoting spiritual transformation and transcendence in such situations. He states that "it has been empirically shown that caring and the provision of spiritual care is not only possible within the technological world of emergency nursing, but it can be positively enhanced by the mastery of the technological environment" (Locin, 1995; Little, 2000) (p. 768). McBrien also comments that "the culture of emergency nursing has become less personal, with an increasing emphasis on the technical aspects of care . . . a more holistic approach to care should be adopted which would entail training and education on spiritual care"(p. 772).

Ziel, Kautz, Marquette, and Greensboro (2009) concur with the earlier statement made by O'Brien (2011) (see section on Serious, Life-Threatening Illness and Spirituality), going so far as to say that the *highest* priority in the ER may be a client's spiritual needs. Ziel and colleagues illustrate this point by discussing a case study of a 70-year-old man who had multiple and serious issues as a result of a fall. He was transferred to an ER from another facility about 2 hours away, and, on arrival to the ER, was intubated and unresponsive. The chaplain at the referring facility contacted the ER nurse, who was told that the client was Roman Catholic, and had not been anointed before leaving the transferring facility. The client's family was quite concerned about this situation. The ER nurse, assessing the man's chances for survival, concluded that one of the most important interventions of the trauma team was to meet the client's and family's spiritual needs—that the client be anointed. While the man was being resuscitated, a Catholic chaplain joined the team, the man was anointed, and the family was informed. The news greatly relieved their distress. The conclusion drawn from this case was that, if faith issues are important to clients/families and death may be imminent, then addressing such issues as a priority is an important intervention that can bring comfort and hope to clients and families.

Reflection 7.2

Reflect on the characteristics of today's ER setting as discussed and perhaps as experienced in your own nursing practice. What are your ideas regarding how to achieve what O'Brien is advocating for in terms of providing spiritual care in the ER context? What would have to change, and who might be involved in creating this change? (Think broadly in reflecting on this question.)

Spirituality and Intensive Care Nursing

O'Brien (2011) discusses the centrality of attending to spirituality in the intensive care unit (ICU) setting, stressing the importance of spiritual assessment and spiritual care for the family as well as clients. As Holt-Ashley (2000) states, "In the critical care unit where patients and their families face an abundance of uncertainty and life-threatening problems, it seems appropriate to believe that their spiritual needs come into play fairly early in the hierarchy of needs" (p. 63). It is also essential to realize that clients can have spiritual experiences in a critical care setting. As one client, who was "unresponsive" during her stay in the ICU, said about her experience:

> I realized that my body was almost dead but my spirit was alive and well. I had no interest whatsoever in all the voices and activity that had surrounded me for these tense days. However, my spirit responded when something of spiritual significance was happening and I remember every detail of these experiences. (Bardanouve, 1994, p. 29)

Nussbaum (2003) identifies the critical care environment as being a place of vulnerability for clients due to the intensity of illness in this setting. She argues for a more humanistic approach to care in such a setting where technology can easily become prominent.

Such an approach should attend to all needs of clients and their families, including spiritual needs. Generic spiritual care activities such as listening and presence should also be characteristic of care in this setting.

Timmins and Kelly (2008) discuss the use of spiritual assessment in critical care. However, they question whether a qualitative approach to assessment is appropriate in this setting: an approach where the nurse converses with the client, asking open-ended and, perhaps, in-depth questions. Timmins and Kelly maintain that there is no spiritual assessment tool specifically focused on spiritual assessment in an ICU or coronary care unit (CCU) context, but say that spiritual assessment "might be a useful adjunct to care delivery in ICU/CCU area, particularly given the potential for patients to have spiritual experiences during their stay" (p. 129). Although the target of the assessment is the client, the assessment may be obtained from the family if the acuity level of the client is compromised. Of course, the spiritual needs of the client's family should also be assessed.

Nussbaum (2003) discusses care for the whole body as constituting spiritual care, which is in keeping with the use of interventions related to generic spiritual care as discussed earlier. In fact, Nussbaum maintains that compassion in the ICU is the quality that makes nurses professionals, rather than technicians. She includes a quote from Norman Cousins, who wrote a landmark book called *Anatomy of an Illness* after recovering from a life-threatening illness. Speaking of his experience with respect to technology and the need for compassion, Cousins stated:

> And there was the utter void created by the longing—ineradicable, unremitting, pervasive—for warmth of human contact. A warm smile and an outstretched hand were valued even above the offerings of modern science, but the latter were far more accessible than the former. I became convinced that nothing a hospital could provide in the way of technological marvels was as helpful as an atmosphere of compassion. (Cousins, 1979, p. 154)

Reflection 7.3

Reflect on the quote by Cousins. Do you agree with his appraisal of the health care system? What place does compassion play in your own nursing practice, particularly with critically ill clients and their families? What have you observed in terms of the impact on clients about nurses who are compassionate versus those who are not?

Specific spiritual care interventions discussed in Chapter 6 (see section on Spiritual Care Interventions) have also been identified as helpful in an ICU/CCU setting. For example, with the help of a music therapist, Heiderscheit, Chlan, and Donley (2011) instituted a music listening intervention in the care of critically ill clients receiving mechanical ventilation, as a way to manage anxiety associated with this stressful situation. Outcomes of the intervention indicate that anxiety decreased, and pleasure increased. Having a sense of control over the type of music and when it was played contributed to self-care agency. Lundberg and Kerdonfag (2010) conducted a study of Thai ICU nurses to identify spiritual care provided by these nurses. In addition to spiritual assessment, the nurses gave emotional support and comfort, communicated with clients/families, facilitated religious rituals and beliefs, and showed respect for clients and families. In the Thai study, spiritual care was largely of a generic nature.

Holt-Ashley (2000), a nurse manager, writes of the use of prayer and spirituality as "complementary therapy" in the ICU setting. As seen from her earlier quote in this section, Holt-Ashley sees spiritual needs coming to the forefront early in the hierarchy of needs due to the possibility of death. She maintains that anxiety of clients and families may be relieved by prayer. In her experience, many critically ill clients and their families elicit "prayer vigils" from their churches or spiritual leaders. However, she cautions that prayer for clients must be at their request or as a result of a spiritual assessment that confirms that prayer is important to the client/family. Prayer should never be forced on clients/families and should be discussed with them beforehand. If the client or family requests that a nurse pray with them, and the nurse does not feel comfortable doing so, then referral to a spiritual care professional/chaplain is warranted.

Holt-Ashley also discusses how nurses, themselves, use prayer to cope with the stresses of working in an ICU setting. Others have studied the place of spirituality in caring for oneself from the perspective of nurses who work in the ICU setting. For example, Campbell (2013) stresses the importance of nurses working in critical care attending to their own spiritual well-being in order to manage their stress. Moreover, Dezorzi and Crossetti (2008) found that nurses in their sample engaged in spiritual practices daily (e.g., connecting with nature, God, or a higher power, and prayer). Dezorzi and Crossetti also found that the nurses' work stimulated them to reflect on existential questions about life, and they sought meaning in caring for themselves, which, in turn, enabled them to better care for clients/families. Such findings are in keeping with the idea of spiritual care being a journey for the nurse as well as the client/family.

Reflection 7.4

Reflect on what has been said about the place of spirituality in the intensive care setting. To what aspects of the discussion can you relate from your own nursing practice? How has the discussion expanded your knowledge about including spirituality in critical care contexts?

SPIRITUAL CARE IN SERIOUS AND LIFE-THREATENING ILLNESS

Many aspects of spiritual care within the context of serious and life-threatening illness are similar to those in spiritual care generally. For example, assessment of a client's/family's spirituality, spiritual history, and spiritual well-being is critical. However, in the case of serious illness, the client may not be able—at least initially—to communicate aspects related to spirituality/spiritual concerns and issues. In this case, the family can speak on behalf of the client. Families can also have a powerful impact on the outcome of the client's experience and also on how he or she perceived his or her illness. Therefore, families need to be included in the care of the client and be allowed access to the client, who can benefit from being near loved ones (Callahan, 2003; Weiland, 2010).

Nurses will need to be comfortable in discussing a wide range of spiritual beliefs and practices with clients in keeping with the notion of spirituality being personally identified and experienced. Encouraging clients and families to reflect on their situation and increasing their awareness of spiritual/religious coping resources is warranted. Generic spiritual care is paramount, that is care focused on such activities as active listening, being empathetic, and being open and approachable. As Dombeck (1996) maintains, often in life-threatening illness the most consistent part of a client's experience is contact with a nurse who is present with the client 24 hours a day. This presence provides ample opportunity to assess clients'/families' spiritual needs and address their spiritual concerns. At times, specific spiritual or religious care interventions may also be needed, for example, the use of prayer or referring a client to a spiritual care professional or spiritual/religious leader.

Spiritual care has been addressed in relation to children with life-threatening illness. For example, Caldcira and Hall (2012) discuss issues related to spirituality in the neonatal ICU setting, stating that such a setting "is a place of intense emotions related to life and death and exploration of meaning where the health team are all constantly confronted by hope and suffering" (p. 1073). Caldeira and Hall argue for a nursing approach that pays attention to spirituality, including spiritual assessment and spiritual and religious support of parents/families. Foster, Whitehead, Maybee, and Cullens (2013) reviewed qualitative research from 1998 to 2011 that was focused on family-centered care in the context of pediatric critical care settings. Salient findings related to spirituality and spiritual care included the following:

- A variety of spiritual needs were identified as well as factors related to meeting those needs.

- Spiritual and religious practices were used to cope with the situation at hand, for example, prayer, rituals, and meditation.

- A crisis of faith could cause spiritual distress or, alternatively, lead to new meanings.

- Interventions such as memorials and hope-building interventions were helpful.

- Generic spiritual care interventions by health care professionals were helpful.

Reflection 7.5

In your experience working with clients who are experiencing serious/life-threatening illness, have you noted whether any of them have developed "positive meanings" in their illness? Compare such clients with those for whom the illness is associated with "negative meanings." What differences exist between these two groups of clients? How can you assist clients to develop "positive meanings?"

SPIRITUALITY AND CHRONIC ILLNESS

The World Health Organization (2002) defines chronic health conditions as "health problems that require ongoing management over a period of years or decades" (p. 11). Thus, the person who is experiencing a chronic health problem has to contend with the additional dimension of longevity of the problem. Long-term support is needed. This will have significant impact for the family of the affected person, who may be in a caregiving as well as a supportive role with the person. Self-esteem, self-worth, and self-concept are all usually impacted by a chronic health problem in some way or another; and at times, considerably so. Social relationships are usually impacted, including relationships within the family. The person's plans and dreams for the future are often altered, or may need to change entirely. Quality of life is affected and a constant reminder of one's mortality may be present. The course of a chronic health problem can be unpredictable. Symptoms associated with chronic illness can vary from mild to severe, and remissions and exacerbations of the problem are common. Preventing and managing medical crises, managing therapeutic regimes, and controlling symptoms are the norms. Stress is also common, both within the person with the chronic health problem and within the family. Chronic pain may also be present and at times the person may need to be hospitalized. Adjusting and adapting to a chronic health problem is difficult but essential to spiritual well-being (Hampton & Weinert, 2006; Landis, 1996; O'Brien, 2011; Stanhope, Lancaster, Jessup-Falcioni, & Viverais-Dresler, 2011).

A diagnosis of a chronic illness can bring about a crisis in a person's life in which disharmony of body, mind, and spirit occurs. Spiritual well-being can be compromised. If a person believes in and has a relationship with God or a higher power, this relationship can devolve into disharmony. Spiritual distress is not uncommon as disorganization and disruption occur. A search for meaning may be present and evident in a person's life. The chronic illness itself can become a spiritual encounter. If the normative spiritual need for hope is met, then this can provide the spiritual strength the client needs to face the disease (Narayanasamy, 1995). A perusal of the literature indicates that spiritual growth and enhanced spiritual well-being can occur as the chronically ill person examines his or her life values, beliefs, and hopes—and the person can emerge with a higher sense of spiritual well-being than was the case before the chronic health problem occurred. For example, as discussed earlier, spirituality is a known protective factor in the development of resilience. The positive adaptation and growth of resilience is a goal of care for the person with a chronic health problem, and nurses are in a unique position to help clients achieve this goal. The nurses may also be of assistance to any caregivers of persons with chronic health problems, as they, too, may exhibit spiritual needs and concerns.

O'Brien (2011) notes that spiritual needs can be manifested by a variety of symptoms in the person experiencing chronic health problems. O'Brien highlights as a priority that nurses support those with chronic health conditions and points out the need for creativity in meeting the spiritual needs of such a population. For example, if physical disabilities are present, and these may impact on the client's ability to participate in various spiritual or religious practices, then the nurse may have to resort to creative methodologies to allow the client to engage in such practices.

For those diagnosed with chronic illnesses, spirituality and religion have been noted to be significant resources for coping with the physical and mental stress present in such illnesses as well as managing other effects of the chronic illnesses (Bowes, Tamlyn, & Butler, 2001; Hampton & Weinert, 2006; Hermanns, Deal, & Haas, 2012; Naghi, Philip, Phan, Cleenewerck, & Schwarz, 2012; O'Brien, 2011; Vance, Struzick, & Raper, 2008).

O'Brien (2011) draws on the work of a number of researchers and states about spiritual/religious practices/beliefs plus their connection to chronic illness: "For many persons, living with chronic illness, transcendent belief and experience provide the impetus to live and to love in the midst of significant pain and suffering" (p. 196).

A number of positive biopsychosocial outcomes have been associated with spirituality in a variety of chronic health conditions (Vance et al., 2008). Examples of some specific chronic health problems include heart failure (Beery, Baas, Fowler, & Allen, 2002), rheumatoid arthritis (Potter & Zauszniewski, 2000), polio (Smith, 1995), bipolar disorder (Mitchell & Romans, 2003), cancer (Fehring, Miller, & Shaw, 1997), and diabetes (Landis, 1996). The outcomes associated with spirituality/religion and some of these specific chronic health problems are discussed later in this chapter.

There are specific spiritual and religious beliefs and practices that have been noted to be useful to people to help them cope with a chronic health problem. For example, Hampton and Weinert (2006) found in their study of women experiencing a variety of chronic health problems that almost all of the women relied on faith to deal with their illnesses. Prayer, sharing and relying on God or a higher power, and reading the Bible and other sacred writings were all activities found to be helpful to these women. Spiritual connection provided the women with a sense of transcendence and was helpful in assisting them to find meaning in their lives. Narayanasamy (1995) found that, for those experiencing chronic illness, prayer was important in providing a number of positive outcomes: comfort, a sense of relief, a sense of well-being, confidence, strength, help, guidance, and a sense of "being lifted." In a later study, Narayanasamy (2002) found that not only prayer but also connection to others was significant to the healing process in chronically ill clients. Bonadonna (2003) identified meditation as a practice that positively impacts on the experience of chronic illness—and particularly in terms of the psychological and physiological symptoms associated with such illnesses.

Many clients with chronic health problems are involved in some kind of rehabilitative therapy. Reig, Mason, and Preston (2006) maintain that clients undergoing rehabilitation have significant spiritual needs that are related to their conditions and for which intervention is appropriate. Faith is seen by Reig and colleagues as a resource for strengthening beliefs and hope during rehabilitation. Feelings associated with the loss accompanying disability may stimulate clients to reflect on spirituality, question their spiritual beliefs, and also turn to their faith as a resource. Struggling with meaning can occur as the client tries to integrate the old self into the new self. Through the use of the nursing process, Reig and colleagues illustrate how to address spirituality with clients in rehabilitation.

Reflection 7.6

Reflect on the issues that persons with chronic health problems can experience. Have you seen evidence of such issues in yourself if you have a chronic health condition, or in others who have chronic health problems? What has been the impact of spirituality on your own chronic health problem or another person's chronic health problem? What was helpful/not helpful to you or the other person in terms of having spiritual needs met and why/why not?

There are far too many serious/life-threatening and chronic illnesses to address them all in this chapter. The following discussion about some selected common illnesses illustrates and confirms much of what has been said generally about the connection between spirituality and serious/life-threatening illnesses and chronic illnesses/health problems. Remember also that many illnesses can be serious, life-threatening, and/or chronic, depending on how they present in any given person.

SPIRITUALITY AND CANCER

Oncology is one specialty area that acknowledges spirituality as an important factor in providing care to clients (Delgado, 2007; Grant, 2004). In fact, Nixon, Narayanasamy, and Penny (2013) assert that spiritual care continues to grow in this area of practice.

Cancer can be both a life-threatening illness and a chronic illness. If it is a chronic condition, then attention to the spiritual dimension can help the client cope with significant adjustments and enhance quality of life. If a person with chronic cancer experiences spiritual distress, then the spiritual need for hope can be explored, which can, in turn, be helpful in the person's search for meaning in the illness and in life itself. Strengthening connection to self, others, nature, and the transcendent can enhance spiritual well-being. The cancer experience can be integrated and interpreted in new ways over time, which may improve self-esteem and spiritual connection (Doka, 2009; Stewart, 2014). As Stewart (2014) states:

> The cancer continuum is riddled with crises and spiritual resources are often an essential aspect of healthy coping. A useful way to approach spirituality is to view it as another relationship, good or bad, simple or complex, in the patient's life. Affirming the relevance of exploring spirituality with patients promotes a comprehensive and patient-centered model of care that considers the whole person. This is applicable whether a patient identifies as spiritual, religious, atheist or agnostic. The [nurse] will be able to better assist people with chronic cancer adjust to and make sense of their illness experience as it is perceived through their unique frameworks of understanding. (pp. 60–61)

Cancer is a disease that is feared by many people, and a diagnosis of cancer can precipitate a spiritual crisis as clients ponder their own mortality. Being diagnosed with cancer can cause spiritual disequilibrium as well, not only because it can be a life-threatening illness, but also because, at least for a while, it can disrupt a person's functioning and sense of coherence. Challenges to a client's faith and spiritual/religious beliefs may also occur. However, a diagnosis of cancer has been shown to cause clients to focus increasingly on religion and spirituality, especially as their illness becomes more acute. Searching for meaning is also common. Spirituality and spiritual well-being are often associated with quality of life in persons with cancer. Spiritual well-being is also known to be a protective factor against depression and despair, which can be associated with cancer, especially when death is imminent (Brady, Peterman, Fitchett, Mo, & Cella, 1999; Burkhart, Schmidt, & Hogan, 2011; Flannelly, Flannelly, & Weaver, 2002; McClain, Rosenfeld, & Breitbart, 2003; Miller et al., 2012; Swinton, Bain, Ingram, & Heys, 2011; Vachon, 2008).

Various types of cancer have been studied in terms of their relationship with spirituality, for example, ovarian cancer (Ferrell, Smith, Juarez, & Melancon, 2003), gynecologic cancer (Lopez, McCaffrey, Griffin, & Fitzpatrick, 2009), and breast cancer.

Breast cancer, the most common cancer for women worldwide (Swinton et al., 2011), has frequently been a focus for studies on spirituality in cancers that affect women. For example, it has been noted that, for breast cancer survivors, their spiritual worldview impacts how the rest of their lives are viewed. For survivors who believe in God, psychological well-being, distress levels, and use of coping strategies are impacted by how God is viewed (e.g., engaged or angry; Ano & Vasconcelles, 2005; Ferrell, Paice, & Koczywas, 2008; McCabe & Jacobs, 2008; Schreiber, 2011, 2012). Living a meaningful life and feeling connected to a higher power have also been found to buffer stress in breast cancer survivors (Bauer-Wu & Farran, 2005). Religious practices, in particular prayer, have been noted to facilitate acceptance of body image and improve some aspects of quality of life (Paiva et al., 2013). Enhanced spiritual awareness can also occur (Coward, 1997; Taylor, 2000).

A study by Kristeller, Sheets, Johnson, and Frank (2011) found in clients adjusting to cancer that those with the highest levels of positive religious involvement and spiritual well-being experienced a good adjustment to cancer. Even if clients had low religious involvement, those who still had a moderately high sense of meaning and peace also tended to experience a good adjustment to cancer. Kristeller and colleagues stress the importance of health care professionals exploring religious and spiritual resources with cancer clients as well as exploring their spiritual or religious concerns.

The interrelations of cancer and spirituality have been studied from a variety of perspectives—clients, their families/caregivers, and nurses. Some examples of salient findings related to spirituality and cancer from these perspectives illuminate the importance of spirituality to cancer care.

Nurses' Perspectives

Bahrami (2011) found that oncology nurses in Australia identified spirituality as one factor contributing to quality of life for clients with cancer. In fact, spirituality was seen by these nurses as a "pervasive aspect of patients' lives" (p. 78). Findings from this study also indicated that the need for spiritual connection may develop to a deep level for clients who are living with cancer. In a study by Nixon and colleagues (2013), nurses identified the spiritual needs of neurooncology clients to be the need to discuss spiritual concerns, religious-oriented needs, and emotional needs. The spiritual needs of family members included: support in the midst of end-of-life decisions; emotional needs related to their experience with a relative who has cancer; exploring the meaning of life; and the need to talk about their experiences. Strategies to meet the needs of both clients and family members included generic spiritual activities and religious support.

Corso (2012) identified the nurse's awareness of his or her personal woundedness and an understanding of the connection between body, mind, and spirit (self-care) to contribute to the level of compassion in oncology nurses. This awareness also insulated the nurses against the stressors inherent in this type of nursing practice.

Clients'/Family Caregivers' Perspectives

Watts (2009) found that cancer survivors identified relationships as providing meaning in their lives. Engaging in community activities also affirmed their self-worth and sense of purpose. Watts concluded that data from her study suggested:

[O]ne important component of spirituality for those living with cancer, is the maintenance of a consistent or congruent "self". For a majority of participants, this congruence involved the maintenance of an active *social* as well as an *individual* self, with secular and humanistic spiritualties common amongst them. (p. 91)

The participants in this study found increasing stress associated with engaging in civic activities due to physical discomfort and fatigue. However, Watts concluded: "Community participation seemed to mediate the effects of the ontological transition from wellness to illness acting as a spiritual buffer against the realities presented by an uncertain cancer trajectory" (p. 92).

Prayer has been the topic of interest in cancer care due to the widespread use of prayer as a spiritual practice by those with cancer. For example, Balboni and colleagues (2011) found that a majority of the sample of oncology clients, oncology nurses, and oncology physicians in their study identified prayer as an important spiritual intervention, at least occasionally. Prayer that was patient initiated, and between the patient and the practitioner, was particularly helpful. The majority of clients also indicated that a practitioner praying with them would be spiritually supportive. It is important that patient–practitioner prayer be specific to each client, which, in turn, emphasizes the need for careful assessment. Perez and colleagues (2011) also found that prayer was helpful, and that specific types of prayer had varying impact on depressive symptoms in clients with cancer. Prayers of adoration, reception, and thanksgiving and for the well-being of others were significantly related to lower depressive symptoms. Furthermore, depressive symptoms may be reduced for those who pray with thanksgiving because ruminative self-focus is decreased and positive emotions are at play. In a similar fashion, the social support perceived to be present when clients with cancer pray for others resulted in less negative effects. Perez and colleagues suggest that nurses and other care providers encourage the use of prayers that are positively associated with well-being, if prayer is congruent with the client's worldview.

Several resources in the nursing literature focus on not only the spirituality of clients but also the spirituality of their family caregivers. For example, Taylor (2006) conducted a study of the spiritual needs of clients with cancer as well as the spiritual needs of their family caregivers. She found the most important spiritual needs were: keeping a positive perspective; loving others; finding meaning; and understanding God or relating to God. The spiritual needs of clients and family caregivers were similar. The strain of the illness (at least incurable illness) was found to be linked to an increase in the importance of spiritual needs. An important finding was that the greater the importance of spiritual needs to the client, the greater the desire for spiritual care from nurses. Religious clients also desired spiritual care from nurses.

In a sample of clients with cancer (and their family caregivers), Taylor and Mamier (2005) found that expectations of the clients and caregivers varied widely in terms of nurses providing spiritual care; although the desire for spiritual care was similar for both groups. The spiritual care therapeutics most desired by participants in this study were those that allowed for independent personal spiritual development, for example, informing clients about spiritual resources. Humor was also important to the participants. In general, less intimate, commonly used, and not overtly religious therapeutics were most desired (other than the religious practices of prayer). As found in other studies, Taylor and Mamier stressed the importance of individual assessment of clients and family caregivers prior to providing spiritual care.

Ferrell and Baird (2012), recognizing the importance of family caregivers of clients with cancer, conclude from a review of the literature on spiritual care of family caregivers that there is ample evidence for the need of such care. Ferrell and Baird state the following about the spiritual needs identified in the literature for family caregivers:

[T]here are . . . profound spiritual needs as caregivers wrestle with their faith, their ability to believe in a God or higher being who could allow cancer in a loved one, the experience of witnessing pain and suffering, and the struggle to maintain hope and faith when life now includes one of the most dreaded threats to life, a cancer diagnosis. (pp. 256–257)

Ferrell and Baird also emphasize the importance of spiritual assessment of family caregivers and identify core spiritual interventions that nurses can use with such caregivers: presence; deep listening; "bearing witness" and accompanying or being with the persons in their journey; and compassion that is action oriented. Ferrell and Baird also point out the fact that caregiving can also be a time for growth for caregivers, providing meaning for them.

Taylor (2005) explored the efficacy of three spiritual complementary therapies often used by clients with cancer: spiritual healing, prayer, and meditation. Taylor concluded from the research that all three therapies can result in positive outcomes for clients, for example, decreasing anxiety, depression, pain, and stress. Positive emotions were also created from the use of such therapeutics. Taylor stresses the importance of assessing what spiritual activities are used by clients and facilitating those that are helpful to them. She also stresses the importance of exploring any distress related to a perceived lack of positive outcomes from engaging in such activities.

In a sample of men with prostate cancer, Walton and Sullivan (2004) found that these men saw spirituality as permeating all aspects of their cancer experience and of their lives. Spirituality was seen as transcending all other domains of personhood. The importance of prayer in providing comfort, strength, and assurance during their experience was verbalized. Receiving support from family, friends, and the community also caused the men to feel loved and cared for. Using spirituality to cope with cancer helped the men face it, choose treatment modalities, and trust themselves and God. Living day by day, finding meaning, and reconnecting to loved ones were also seen as important aspects.

In keeping with the previous comments about a cancer experience involving spiritual growth, Vachon (2008) maintains that some cancer survivors find that their disease results in spiritual transformation and a new meaning, both of which contribute to their sense of well-being. Therefore, Vachon advocates for nurses to encourage cancer survivors to engage in activities that may promote meaning and spirituality, and also to discuss the meaning of their illness.

There are many more resources in the literature focusing on specific aspects of spirituality in cancer: for example, the process of spiritual development (Halstead & Hull, 2001); the positive outcomes of hematological malignancies from a spiritual perspective (McGrath, 2004); and the need for and process of forgiveness (Mickley & Cowles, 2001). How nurses can attend to spirituality in the care of clients with cancer and their families is also a focus in the literature. Examples include the spiritual assessment of clients with cancer (Stewart, 2014) and helping clients find new meaning at various turning points in the cancer trajectory (Coward, 1997). Much has also been written about spirituality and the cancer experience for children and their families, for example, Brody and Simmons (2007) who identified faith communities and faith in God as a source of resilience in fathers of children with cancer. Referencing these sources provides further information.

Reflection 7.7

- Reflect on the various responses that you have witnessed in clients with cancer. What positive responses have you witnessed and to what do you attribute such responses? What negative responses have you witnessed, and again, to what do you attribute these responses?
- Review the findings of studies on spirituality and cancer as just presented. Itemize these findings. Which "ring true" in terms of your clinical experience with clients and their families? How can the findings inform your clinical practice?

SPIRITUALITY AND CARDIAC DISEASE

Cardiac disease is a common health problem in Western society today. Cardiac disease has physical, psychological, social, economic, and spiritual impacts on individuals affected and their families. It can be a serious and life-threatening illness, and/or it can be a chronic condition.

Villagomeza (2006) reviewed the research from 1991 to 2004 on the role of spirituality in cardiac illness. Examples of significant findings from this review include the following:

- Clients found prayer to be a helpful practice.

- Spirituality was influential in recovering from and adapting to cardiac disease, providing such outcomes as courage, inner strength, and enhanced coping.

- Spirituality/religiosity may lower blood pressure (directly or indirectly).

- High spiritual well-being scores resulted in the greatest amount of regression of coronary obstruction, whereas low spiritual well-being scores were associated with the most progression of coronary obstruction.

Villagomeza provides a summary of the studies analyzed, including their purpose, instruments used, and the outcomes (pp. 173–180). Based on the literature review, Villagomeza proposes a conceptual model of spirituality that includes seven key constructs (p. 184). Reference to the model is recommended.

Naghi and colleagues (2012) maintain that the suffering experienced by clients with chronic heart failure (and the suffering by their families) may lead them to question their faith in a higher power, which can be a significant spiritual struggle. They review the evidence that indicates that spirituality can enhance coping and contribute to quality of life in late and terminal stages of heart failure, offering peace, the ability to accept the situation, a sense of meaning, and a decrease in stress, symptom burden, and depression.

Focusing on a sample of clients in recovery from myocardial infarction, Walton (2002) found that their spirituality was nurtured by their relationship with God and by their connection with nature, friends, family, and community. The presence of family was noted to be especially calming for these clients during the acute stage—an important finding for nursing. The clients' spirituality was based on the development of their faith, their discovery of meaning and purpose in the midst of their illness, and by giving of themselves to others. Walton also found that the presence of nurses was integral to the decrease of fear in these clients, as well as in the fostering of hope.

A number of spirituality-focused interventions with positive results have been employed in the context of care of clients with cardiac disease. For example, Delaney and Barrere (2008) conducted a quasi-experimental study to assess the efficacy of a spirituality-based music/imagery intervention. The findings indicated that there was a positive relationship between the intervention and psychological outcomes, for example, less anxiety. Spiritual outcomes were also noted, such as an increase in focus on spirituality. The clients reported that the intervention calmed them and gave them a sense of relaxation and tranquility, all of which enabled them to better cope with their situations. They also reported that the intervention facilitated the process of "meaning making" as they found a deeper meaning in the words of the imagery script. Delaney and Barrere also assessed the impact of a spirituality-based ecospiritual meditation intervention for clients with cardiovascular disease (Delaney & Barrere, 2009). This intervention resulted in a heightened awareness of and connection to the environment, feelings of peace and solace, and a positive, transforming change within the clients' internal environments. Delaney and Barrere (2009) conclude that the clients' ecospirituality had been enhanced as a result of this intervention.

SPIRITUALITY AND HIV/AIDS

The connection between spirituality and HIV and AIDS has been extensively explored in the health care literature. Such literature points to the centrality of spirituality in clients with HIV infection. For example, Pargament and colleagues (2004) concluded from a review of the literature on religion and coping in HIV-infected persons that there is empirical evidence that religion and spirituality are important to their health and well-being. Conversely, it has also been found that religion and spirituality can bring pain, suffering, and struggle to such persons because of the religious stigma that can be associated with HIV infection; and also because of the challenge the illness poses to one's basic worldview.

Spirituality has been noted to be of benefit in various contexts associated with HIV/AIDS. For example, Peltzer and Leenerts (2007) note that spirituality was particularly important to a group of women with HIV infection who had abuse histories. Spirituality helped them regain connectedness to themselves, thus empowering them to adopt self-care behaviors that promoted their health. Pargament and colleagues (2004) describe in detail an 8-week spiritual intervention for women with HIV infection (pp. 1202–1207), noting that this intervention provided a means for spiritual resources and struggles to be addressed. Vance and colleagues (2008) discuss the power of spirituality to assist people to deal with the challenges of aging with HIV infection, due to the positive impact of spirituality on biopsychosocial functioning in aging. Chaudoir and colleagues (2012) found that spiritual peace was a factor in counteracting the depression associated with the stigma of HIV/AIDS. Spiritual peace was described by these authors as "the degree to which spiritual beliefs provide a sense of peace and meaning . . . a specific resource that may be effective in coping with HIV stigma" (p. 2383). Haddad (2011) wrote a book focused on religion (and in particular African traditional religions) and its role in HIV infection. Although set in South Africa, Fray (2012) comments that the information in Haddad's book may be relevant beyond South Africa "because religion casts a wide net, shaping beliefs and cultural practices universally" (p. 271).

Various spiritual and religious practices/beliefs have been noted to be efficacious in those living with HIV infection. For example, Dalmida, Holstad, DiIorio, and Laderman (2011) found that spiritual beliefs and existential well-being were important to health-related quality of life in a group of African American women with HIV infection. Private religious practices, such as prayer, were commonly used by these women. Coleman and colleagues (2006) also found prayer was used to deal with various symptoms of HIV infection in an ethnically diverse sample of HIV-infected people. African Americans and Hispanics were found to be more likely to use prayer than other ethnic groups. Scarinci, Griffin, Grogoriu, and Fitzpatrick (2009) found that prayer, helping others, and listening to music were the three most frequently used spiritual practices of a group of women with HIV infection. Sowell and colleagues (2000) found in a study of women with HIV infection that, as spiritual activities increased (e.g., prayer, manifestations of spiritual beliefs), emotional distress decreased. As Slomka, Lim, Gripshover, and Daly (2013) state in reporting on their study of adults with HIV infection:

> A majority of participants attributed a large part of their health and ability to cope with challenges of living with HIV to religious and/or spiritual beliefs. Faith, prayer, and spirituality were seen as helping with physical and emotional healing, especially during an illness crisis. (p. 455)

SPIRITUALITY AND RENAL DISEASE

Mattison (2006) identifies the chronic nature of renal disease as important to consider in the care of clients as it demands that clients find ways to live with and to cope with the disease over time. Mattison identifies the spiritual struggles of those with renal disease to be powerlessness, a negative self-concept, hopelessness, meaninglessness, and isolation and loneliness. Mattison advocates for the inclusion of "transpersonal medicine" (p. 31) in the care of such clients, an approach "that incorporates a spiritual dimension and defines health in terms of balance and meaning" (p. 31). Mattison identifies spirituality as a factor that can enable people to be well despite their disease, providing capacity and potential for well-being. Spirituality-based practice encourages a client's internal experience to transform an external situation: "a way to rise above the challenges of renal disease and see it from a different perspective" (p. 31).

In a qualitative study by Walton (2002), clients on hemodialysis due to renal disease described spirituality as finding a balance of body, mind, and spirit in life. Walton used a balancing scale as a metaphor to portray this description of spirituality (p. 448). In the diagram of the balancing scale, spiritual concepts that clients identified as important to their spirituality included faith (beliefs, religion, and relationship to God); the presence of God, others, community, and nature; and receiving help and giving back to others. Walton provides quotes from participants in the study to not only illustrate these three spiritual concepts but also to illustrate phases of finding a balance.

In another qualitative study, Tanyi and Werver (2008) found that spirituality was extremely important to a sample of women dealing with end-stage renal disease and dialysis. Spirituality was characterized by these women as "an inner force that engendered insights and allowed them to question, understand, and learn from their illness" (p. 41). Spirituality provided these women with strength to endure and to accept the diagnosis, the treatment, themselves, and their lives. It also helped them face mortality, accept living day by day, buffer negative emotions, and allow more positive emotions to emerge, thus fostering coping.

Clients who are having dialysis form close relationships with their nurses over time. Therefore, these nurses are in a prime position to assess the spirituality of clients and to provide spiritual care. As alluded to in the discussion so far, there is an acknowledgment of the centrality of spirituality in the lives of people who are on dialysis as it is capable of helping them cope with their situation (Al-Arabi, 2006; Berman et al., 2004; Deal & Grassley, 2012; Tanyi, Werner, Recine, & Sperstad, 2006). Deal and Grassley (2012) maintain that nephrology nurses can also encounter clients' anger, which is sometimes present in the dialysis process, and nurses may need to offer assistance to clients in dealing with this anger. Deal and Grassley found that spiritual care offered by the nephrology nurses in her study was intricately connected to generic spiritual care.

SPIRITUALITY AND PARKINSON'S DISEASE (PD)

Perusal of the health care literature yields a number of works that describe disease-related alterations in religiosity in those with Parkinson's disease (PD), for example, Butler, McNamara, and Durso (2010a, 2010b) and Butler, McNamara, Ghofrani, and Durso (2011). Such articles discuss changes in religiosity that are attributed primarily to prefrontal neuropsychological functioning in clients with PD. However, the discussion in this section relates primarily to the experiences of those with PD and how they are connected to spirituality.

Stanley-Hermanns and Engebretson (2010) conducted a study that had as its aim to understand the experience of people with PD. The metaphor "sailing the seas in the eye of the storm" (p. 350) was used to conceptualize the journey of those living with PD. Stanley-Hermanns and Engebretson say that this metaphor

> . . . reflects a sense of adventure, challenge, and unpredictability that is similar to how persons with PD described their illness experience while performing daily negotiations in the management of PD. Parkinson's disease requires participants to embark on a one-way journey into the stormy seas. The storm, PD, an unpredictable, fluctuating and complicated voyage provides those affected with no chart or clear course. Their voyage remains stormy; a one-way journey with no return. (p. 351)

Participants in the study by Stanley-Hermanns and Engebretson described the need to construct meaning in the illness experience, a process that was often facilitated by their spiritual faith. They also described making meaning of the present self in terms of reconstructing the self, and also making meaning in the individual sense of personhood. Some participants described surrendering to God or a higher power, which enabled them to release aspects of the former self, such as dreams, expectations, and plans. All participants indicated that they had a strong faith in God. Elaborating on the findings in this study, Hermanns (2011) states:

> For most, their active expression of their spiritual faith in God was identified as the process by which they came to terms with PD. It was as if the participants recognized their physical, psychological, and spiritual limitations and allowed God to take control of the helm. More specifically, their inner strength, perseverance, and strong faith were seen as an impetus toward acknowledging that they will never be the persons they were, persons without PD . . . . In their quest to discover a deeper meaning of self, many relied on their spiritual faith. (p. 81)

Bingham and Habermann (2006) also found that belief and faith helped the participants with PD in their study deal with the disease. Believing that there was meaning and purpose in the disease also facilitated acceptance of the consequences of the disease. Prayer, connecting with others, and adopting a sense of gratitude and hope were also important in managing the disease. These findings were also true with respect to their family members. Hope, an identified spiritual need, has also been found by others to be important to those living with PD in terms of it promoting health and spiritual growth and in terms of interpersonal relationships (Fowler, 1997).

Giaquinto, Bruti, Dall'Armi, and Spiridigliozzi (2010) concluded from a study of clients with PD that they maintained their faith in spite of the severity of the disease. This finding suggests that religious coping can be a way for those with PD to cope with their illness over the long term.

Hermanns and colleagues (2012) found in a review of research studies of clients with PD that aspects of spiritual experience in the form of music and complementary mind–body interventions such as yoga were used to help clients with PD. Meaning making was also identified as an important aspect. Based on the review, Hermanns and colleagues conclude that there is a gap in the scientific literature on spiritual approaches to care of clients with PD. They identified the need for further research in this area given the complex, multifaceted impact of PD in a person's life.

In addition to the illnesses just described, spirituality has been connected to and discussed in relation to a variety of other illnesses. For example:

- Lin, Gau, Lin, and Lin (2011) reviewed the research literature exploring spiritual well-being in people with rheumatoid arthritis.

- Anema, Johnson, Zeller, Fogg, and Zetterlund (2009) explored spiritual well-being in a sample of people with fibromyalgia syndrome.

- Pierce, Steiner, Havens, and Tormoehlen (2008) explored spirituality as expressed by adult caregivers of stroke survivors.

- Giaquinto, Spiridigliozzi, and Caracciolo (2007) focused on the stroke survivors themselves, examining the relationship between spirituality and depression in these people.

- Pollock and Sands (1997) focused on meaning in suffering for those with multiple sclerosis.

- Landis (1996), Green (2004), and Polzer (2007) all focused on spirituality and diabetes. Landis explored spiritual well-being as a resource for dealing with diabetes. Green focused on the importance of considering clients' religious backgrounds in diabetic education. Polzer explored the importance of the spirituality/religiosity of the health care provider to a sample of African Americans with diabetes. Referencing these resources provides further elaboration of their findings.

Reflection 7.8

Reflect on the discussion of spirituality in the illnesses described in this chapter. How can this discussion encourage you to be more intentional about incorporating spirituality into your nursing practice? What further information might you need?

This chapter has focused on the place of spirituality in serious, life-threatening illness as well as in chronic illness. As can be surmised from the discussion, spirituality and religion are intricately connected to such illnesses. Given the potential struggles and issues connected with spirituality or religion that those with such illnesses can encounter, as well as the fact that spirituality and religion are resources to deal with the illnesses, nurses need to be vigilant in assessing clients' spirituality and in providing spiritual care. Consulting the following case studies and reflecting on the directives given with respect to these cases provide an opportunity to further explore how you might include the spiritual dimension of care in those with serious/life-threatening illness and chronic illness.

Taking It Further

1. Read the case study of Terry in Highfield (1997, pp. 239–240, including Tables 2 and 3).

   a. Review the stages of Terry's journey with cancer as recorded in the case study. Picture the descriptors in each stage as a statement from Terry to you as a nurse. Use what you know about spiritual assessment and spiritual conversations, and for each statement, formulate a response to Terry (in actual words).

   b. What insights did you gain from this exercise?

   c. Share your statements with a colleague/peer and together, appraise the value of each statement in terms of its potential helpfulness to Terry.

2. Read the five case studies in Carson (2008, pp. 126–127).

   a. What spiritual needs might be identified in each of the case studies and what information is given to support each of the spiritual needs identified?

   b. Which of these case studies would you find most challenging; and why?

    c. What client statements would you want to explore further to conduct a more thorough assessment? How would you proceed from the statements given? What possible responses might you make to each statement to encourage further disclosure from the clients?

    d. What spiritual care interventions might you hypothesize that could be beneficial to each client?

3. Model, borderline, and related and contrary case studies of spiritual distress in adult cancer clients are provided in Villagomeza (2005, p. 289; pp. 291–292).

    a. Read each case study, but before reading the author's commentary on each, identify cues to spiritual distress (or lack thereof) as presented in the case study using the defining attributes and empirical referents of spiritual distress and the antecedents of spiritual distress in persons with cancer as presented by Villagomeza (p. 290). Compare the cues that you identify with those of the author.

    b. If you were the nurse caring for each of these clients, what interventions might you employ and why?

    c. What feelings were evoked within you as you were reading each of the case studies? Reflect on the possible reasons for your feelings. Is there some "work" that you need to do in terms of future provision of spiritual care with clients?

4. Read the case studies of Mr. Jones, a man who is in the ICU with a myocardial infarction, in Kim-Godwin (2013, p. 212).

    a. Answer the questions posed in the article at the end of the case study.

    b. How would you facilitate the expression of Mr. Jones's feelings regarding his perception that he will die?

5. Read the case study of John, who suffered multiple injuries from a fall and was admitted to the ER, in Zeil and Kautz (2009, p. 50).

    a. What information in the case study points to spiritual/religious needs?

    b. Research information about the practice of anointing the sick/dying in the Roman Catholic faith. Why was this so important to the family?

    c. If you were Ruth, the admitting nurse in the emergency room, how might you have felt in this situation; and why?

    d. How can insights from this case study inform your nursing practice?

6. Read the case study of Laura Miller, who experienced necrotizing fasciitis, in Moorman (2010, pp. 18–19; pp. 22–24).

    a. What indication(s) of spiritual needs is found in this case study?

    b. Read Moorman's personal philosophy as a Christian nurse (p. 20). Can you relate to any of the perspectives that she holds; and if so, which aspect(s)?

    c. How was Moorman's personal philosophy operationalized in her care of Laura Miller?

    d. Write a statement of your own personal spiritual philosophy. How does your philosophy impact your care of clients?

7. Read the case study of Jane, a woman who is HIV positive, in Martsolf and Mickley (1998, p. 295).

    a. What information is in the case study that is linked to the meaning of this disease for Jane and her husband, including for their relationship? How might you explore this aspect of spirituality further with Jane (and perhaps her husband also)? What benefit might there be from such an exploration?

    b. If you were to make a diagnosis of spiritual distress in this situation, what data would support your diagnosis?

    c. How is Jane's interrelationship with her work/family/environment impacted by being HIV positive? How is the spiritual dimension impacted?

8. Read the case study of Mr. Ahmad, a Muslim client on a cardiology unit, in Lawrence and Rozmus (2001, pp. 228–233).

    a. What do you know of the Muslim religion? Research information about this religion if you are not aware of its basic tenets and also of the beliefs, values, and practices that might impact health and illness.

    b. If you were encountering Mr. Ahmad in your nursing practice, how would you go about learning about his faith? What resources might be available to you?

    c. As a nurse, how would you feel about the constant presence of Mr. Ahmad's family at his bedside? What is your understanding of why this is so, from both a cultural and perhaps a religious practice? How might this impact your nursing care of Mr. Ahmad?

    d. What aspects of Mr. Ahmad's faith were operant in his care (as discussed in the case study)? Who needed to be involved to ensure that these aspects were incorporated into his nursing care?

    e. In the case study, it states that Mr. Ahmad believed that his illness was God's will. What are the implications of such a belief for spiritual care? What are the implications, in particular, in terms of the need to develop meaning in the illness?

    f. What insights have you gained from this case study about the care of Muslim clients? What insights have you gained about your own education with respect to the religious care of clients? Where will you proceed from here in this regard?

9. Read the case study of a woman, Judy, who was hospitalized for a surgical procedure, in Dameron (2012, p. 201).

a. How does this case study illustrate the use of presence as a nursing intervention? What specific actions does the nurse employ that illustrates being present with the client?

b. What actions by the nurse indicate that spiritual care is being provided to Judy?

c. Review various definitions of the concept of "presence" in the nursing literature. What aspects of presence from your research are present in this case study?

10. Read the three case studies in Mayer (1992, pp. 37–42): Angela, a client who is having a liver transplant; John, a client with cancer and his wife, Jean, who has severe arthritis/disabilities; and Ruth, who had a liver transplant that has failed.

a. What evidence of spiritual needs is found in each of the case studies? How might you address each?

b. What place, if any, does religion play in each case study?

c. How do these case studies emphasize the importance of corporate dimensions of spiritual care, that is, aspects related to the hospital setting and staff interactions?

d. How was a "controlling, hierarchical model" (p. 47) of care illustrated in the case studies? What is the impact of such a model on spiritual care?

e. What evidence is there of a problem-solving approach to care in the case studies? How might such an approach impact spiritual care?

f. How do these case studies illustrate the importance of viewing spiritual care as more than "a parallel or subordinate adjunct to physical care" (p. 48)?

11. Read the two case studies in Laukhuf and Werner (1998) of Greg, a client with a subarachnoid hemorrhage; and Les, a client with a metastatic brain tumor.

a. What spiritual care was offered in each of the case studies? How was the spiritual care tailored to each client?

b. In the case of Les, how did the nurse broach the topic of spirituality? What needs/issues/strengths arose from the nurse's initial inquiry?

c. What did Les's wife say about the place of prayer in their lives? Why is it important to ask clients not only if they pray, but also what the outcomes of their prayers might be?

d. How does Les's statement that "it was the little things" (speaking of spiritual care) impact on how you might relate to clients in the future, especially in terms of spiritual care?

e. How do nurses benefit from engagement in spiritual care with clients?

12. Read the three case studies in Sawatzky and Pesut (2005): Nurse A used to illustrate the importance of transcendent awareness in nurses as an antecedent to spiritual care; Nurse B used to illustrate the willingness needed by nurses to

overcome fears and anxieties about engaging in spiritual care; and Mrs. M. used to illustrate the appropriate sharing of the nurse's own spiritual beliefs with clients.

For Nurse A:

    a. Can you identify with Nurse A in terms of your own spiritual positioning?

    b. How does Nurse A's spiritual positioning impact her sensitivity to the client?

    c. Appraise the appropriateness of prayer as a spiritual intervention in this case study.

    d. What were the outcomes of the spiritual care provided for both the nurse and the client?

For Nurse B:

    a. Can you identify with Nurse B in terms of encountering clients with spiritual/religious beliefs that are different from your own?

    b. If you were Nurse B and you engaged in dialogue with the client, then how might you initiate a conversation about spirituality with this client?

    c. How do the differing views of spirituality/religion of the nurse and client impact spiritual care?

For Mrs. M:

    a. Have you encountered clients with similar fears as Mrs. M in your nursing practice? How does such a situation impact you?

    b. Appraise the appropriateness of the nurse sharing her own spiritual beliefs with the client.

    c. What guidelines are necessary to follow in terms of nurses sharing their own spiritual beliefs with clients?

REFERENCES

Al-Arabi, S. (2006). Quality of life: Subjective descriptions of challenges to patients with end stage renal disease. *Nephrology Nursing Journal, 33*(3), 285–292.

Anema, C., Johnson, M., Zeller, J. M., Fogg, L., & Zetterlund, J. (2009). Spiritual well-being in individuals with fibromyalgia syndrome: Relationships with symptom pattern variability, uncertainty, and psychosocial adaptation. *Research and Theory for Nursing Practice: An International Journal, 23*(1), 8–22. doi:10.1891/1541-6577.23.1.8

Ano, G. G., & Vasconcelles, E. B. (2005). Religious coping and psychological adjustment to stress: A meta-analysis. *Journal of Clinical Psychology, 61*(4), 461–480. doi:10.1002/jclp.20049

Bahrami, M. (2011). Meanings and aspects of quality of life for cancer patients: A descriptive exploratory qualitative study. *Contemporary Nurse, 39*(1), 75–84. doi:10.5172/conu.2011.39.1.75

Balboni, M. J., Babar, A., Dillinger, J., Phelps, A. C., George, E., Block, S. D., . . . Balboni, T. A. (2011). "It depends": Viewpoints of patients, physicians, and nurses on patient-practitioner prayer in the setting of advanced cancer. *Journal of Pain and Symptom Management, 41*(5), 836–847. doi:10.1016/j.jpainsymman.2010.07.008

Baldacchino, D. R., Borg, J., Muscat, C., & Sturgeon, C. (2012). Psychology and theology meet: Illness appraisal and spiritual coping. *Western Journal of Nursing Research, 34*(6), 818–847. doi:10 .1177/0193945912441265

Bardanouve, V. E. (1994). Spiritual ministry in the ICU. *Journal of Christian Nursing, 11*(4), 28–29.

Bauer-Wu, S., & Farran, C. J. (2005). Meaning in life and psycho-spiritual functioning: A comparison of breast cancer survivors and healthy women. *Journal of Holistic Nursing, 23*(2), 172–190. doi:10.1177/0898010105275927

Beery, T. A., Baas, L. S., Fowler, C., & Allen, G. (2002). Spirituality in persons with heart failure. *Journal of Holistic Nursing, 20*(1), 5–25. doi:10.1177/089801010202000102

Berman, E., Merz, J. F., Rudnick, M., Snyder, R. W., Rogers, K. K., Lee, J., . . . Lipschutz, J. H. (2004). Religiosity in a hemodialysis population and its relationship to satisfaction with medical care, satisfaction with life, and adherence. *American Journal of Kidney Disease, 44*(3), 488–497. doi:10.1053/j .ajkd.2004.05.027

Bingham, V., & Habermann, B. (2006). The influence of spirituality on family management of Parkinson's disease. *Journal of Neuroscience Nursing, 38*(6), 422–427.

Bonadonna, R. (2003). Meditation's impact on chronic illness. *Holistic Nursing Practice, 17*(6), 309–319. doi:10.1097/00004650-200311000-00006

Bowes, D. E., Tamlyn, D., & Butler, L. J. (2001). Women living with ovarian cancer: Dealing with an early death. *Health Care Women International, 23*(2), 135–148. doi:10.1080/0739933 02753429013

Brady, M. J., Peterman, A. H., Fitchett, G., Mo, M., & Cella, D. (1999). A case for including spirituality in quality of life measurement in oncology. *Psycho-Oncology, 8*(5), 417–428. doi:10.1002/ (SICI)1099-1611(199909/10)8:5<417::AID-PON398>3.0.CO;2-4

Brody, A. C., & Simmons, L. A. (2007). Family resilience during childhood cancer: The father's perspective. *Journal of Pediatric Oncology, 24*(3), 152–165. doi:10.1177/1043454206298844

Burkhart, L., Schmidt, L., & Hogan, N. (2011). Development and psychometric testing of the Spiritual Care Inventory instrument. *Journal of Advanced Nursing, 67*(11), 2463–2472. doi:10.1111/ j.1365-2648.2011.05654.x

Butler, P. M., McNamara, P., & Durso, R. (2010a). Side of onset in Parkinson's disease and alterations in religiosity: Novel behavioral phenotypes. *Behavioral Neurology, 24*(2), 133–141. doi:10.3233/ BEN-2011-0282

Butler, P. M., McNamara, P., & Durso, R. (2010b). Deficits in the automatic activation of religious concepts in patients with Parkinson's disease. *Journal of the International Neuropsychological Society, 16*(2), 252–261. doi:10.1017/S1355617709991202

Butler, P. M., McNamara, P., Ghofrani, J., & Durso, R. (2011). Disease-associated differences in religious cognition in patients with Parkinson's disease. *Journal of Clinical and Experimental Neuropsychology, 33*(8), 917–928. doi:10.1080/13803395.2011.575768

Caldeira, S., & Hall, J. (2012). Spiritual leadership and spiritual care in neonatology. *Journal of Nursing Management, 20*(8), 1069–1075. doi:10.1111/jonm.12034

Callahan, H. E. (2003). Families dealing with advanced heart failure: A challenge and an opportunity. *Critical Care Nurse, 26*(3), 230–245.

Campbell, D. (2013). Spirituality, stress, and retention of nurses in critical care. *Dimensions of Critical Care Nursing, 32*(2), 78–83. doi:10.1097/DCC.0b013e31828083a4

Carson, V. B. (2008). Spirituality: Identifying and meeting spiritual needs. In V. B. Carson & H. G. Koenig (Eds.), *Spiritual dimensions of nursing practice* (Rev. ed., pp. 125–153). West Conshohocken, PA: Templeton Foundation.

Chaudoir, S. R., Norton, W. E., Earnshaw, V. A., Moneyham, L., Mugavero, M. J., & Hiers, K. M. (2012). Coping with HIV stigma: Do proactive coping and spiritual peace buffer the effect of stigma on depression? *AIDS and Behaviour, 16*(8), 2382–2391. doi:10.1007/s10461-011-0039-3

Coleman, C. L., Eller, L. S., Nokes, K. M., Bunch, E., Reynolds, N. R., Corless, I. B., . . . Holzerner, W. L. (2006). Prayer as a complementary health strategy for managing HIV-related symptoms among ethnically diverse patients. *Holistic Nursing Practice, 20*(2), 65–72. doi:10.1097/00004650 -200603000-00006

Corso, V. M. (2012). Oncology nurse as wounded healer: Developing a compassion identity. *Clinical Journal of Oncology Nursing, 16*(5), 448–450.

Coward, D. D. (1997). Constructing meaning from the experience of cancer. *Seminars in Oncology Nursing, 13*(4), 248–251. doi:10.1016/S0749-2081(97)80019-8

Dalmida, S. G., Holstad, M. M., DiIorio, C., & Laderman, G. (2011). Spiritual well-being and health-related quality of life among African American women with HIV/AIDS. *Applied Research in Quality of Life, 6*(2), 139–157. doi:10.1007/s11482-010-9122-6

Dameron, C. M. (2012). Presence. *Journal of Christian Nursing, 29*(4), 201. doi:10.1097/CNJ .0b013e31826804cc

Deal, B., & Grassley, J. S. (2012). The lived experience of giving spiritual care: A phenomenological study of nephrology nurses working in acute and chronic hemodialysis settings. *Nephrology Nursing Journal, 39*(6), 471–496.

Delaney, C., & Barrere, C. (2008). Blessings: The influence of a spirituality-based intervention on psychospiritual outcomes in a cardiac population. *Holistic Nursing Practice, 22*(4), 210–219. doi:10.1097/01.HNP.0000326004.57687.74

Delaney, C., & Barrere, C. (2009). Ecospirituality: The experience of environmental meditation in patients with cardiovascular disease. *Holistic Nursing Practice, 23*(6), 361–369. doi:10.1097/ HNP.0b013e3181bf381c

Delgado, C. (2007). Meeting clients' spiritual needs. *Nursing Clinics of North America, 42*(2), 279–293. doi:10.1016/j.cnur.2007.03.002

DeWit, S. C., & Kumagai, C. K. (2013). Caring for medical-surgical patients. In S. C. DeWit & C. K. Kumagai (Eds.), *Medical-surgical nursing: Concepts & practice* (2nd ed., pp. 7–11). St. Louis, MO: Elsevier Mosby.

Dezorzi, L. W., & Crossetti, M. O. (2008). Spirituality in self-care for intensive care nursing professionals. *Revista Latino-Americana de Enfermagem, 16*(2), 212–217. doi:10.1590/S0104-11692008 000200007

Doka, K. (2009). *Counseling individuals with life-threatening illness.* New York, NY: Springer Publishing Company.

Dombeck, M. B. (1996). Chaos and self-organization as a consequence of spiritual disequilibrium. *Clinical Nurse Specialist, 10*(2), 69–73.

Dzul-Church, V., Cimino, J. W., Adler, S. R., Wong, P., & Anderson, W. G. (2010). "I'm sitting here by myself . . .": Experiences of patients with serious illness at an urban public hospital. *Journal of Palliative Medicine, 13*(6), 695–701. doi:10.1089/jpm.2009.0352

Fehring, R. J., Miller, J. F., & Shaw, C. (1997). Spiritual well-being, religiosity, hope, depression, and other mood states in elderly people coping with cancer. *Oncology Nursing Forum, 24*(4), 663–671.

Ferrell, B. R., & Baird, P. (2012). Deriving meaning and faith in caregiving. *Seminars in Oncology Nursing, 28*(4), 256–261. doi:10.1016/j.soncn.2012.09.008

Ferrell, B., Paice, J., & Koczywas, M. (2008). New standards and implications for improving the quality of supportive oncology practice. *Journal of Clinical Oncology, 26*(23), 3824–3831. doi:10.1200/ JCO.2007.15.7552

Ferrell, B. R., Smith, S. L., Juarez, G., & Melancon, C. (2003). Meaning of illness and spirituality in ovarian cancer survivors. *Oncology Nursing Forum, 30*(2), 249–257. doi:10.1188/03.ONF.249-257

Flannelly, L. T., Flannelly, K. J., & Weaver, A. J. (2002). Religious and spiritual variables in three major oncology nursing journals, 1990–1999. *Oncology Nursing Forum, 29*(4), 679–685. doi:10 .1188/02.ONF.679-685

Foster, M. J., Whitehead, L., Maybee, P., & Cullens, V. (2013). The parents', hospitalized child's, and health care providers' perceptions and experiences of family centered care within a pediatric critical care setting: A metasynthesis of qualitative research. *Journal of Family Nursing, 19*(4), 431–468. doi:10.1177/1074840713496317

Fowler, S. (1997). Hope and a health-promoting lifestyle in persons with Parkinson's disease. *Journal of Neuroscience Nursing, 29*(2), 111–116.

Fray, B. M. (2012). Religion and HIV and AIDS: Charting the terrain. *Journal of the Association of Nurses in AIDS Care, 23*(3), 268–271. doi:10.1016/j.jana.2012.01.007

Frybeck, P. B., & Reinert, B. R. (1999). Spirituality and people with potentially fatal diagnoses. *Nursing Forum, 34*(1), 13–22. doi:10.1111/j.1744-6198.199.tb00231.x

Giaquinto, S., Bruti, L., Dall'Armi, V., & Spiridigliozzi, C. (2010). Religious and spiritual beliefs in outpatients suffering from Parkinson's disease. *International Journal of Geriatric Psychiatry, 26*(9), 916–922. doi:10.1002/gps.2624

Giaquinto, S., Spiridigliozzi, C., & Caracciolo, B. (2007). Can faith protect from emotional distress after stroke? *Stroke, 38*(3), 993–997. doi:10.1161/01.STR.0000257996.26950.59

Grant, D. (2004). Spiritual interventions: How, when, and why nurses use them. *Holistic Nursing Practice, 18*(1), 36–41.

Green, V. (2004). Understanding different religions when caring for diabetes patients. *British Journal of Nursing, 13*(11), 658–662. doi:10.12968/bjon.2004.13.11.13224

Haddad, B. (2011). *Religion and HIV and AIDS: Charting the terrain*. Scottsville, South Africa: UKZN Press.

Halstead, M. T., & Hull, M. (2001). Struggling with paradoxes: The process of spiritual development in women with cancer. *Oncology Nursing Forum, 28*(10), 1534–1544.

Hampton, J. S., & Weinert, C. (2006). An exploration of spirituality in rural women with chronic illness. *Holistic Nursing Practice, 20*(1), 27–33.

Heiderscheit, A., Chlan, L., & Donley, K. (2011). Instituting a music listening intervention for critically ill patients receiving mechanical ventilation: Exemplars from two patient cases. *Music and Medicine, 3*(4), 239–245.

Hermanns, M. (2011). Weathering the storm: Living with Parkinson's disease. *Journal of Christian Nursing, 28*(2), 76–82. doi:10.1097/CNJ.0b013e31820b8d9f

Hermanns, M., Deal, B. J., & Haas, B. K. (2012). Biopsychosocial and spiritual aspects of Parkinson disease: An integrative review. *Journal of Neuroscience Nursing, 44*(4), 194–205. doi:10.1097/JNN.0b013e3182527593

Highfield, M. F. (1997). Spiritual assessment across the cancer trajectory: Methods and reflections. *Seminars in Oncology Nursing, 13*(4), 237–241. doi:10.1016/S0749-2081(97)80017-4

Hilbers, J. M., Haynes, A. S., & Kivikko, J. G. (2010). Spirituality and health: An exploratory study of hospital patients' perspectives. *Australian Health Review, 34*(1), 3–10. doi:10.1071/AH09655

Holt-Ashley, M. (2000). Nurses pray: Use of prayer and spirituality as a complementary therapy in the IC setting. *Maternal Child Nursing Clinical Issues: Advanced Practice in Acute and Critical Care, 11*(1), 60–67.

Johnson, K. S., Tulsky, J. A., Hays, J. C., Arnold, R. M., Olsen, M. K., Lindquist, J. H., & Steinhauser, K. E. (2011). Which domains of spirituality are associated with anxiety and depression in patients with advanced illness? *Journal of Internal Medicine, 26*(7), 751–758. doi:10.1007/s11606-011-1656-2

Kaplow, R. (2003). AACN Synergy Model for Patient Care: A framework to optimize outcomes. *Critical Care Nurse, 23*(Suppl.), 27–30.

Kim-Godwin, Y. (2013). Prayer in clinical practice: What does evidence support? *Journal of Christian Nursing, 30*(4), 208–215. doi:10.1097/CNJ.0b013e31826c2219

Kristeller, J. L., Sheets, V., Johnson, T., & Frank, B. (2011). Understanding religious and spiritual influences on adjustment to cancer: Individual patterns and differences. *Journal of Behavioral Medicine, 34*(6), 550–561. doi:10.1007/s10865-011-9335-7

Landis, B. J. (1996). Uncertainty, spiritual well-being and psychosocial adjustment to chronic illness. *Issues in Mental Health Nursing, 17*(3), 217–231. doi:10.3109/01612849609049916

Laukhuf, G., & Werner, H. (1998). Spirituality: The missing link. *Journal of Neuroscience Nursing, 30*(1), 60–67. doi:10.1097/01376517-199802000-00007

Lawrence, P., & Rozmus, C. (2001). Culturally sensitive care of the Muslim patient. *Journal of Transcultural Nursing, 12*(3), 228–233. doi:10.1177/104365960101200307

Lin, W., Gau, M., Lin, H., & Lin, H. (2011). Spiritual well-being in patients with rheumatoid arthritis. *Journal of Nursing Research, 19*(1), 1–11. doi:10.1097/JNR.0b013e31820b0f8c

Lopez, A. J., McCaffrey, R., Griffin, M. T. Q., & Fitzpatrick, J. J. (2009). Spiritual well-being and practices among women with gynecologic cancer. *Oncology Nursing Forum, 36*(3), 300–305. doi:10.1188/09.ONF.300-305

Lundberg, P. C., & Kerdonfag, P. (2010). Spiritual care provided by Thai nurses in intensive care units. *Journal of Clinical Nursing, 19*(7–8), 1121–1128. doi:10.1111/j.1365-2702.2009.03072.x

Martsolf, D. S., & Mickley, J. R. (1998). The concept of spirituality in nursing theories: Differing world-views and extent of focus. *Journal of Advanced Nursing, 27*(2), 294–303. doi:10.1046/j.1365-2648.1998.00519.x

Mattison, D. (2006). The forgotten spirit: Integration of spirituality in health care. *Nephrology News & Issues, 20*(2), 30–32.

Mayer, J. (1992). Wholly responsible for a part, or partly responsible for a whole? The concept of spiritual care in nursing. *Second Opinion, 17*(3), 26–55.

McBrien, B. (2008). Emergency nurses should be careful not to neglect their patients' spiritual needs. *Emergency Nurse, 16*(4), 39.

McBrien, B. (2009). Nurses' provision of spiritual care in the emergency setting—An Irish perspective. *International Emergency Nursing, 18*(3), 119–126. doi:10.1016/j.ienj.2009.09.004

McBrien, B. (2010a). Emergency nurses' provision of spiritual care: A literature review. *British Journal of Nursing, 19*(12), 768–773. doi:10.12968/bjon.2010.19.12.48655

McBrien, B. (2010b). Nurses' provision of spiritual care in the emergency setting: An Irish perspective. *International Emergency Nursing, 18*(3), 119–126. doi:10.1016/j.ienj.2009.09.004

McCabe, M. S., & Jacobs, L. (2008). Survivorship care: Models and programs. *Seminars in Oncology Nursing, 24*(3), 202–207. doi:10.1016/j.soncn.2008.05.008

McClain, C., Rosenfeld, B., & Breitbart, W. (2003). Effect of spiritual well-being on end-of-life despair in terminally ill cancer patients. *Lancet, 361*(9369), 1603–1607. doi:10.1016/S0140-6736(03)13310-7

McCord, G., Gilchrist, V. J., Grossman, S. D., King, B. D., McCormick, K. F. Oprandi, A. M., . . . Srivastava, M. (2004). Discussing spirituality with patients: A rational and ethical approach. *Annals of Family Medicine, 2*(4), 356–361. doi:10.1370/afm.71

McGrath, P. (2004). Positive outcomes for survivors of hematological malignancies from a spiritual perspective. *International Journal of Nursing Practice, 10*(6), 280–291.

Mickley, J. R., & Cowles, K. (2001). Ameliorating the tension: Use of forgiveness for healing. *Oncology Nursing Forum, 28*(1), 31–37.

Miller, L., Wickramaratne, P., Gameroff, M. J., Sage, M., Tenke, C. E., & Weissman, M. M. (2012). Religiosity and major depression in adults at high risk: A ten-year prospective study. *The American Journal of Psychiatry, 169*(1), 89–94. doi:10.1176/appi.ajp.2011.10121823

Mitchell, L., & Romans, S. (2003). Spiritual beliefs in bipolar affective disorder: Their relevance for illness management. *Journal of Affective Disorders, 75*(3), 247–257. doi:10.1016/S0165-0327(02)00055-1

Molzahn, A. E., & Sheilds, L. (2008). Why is it so hard to talk about spirituality? *Canadian Nurse, 104*(1), 25–29.

Molzahn, A., Sheilds, L., Bruce, A., Stajduhar, K., Makaroff, K. S., Beuthin, R., & Shermak, S. (2012). People living with serious illness: Stories of spirituality. *Journal of Clinical Nursing, 21*(15–16), 2347–2356. doi:10.111/j.1365-2702.2012.04196.x

Moorman, S. (2010). Surviving life-threatening illness: Keys to optimal care. *Journal of Christian Nursing, 27*(1), 18–24. doi:10.1097/01.CNJ.0000365985.95141.3d

Naghi, J. J., Philip, K. J., Phan, A., Cleenewerck, L., & Schwarz, E. R. (2012). The effects of spirituality and religion on outcomes in patients with chronic heart failure. *Journal of Religion & Health, 51*(4), 1124–1136. doi:10.1007/s10943-010-9419-7

Narayanasamy, A. (1995). Spiritual care of chronically ill patients. *Journal of Clinical Nursing, 4*(6), 1–2. doi:10.1111/j.1365-2702.1995.tb00042.x

Narayanasamy, A. (2002). Spiritual coping mechanisms in chronically ill patients. *British Journal of Nursing, 11*(22), 1461–1470. doi:10.12968/bjon.2002.11.22.10957

Neuman, B. (1995). *The Neuman systems model* (3rd ed.). Stamford, CT: Appleton & Lange.

Neuman, M. E. (2011). Addressing children's beliefs through Fowler's stages of faith. *Journal of Pediatric Nursing, 26*(1), 44–50. doi:10.1016/j.pedn.2009.09.002

Nixon, A. V., Narayanasamy, A., & Penny, V. (2013). An investigation into the spiritual needs of neuro-oncology patients from a nurse perspective. *BMC Nursing, 12*(2), 2–11. doi:10.1186/1472-6955-12-2

Nussbaum, G. B. (2003). Spirituality in critical care: Patient comfort and satisfaction. *Critical Care Nursing Quarterly, 26*(3), 214–220.

O'Brien, M. E. (2011). *Spirituality in nursing: Standing on holy ground* (4th ed.). Sudbury, MA: Jones & Bartlett.

Paiva, C. E., Paiva, B. S. R., Amaral de Castro, R., dePadua Souza, C., de Paiva Maia, Y., Ayres, J. A., & Michelin, O. C. (2013). A pilot study addressing the impact of religious practice on quality of life of breast cancer patients during chemotherapy. *Journal of Religion & Health, 52*(1), 184–193. doi:10.1007/s10943-011-9468-6

Pargament, K. I., McCarthy, S., Shah, P., Ano, G., Tarakeshwar, N., Wachholtz, A., . . . Duggan, J. (2004). Religion and HIV: A review of the literature and clinical implications. *Southern Medical Journal, 97*(12), 1201–1209. doi:10.1097/01.SMJ.0000146508.14898.E2

Peltzer, J., & Leenerts, M. H. (2007). Spirituality as a component of holistic self-care practices in human immunodeficiency virus-positive women with histories of abuse. *Holistic Nursing Practice, 21*(3), 105–112. doi:10.1097/01.HNP.0000269146.35237.2e

Perez, J. E., Smith, A. R., Norris, R., Canenguez, K. M., Tracey, E. F., & Cristofaro, S. B. (2011). Types of prayer and depressive symptoms among cancer patients: The mediating role of rumination and social support. *Journal of Behavioral Medicine, 34*(6), 519–530. doi:10.1007/s10865-011-9333-9

Pierce, L. L., Steiner, V., Havens, H., & Tormoehlen, K. (2008). Spirituality expressed by caregivers of stroke survivors. *Western Journal of Nursing Research, 30*(5), 606–619. doi:10.1177/0193945907310560

Pollock, S. E., & Sands, D. (1997). Adaptation to suffering: Meaning and implications for nursing. *Clinical Nursing Research, 6*(2), 171–185. doi:10.1177/105477389700600206

Polzer, R. L. (2007). African Americans and diabetes: Spiritual role of the health care provider in self-management. *Research in Nursing and Health, 30*(2), 164–174. doi:10.1002/nur.20179

Potter, M. L., & Zauszniewski, J. A. (2000). Spirituality, resourcefulness, and arthritis impact on health perception of elders with rheumatoid arthritis. *Journal of Holistic Nursing, 18*(4), 311–331. doi:10.1177/089801010001800403

Puchalski, C. (2004). Spirituality in health: The role of spirituality in critical care. *Critical Care Clinics, 20*(3), 487–504. doi:10.1016/j.ccc.2004.03.007

Reig, L., Mason, C., & Preston, K. (2006). Spiritual care: Practice guidelines for rehabilitation nurses. *Rehabilitation Nursing, 31*(6), 249–256. doi:10.1002/j.2048-7940.2006.tb00021.x

Roy, C., & Andrews, H. A. (2009). *The Roy Adaptation Model* (3rd ed.). New York, NY: Pearson.

Sawatzky, R., & Pesut, B. (2005). Attributes of spiritual care in nursing practice. *Journal of Holistic Nursing, 23*(1), 19–33. doi:10.1177/0898010104272010

Scarinci, E. G., Griffin, M. T. Q., Grogoriu, A., & Fitzpatrick, J. J. (2009). Spiritual well-being and spiritual practices in HIV-infected women: A preliminary study. *Journal of the Association of Nurses in AIDS Care, 20*(1), 69–76. doi:10.1016/j.jana.2008.08.003

Schreiber, J. A. (2011). Image of God: Effect on coping and psychospiritual outcomes in early breast cancer survivors. *Oncology Nursing Forum, 38*(3), 293–301. doi:10.1188/11.ONF.293-301

Schreiber, J. A. (2012). Psychometric properties of the image of God scale in breast cancer survivors. *Oncology Nursing Forum, 39*(4), E346–352. doi:10.1188/12.ONF.E346-E352

Slomka, J., Lim, J., Gripshover, B., & Daly, B. (2013). How have long-term survivors coped with living with HIV? *Journal of the Association of Nurses in AIDS care, 24*(5), 449–459. doi:10.1016/j.jana.2012.09.004

Smith, A. R. (2006). Using the synergy model to provide spiritual care in critical care settings. *Critical Care Nurse, 26*(4), 41–47.

Smith, D. W. (1995). Power and spirituality in polio survivors: A study based on Rogers' science. *Nursing Science Quarterly, 8*(3), 133–139. doi:10.1177/089431849500800309

Sowell, R., Moneyham, L., Hennessy, M., Guillory, J., Demi, A., & Seals, B. (2000). Spiritual activities as a resistance resource for women with human immunodeficiency virus. *Nursing Research, 49*(2), 73–82. doi:10.1097/00006199-200003000-00003

Stanhope, M., Lancaster, J., Jessup-Falcioni, H., & Viverais-Dresler, G. A. (2011). *Community health nursing in Canada* (2nd ed.). Toronto, ON, Canada: Elsevier.

Stanley-Hermanns, M., & Engebretson, J. (2010). Sailing the stormy seas: The illness experience of persons with Parkinson's disease. *The Qualitative Report, 15*(2), 340–369. Retrieved from http://www.nova.edu/ssss/QR/QR15-2/stanley-hermanns.pdf

Stewart, M. (2014). Spiritual assessment: A patient-centered approach to oncology social work practice. *Social Work in Health Care, 53*(1), 59–73. doi:10.1080/00981389.2013.834033

Stoll, R. I. (1979). Guidelines for spiritual assessment. *American Journal of Nursing, 79*(9), 1574–1577. doi:10.1097/00000446-197909000-00041

Swinton, J., Bain, V., Ingram, S., & Heys, S. D. (2011). Moving inwards, moving outwards, moving upwards: The role of spirituality during the early stages of breast cancer. *European Journal of Cancer Care, 20*(5), 640–652. doi:10.1111/j.1365-2354.2010.01260.x

Tanyi, R. A., & Werner, J. S. (2008). Women's experience of spirituality within end-stage renal disease and hemodialysis. *Clinical Nursing Research, 17*(1), 32–49. doi:10.1177/1054773807311691

Tanyi, R. A., Werner, J. S., Recine, A. C., & Sperstad, R. A. (2006). Perceptions of incorporating spirituality into their care: A phenomenological study of female patients on hemodialysis. *Nephrology Nursing Journal, 33*(5), 532–538.

Taylor, E. J. (2000). Transformation of tragedy among women surviving breast cancer. *Oncology Nursing Forum, 27*(5), 781–788.

Taylor, E. J. (2005). Spiritual complementary therapies in cancer care. *Seminars in Oncology Nursing, 21*(3), 159–163. doi:10.1016/j.soncn.2005.04.003

Taylor, E. J. (2006). Prevalence and associated factors of spiritual needs among patients with cancer and family caregivers. *Oncology Nursing Forum, 33*(4), 729–735. doi:10.1188/06.ONF.729-735 #sthash.sYYu7J84.dpuf

Taylor, E. J. (Ed.). (2012). *Religion: A clinical guide for nurses.* New York, NY: Springer Publishing Company.

Taylor, E. J., & Mamier, I. (2005). Spiritual care nursing: What cancer patients and family caregivers want. *Journal of Advanced Nursing, 49*(3), 260–267. doi:10.1111/j.1365-2648.2004.03285.x

Timmins, F., & Kelly, J. (2008). Spiritual assessment in intensive and cardiac care nursing. *Nursing in Critical Care, 13*(3), 124–131. doi:10.1111/j.1478-5153.2008.00276.x

Vachon, M. L. S. (2008). Meaning, spirituality, and wellness in cancer survivors. *Seminars in Oncology Nursing, 24*(3), 218–225. doi:10.1016/j.soncn.2008.05.010

Vance, D. E., Struzick, T. C., & Raper, J. L. (2008). Biopsychosocial benefits of spirituality in adults aging with HIV: Implications for nursing practice and research. *Journal of Holistic Nursing, 26*(2), 119–125. doi:10.1177/0898010107310615

Villagomeza, L. R. (2005). Spiritual distress in adult cancer patients: Toward conceptual clarity. *Holistic Nursing Practice, 19*(6), 285–294.

Villagomeza, L. R. (2006). Mending broken hearts: The role of spirituality in cardiac illness: A research synthesis, 1991–2004. *Holistic Nursing Practice, 20*(4), 169–186.

Walton, J. (2002). Finding a balance: A grounded theory study of spirituality in hemodialysis patients. *Nephrology Nursing Journal, 29*(5), 447–457.

Walton, J., & Sullivan, N. (2004). Men of prayer: Spirituality of men with prostate cancer: A grounded theory study. *Journal of Holistic Nursing, 22*(2), 133–151. doi:10.1177/0898010104264778

Watts, J. H. (2009). Meanings of spirituality at the cancer drop-in. *International Journal of Qualitative Studies on Health and Well-Being, 4*(2), 86–93. doi:10.1080/17482620902831185

Weiland, S. A. (2010). Integrating spirituality into critical care: An APN perspective using Roy's Adaptation Model. *Critical Care Nursing Quarterly, 33*(3), 282–291. doi:10.1097/CNQ.0b013e318 1ecd56d

World Health Organization. (2002). Innovative care for chronic conditions: Building blocks for action. Retrieved from http://www.who.int/chp/knowledge/publications/icccglobalreport.pdf?ua=1

Ziel, R., & Kautz, D. D. (2009). The highest priority in the emergency department may be a patient's spiritual needs. *Journal of Emergency Nursing, 35*(1), 50–51. doi:10.1016/j.jen.2008.09.005

8

Spirituality in Mental Health Care

In Chapter 2 (see section on Religion/Spirituality in Health and Illness), there were some general and summary comments on the connection between spirituality/religion and mental health. This chapter provides a more in-depth discussion on the connection between spirituality/religion, mental health, and mental illness.

SPIRITUALITY/RELIGION AND MENTAL HEALTH

As previously mentioned in other chapters, it is easier to study the impact of religion on health compared to the impact of spirituality on health because religion is the outward practice of spirituality through rituals, beliefs, practices, and the living out of various beliefs and values. Common themes in the literature on religion and the impact on mental health indicate that religion and/or spirituality generally have a positive impact on mental health. Some examples include:

- Religion/spirituality can contribute to improved coping ability (Buswell et al., 2006; Koenig, 2009; Phillips & Stein, 2007).

- Religion/spirituality can create a sense of well-being and enhance quality of life in terms of increasing self-esteem, hope, connection to others and to God/higher power, happiness, a higher morale, and satisfaction with life (Koenig 1997, 2005; Sawatzky, Ratner, & Chiu, 2005; Swinton, 2001).

- Religion is a known protective factor against substance misuse/abuse (Huguelet, Borras, Gillieron, Brandt, & Mohr, 2009; Koenig, 2009; Rew & Wong, 2006).

- There is evidence that religious conversion experiences have been beneficial to peoples' mental health, even those with severe mental illness (Koenig, 2005).

- Religion/spirituality provides support and comfort. For example, if a person believes in God and that God is present with him or her in a beneficial way, then this is a comforting belief. Religious/spiritual rituals and a faith community can also be supportive and comforting (Swinton, 2001).

- Religion/spirituality can provide a framework for meaning and purpose in life and also for meaning making in life events (both positive and negative events). It can also provide a framework for hope and for forgiveness (Swinton, 2001).

- Religion/spirituality is a protective factor against anxiety, depression, self-destructive behaviors, and other mental disorders. Religion/spirituality can also function to sustain the mental health of a person (Buswell et al., 2006; Koenig, 2005, 2009).

- Concepts associated with major world religions, such as gratefulness, forgiveness, altruism, and social support, are associated with greater mental well-being (Scharf, 2007).

- The teachings of various world religions can provide a protective factor against divorce and promiscuity, for example, the teachings of the Christian faith. Divorce and promiscuity can impact negatively on relational health as well as overall mental health.

For an in-depth discussion on the relationship between religion and mental health, refer to Koenig (2005). Some of Koenig's discussion may also apply to the impact of the more general concept of spirituality on mental health.

The examples given of the positive impact of religion/spirituality on mental health do not preclude religion/spirituality having a negative impact on mental health (Swinton, 2001). For example, certain religious or spiritual beliefs can cause anxiety and distress, both of which impact a person's mental health. Pieper and van Uden (2012) found in their study of inpatient psychiatric clients that the emphasis placed on feelings of humility and guilt by some religions contributed negatively to the clients' well-being. Neurotic use of religion, such as using religion to control others, can also be detrimental to well-being. This is particularly relevant in the case of those who are emotionally vulnerable. The beliefs and doctrines associated with some religions can actually "reinforce neurotic tendencies, enhance fear or guilt, and restrict life rather than enhance it. In such cases, religious beliefs may be used in primitive and defensive ways to avoid making necessary life changes" (Koenig, 2009, p. 289). In such instances, Koenig (1997) sees such use of religion as evidence of a person's insecurity or mental disturbance:

> [I]t is the misuse and abuse of religion that most neurotic manifestations of it reflect (p. 110) . . . . It is usually the immature forms of religious expression that lend themselves to neurotic use. Mature employments of religion that emphasize love, forgiveness, acceptance, mercy and compassion are difficult to neuroticize. (p. 111)

Koenig makes an important point when he emphasizes the fact the mental health professionals are more likely to see neurotic uses of religion because they see people with mental illness. However, they cannot, on that basis, conclude that religion is a *cause* of pathology or that most people from a particular religion see things in a neurotic manner.

> ### Reflection 8.1
>
> - Reflect on the examples of the impact of religion/spirituality on mental health. Can you identify with any of these outcomes in terms of your own mental health? Are there additional aspects of religion/spirituality that you can identify and that contribute to your own mental health?
> - Have you witnessed misuse and abuse of religion? If so, then what was the impact on the person? What are some cautions for nurses with respect to judging how a person experiences his or her religion?

MENTAL ILLNESS

Before discussing the impact of religion/spirituality on mental illness, a few general comments about mental illness itself are in order. Worldwide, mental illness is a health problem that is increasing in terms of the numbers of people affected by such illness: An estimated 450 million people are affected by mental illness, many of whom are not diagnosed or treated. Depression has been identified in the top 10 causes of disability worldwide (World Health Organization Quality of Life-Spirituality, Religiousness and Personal Beliefs [WHOQOL-SRPB] Group, 2006). It has also been labeled as the "common cold" of mental health problems (Swinton, 2001).

The impact of mental illness on a person is multifaceted. O'Reilly (2004) likens mental illness to "a thief who steals individuals' essential self" (p. 47). Many clients with mental illness, and in particular severe mental illness, find that they face a painful life journey: loneliness; loss of self-esteem; unemployment or underemployment; loss of meaning, purpose, and hope; and unstable living arrangements. Some will also have to deal with ongoing hallucinations, delusions, and paranoia. Others will abuse alcohol or drugs. Some will see their mental illness as a punishment, causing additional stress and anguish (Landeen, Pawlick, Woodside, Kirkpatrick, & Byrne, 2000; Luk, 2011; O'Reilly, 2004; Peterson & Nelson, 1987; Scharf, 2007). Because of the chronicity and emotional distress that often accompany mental illness, O'Reilly states: "Distress of the human spirit can easily be considered a correlative of psychiatric disorders, given the chronicity and emotional anguish of mental illness" (p. 46). She adds:

> The organic, cognitive, and emotional events of mental illness derail the process of becoming; diminish clients' ability to perceive internal and external relatedness; and result in an experience of existential aloneness, helplessness, and pointlessness. Mental illness is thus proposed as a disruption of the body, mind, and spirit that results in pain and impaired functioning in all dimensions of the human experience. (p. 47)

Of course, many factors can affect how a person with a mental illness journeys through life. For example, the degree and severity of the illness determine how it is experienced. Moreover, having a mental illness can create strength and resilience in a person.

SPIRITUALITY, RELIGION, AND MENTAL ILLNESS

The descriptors of the impact of mental illness on a person are infused with allusions to spiritual concepts, such as meaning and purpose, hope, relatedness, and a sense of self. Spirituality, then, is intricately connected to mental illness. As the Mental Health Foundation (1999) puts it:

> The experience of breaking down, becoming depressed, anxious, or psychotic frequently has a spiritual element to it. Many people have described their initial problems . . . of a search for meaning in their lives and that search is often still continuing during the period when their problems become so great that they find themselves diagnosed with a mental illness. (p. 11)

Mohr (2006) agrees with this position, stating: "Suffering in the context of psychiatric-mental health nursing is uniquely multilayered and multileveled, involving body, mind, and spirit, and often challenging personal meaning systems" (p. 174).

Koenig's work regarding the relationship between religion and mental health/mental illness is expansive and illuminative (Koenig, 1997, 2005, 2007, 2009). Koenig uses the word "religion" to refer to institutionalized forms of religion, as well as considering religion to be a multidimensional construct. In this regard, he uses the terms "religion" and "spirituality" synonymously (Koenig, 2009).

Koenig (2009) conducted a review of the research conducted on religion's relationship with/to depression, suicide, anxiety, psychotic disorders, and substance abuse. These mental health problems are discussed in more detail later in this chapter. Koenig acknowledges that religious delusions may be common in psychosis but stresses that even in such a context, "healthy normative religious beliefs and practices appear to be stabilizing and may reduce the tremendous isolation, fear, and loss of control that those with psychosis experience" (p. 289). Koenig points out that religious coping as a means to help patients deal with both physical and mental illness is widespread throughout the world. This is an assertion supported by other researchers (e.g., Pieper & van Uden, 2012). Koenig (2009) proposes that religious coping, as well as sensible religion, can be quite helpful to clients with mental illness because:

> Religious beliefs [and religion itself] provide a sense of meaning and purpose during difficult life circumstances that assist with psychological integration; they usually promote a positive worldview that is optimistic and hopeful; they provide role models in sacred writings that facilitate acceptance of suffering; they give people a sense of indirect control over circumstances, reducing the need for personal control; and they offer a community of support, both human and divine, to help reduce isolation and loneliness. Unlike many other coping resources, religion is available to anyone at any time, regardless of financial, social, physical, or mental circumstances. (Koenig, 2009, p. 285)

Meisenhelder (2002) discusses religious coping in crisis situations, maintaining that people who use positive religious coping strategies see life more broadly. They also try to find meaning in the crisis. Positive religious coping is described by Meisenhelder in these terms: working with God as a partner in dealing with a crisis; looking to God for love and support, strength, and guidance through the crisis; engaging in religious practices, such as worship and prayer; and trying to give spiritual support to others as well as receive it from others. (*Note*: These descriptors assume a particular religious worldview.) An interesting aspect in Meisenhelder's discussion is that when people are in crisis and have no control, and if they look to a greater power such as God perceived as having control, then this seems to foster their sense of control and reassurance for the future.

Spirituality/religion is also known to contribute to peoples' resilience as they cope with mental illness. For example, Edward, Welch, and Chater (2009) identified hope, faith, meaningful relationships, a sense of meaning and purpose, and being spiritual to be important to the resilience of adults with mental illness.

Although Koenig acknowledges that many people are helped by religion/spirituality, not all experience complete relief from mental distress and destructive behavioral tendencies through religious coping. As mentioned earlier, unhealthy forms of religious/spiritual involvement can be present. How does a nurse know if religious beliefs and behaviors are distorted or unhelpful? Consulting a religious leader or spiritual care professional can be helpful. John (1983), in a classic book on spirituality and mental health nursing, gives some criteria for identifying distorted or unhealthy religious beliefs. John maintains that unhealthy religious beliefs are characterized by/and or result in the following:

- Preoccupation with sin as well as an inability to accept forgiveness

- A compulsive lack of freedom, for example, being legalistic or "being driven"

- A magical view of how God intervenes

- Poor self-esteem or, conversely, grandiosity

- A view of suffering as punishment or actually seeking suffering

- Distorted relationships, for example, separating oneself from others or having no individual identity

Refer to John (Chapter 7) for further discussion on each of the points just discussed, including case studies illustrating such points.

Reflection 8.2

- Reflect on religious clients you may have encountered in your practice who were/are experiencing mental illness. Using the criteria given by Shelly and John (1983), judge the "health" of their religious beliefs and behavior.
- How might the nurse assist clients whose religious beliefs and behaviors are distorted or unhealthy?

Although Koenig (2009, 2005) identifies the importance of faith communities in providing support to those with mental illness, many clients with mental illness find themselves estranged from faith communities, and even shunned by them. Scharf (2007) calls upon faith communities to support and care for those who have mental illnesses. Some faith communities are rising to the task, for example, creating educational opportunities about mental illness for their members, and providing individual and group support to people who have a mental illness. Mental health nurses can be advocates for such initiatives by local faith communities. Some faith communities have a long tradition of working with those who suffer with mental illness, for example, The Salvation Army.

Keltner (2005) raises an interesting point when he proposes that spirituality should be part of mental health care due to the etiology of some mental health problems. He acknowledges the biological processes that may be related to mental illness but states: "mental health problems may also be related to behaviors that in previous generations would have precipitated censor from society, shame within individuals and families, and rebuke from religious authorities" (p. 142). Keltner maintains that some people who have mental health problems willfully act in ways that compromise them emotionally. He frames such situations as suffering from a "soul disorder" (p. 142). The prevalence and impact of engaging in pornography and extreme promiscuity may be examples. Keltner discusses four cultural changes that have created a societal environment that is devoid of shame and wary of religion/spirituality: (a) psychiatry's view of religion, which is to consistently diminish it as relevant; (b) the erosion of personal responsibility; (c) a focus on feelings about behavior rather than behavior itself; and (d) the ascension of individualism (pp. 143–144). Keltner asserts that cultural decline has contributed negatively to the population's mental health in terms of the choices that people make. He calls upon mental health professionals to raise awareness of cultural decline and the impact of that decline upon mental health problems. He further recommends addressing such problems from a spiritual framework.

Reflection 8.3

- What do you think about Keltner's assertions regarding (a) the connection between cultural decline and mental health; and (b) that some mental health problems/illnesses are related to "wrong," "immoral," or "sinful" behavior?
- How might such a stance foster an attitude of "judgment" or "victim blaming" in nurses? How can nurses avoid such a stance, even if they agree with Keltner's assertions?

As discussed earlier, religious/spiritual themes may display themselves in clients with severe mental illness. For example, in clients with schizophrenia or bipolar disorder, normative religious beliefs can become distorted. Such clients may believe that God speaks to them audibly, asking them to do harmful things to themselves or others. Preoccupation with religious beliefs and practices that is beyond the normative can also occur. Obsession with real or imagined transgressions can result in severe guilt and/or self-blame. Psychotic distortions that involve religious themes can also be present (Mohr, 2006).

In the health care literature, there is discussion about various spiritual needs and their manifestation in mental illness. As has been reiterated before in this book, Narayanasamy (1999) maintains that spiritual needs come to the forefront during emotional stress and crisis, including mental health crises. Mental illness can impact the need for hope and strength as clients struggle with issues associated with mental illness. The need for love and relatedness can be exacerbated in mental illness as many clients may have poorly developed social skills generally, or have social skills that have deteriorated during their illness. Mental illness itself has been described previously in this chapter as isolating (see section on Mental Illness). The need for forgiveness may also be evident. If forgiveness is not forthcoming, then the result may be guilt and resentment, or even feelings of paranoia, hostility, worthlessness, defensiveness and/or withdrawal (Narayanasamy, 1991). Shelly (1983) discusses three issues related to spiritual needs in a psychiatric setting that can impact assessment of such needs as well as interventions to meet the needs (pp. 59–60):

- The issue of distortion of beliefs due to psychosis, poor self-concept, and/or distorted and confused thinking. Religion can also be used as a manipulative technique by clients.

- The issue of misinterpretation of religious concepts, writings, and symbols by clients. Verifying comments made with respect to their meaning to the client is essential.

- The intensity of spiritual needs, which can prevent nurses from recognizing the needs. For example, loss of meaning and purpose can be so profound that the client has no hope.

There may also be variations in the foundational spiritual needs of people with mental illness. As Thompson (2002) states, "a person's mental health problems might impinge on the usual accommodation of [spiritual] needs" (p. 36). For example, a person may be obsessive about the need to be forgiven for wrongdoings that are not based in reality. A person may also have experienced repeated rejections from a variety of people, or felt "used" by people, creating difficulties in meeting the normative need for love and relatedness (Peterson & Nelson, 1987).

Folkman (2008) identifies coping that is meaning focused as providing positive emotions, which can coexist with negative emotions during stressful situations. Folkman draws on the work of Park and Folkman (1997) and Aldwin (2007) in describing meaning-focused coping as coping that draws on a person's beliefs, values, and existential goals not only to motivate the person to cope but also to sustain coping and well-being during times of difficulty and stress. Folkman raises a key question with respect to positive emotions: Which religious and spiritual coping processes are related primarily to positive emotions? The answer to this question is important for nurses when working with clients experiencing stress. Exploration and attention to the sources of emotions can assist nurses in generating and sustaining these positive emotions in clients.

> ### Reflection 8.4
>
> - Do you know people (personally and/or professionally) who have been impacted by mental illness? What aspects of their lives have been impacted by their illness, both negatively and positively?
> - Reflect on the place of spirituality/religion in mental illness, in particular in terms of evident spiritual needs; and also in terms of spirituality/religion as a resource for those dealing with mental illness. What spiritual needs have you witnessed in those with mental illness? What spiritual/religious resources have they used and what has been the impact?

SPIRITUALITY/RELIGION IN VARIOUS MENTAL HEALTH CONDITIONS

To obtain a more expansive knowledge of how spirituality/religion intersects with mental illness, it is appropriate to engage in a brief discussion of this connection with respect to various mental illnesses. Many of the studies on spirituality/religion and mental illness focus on these particular illnesses.

ANXIETY, DEPRESSION, AND SUICIDE

Anxiety and depression are common mental health problems in today's Western society. With respect to anxiety, Koenig (2009) identifies that religious beliefs and practices are helpful to people who are anxious or fearful, increasing their sense of control, enhancing feelings of security, and increasing their self-confidence and/or their confidence in the divine beings. In his review of studies focusing on religion/spirituality in anxiety, Koenig observed that almost half of the observational studies found significantly less anxiety and fear in those clients who were more religious. The majority of studies examining the impact of religious interventions on clients with anxiety also found that in the case of religious clients, religious interventions reduced anxiety levels more quickly than secular interventions. Bowen, Baetz, and D'Arcy (2006) found in a sample of clients with panic disorder that a self-reported importance of religion was a significant predictor of improvement in panic symptoms, as well as lower perceived stress.

With respect to depression, Swinton (2001) sees it as a condition that impacts the entire person, "producing a deep spiritual, existential, physical, psychological and relational crisis" (p. 131). Swinton elaborates further:

> As one reflects upon the nature of depression it becomes clear that it is a profoundly spiritual experience that cannot be understood and dealt with through drugs and therapy alone. Its central features of profound hopelessness, loss of meaning in life, perceived loss of relationship with God or higher power, low self-esteem and general sense of purposelessness, all indicate a level of spiritual distress. (pp. 95–96)

Swinton concludes from the findings in his study on the lived experience of depression that "Depression is a profoundly spiritual experience" (p. 131). He also points out that the findings also indicate that depression can be a "catalyst for a degree of positive change. Despite the soul-destroying experience of depression, for some, the journey through darkness brought about new spiritual insights and fresh possibilities even in the midst of deep sadness" (p. 122). Swinton challenges mental health professionals to reframe depression from a spiritual perspective. Such a perspective can help such professionals uncover "new priorities and fresh possibilities for interventions that do not fall within the remit of purely materialistic psychiatry" (p. 170). In this manner, the client's situation can be reframed from one of loss to "the possibility of hope, purpose and a meaningful existence, even in the midst of severe psychological disturbance" (p. 170).

Koenig, McCullough, and Larson (2001) found that the majority of studies focusing on the relationship between religion and depression indicated that the more religious clients had lower rates of depressive disorder, fewer depressive symptoms, and faster symptom improvement. The more recent review by Koenig (2009), especially of studies examining religion and depression in clients with physical illness, indicated that religious involvement helped these people cope. Pesut, Clark, Maxwell, and Michalak (2011) make the following statement about Koenig's 2009 review:

> Koenig's 2009 review of the interface between religion, spirituality and mental health reported that over 100 quantitative studies had examined the relationship between religion and unipolar depression prior to the year 2000 and that this body of work is developing apace. Findings from the review suggested that religion may play a beneficial role for individuals experiencing depression. (pp. 792–793)

Ameling and Povilonis (2001) also found in their review of the literature on spirituality and mental illness that spiritual interventions helped to alleviate the symptoms of depression and anxiety.

Focusing on bipolar disorder, Michalak, Yatham, Kolesar, and Lam (2006) found in their qualitative study that religion/spirituality was a resource for clients with this disorder, important to their quality of life. Pesut and colleagues (2011) point out that religion and spirituality may be of particular concern to people with bipolar disorder because many such clients may have religious or spiritual delusions. Clients with bipolar illness may find it challenging "to maintain a supportive [religious/spiritual] perspective amidst the variability of their illness" (Pesut et al., p. 792). An example of such a challenge would be their participation in a faith community. Pesut and colleagues also point to the potential barriers between clients with bipolar disorder and health care providers when care involves religion and spirituality. For example, how clients perceive and explain their illness and treatment may cause conflict with health care professionals because of the clients' religious or spiritual beliefs. Yet, as Pesut and colleagues indicate, the importance of including religion/spirituality to positively impact coping and decision making should not be ignored. They call for more longitudinal qualitative and quantitative studies on religion/spirituality in bipolar disorder. Such studies have the potential to not only account for spiritual/religious transformations in clients over time, but also contribute to a more in-depth understanding of how religion/spirituality interfaces with bipolar disorder. How religion/spirituality is effectively and ethically incorporated into clients' therapeutic regimes is also important to understand. Reference to the article by Pesut and colleagues provides a more in-depth discussion of the research on religion/spirituality in bipolar disorder.

Ward (2011) described the lived experience of adults with both bipolar disorder and substance use disorder. The importance of spiritual support emerged as a significant theme in the study. Spiritual support was described by participants in this study as "perceived personally supportive components of their relationship with God" (p. 24). This sense of spiritual support was very important as the participants exhibited several spiritual needs significant to those struggling with mental illness:

- The need for love and relatedness: Many of the participants had moved frequently and had experienced torn relationships with family and loved ones (which they considered to be the most devastating consequence of living with bipolar disorder and substance abuse).

- The need for hope, meaning, and purpose: Participants described living with pain, failed life expectancies, depression, and suicide attempts, all of which engendered loss of hope and loss of meaning and purpose.

- The need for forgiveness: Participants wanted to be heard, accepted, and forgiven and felt that this would help them recover and have an opportunity to be productive, thereby finding meaning and purpose.

All participants were actively involved in a 12-step program that included spiritual aspects. Activities such as daily connecting with God, seeking forgiveness, reading the Bible, and worshipping at a local church were identified by participants as providing support and strength. Prayer and meditation also enabled them to meet life's challenges. Their belief that God was there for them no matter what provided them with not only motivation but also support. Also, the belief that God listened to them was important as it contrasted with feelings of not being heard by others. Two of the participants said:

> I get on my knees and I really, I really get down and pray and it helps me. I do believe that He is up there looking after me. Anytime I get in a tight situation or whatever, I can go to God. It helps me for some reason; it calms me down where I can be able to function. (Ward, 2011, p. 25)

> I pray a lot. God is everything. He's everything. I pray a lot. I thank Him for waking me up in the morning and I pray every morning. I have suffered a lot; God eases it from my life. (Ward, 2011, p. 25)

In the case of clients with suicidal ideation, hopelessness is a significant issue. However, Jones (2010) identifies that within the suicidal person there is "a strange kind of 'hope'—the perverse belief that by the most extreme act, suffering may finally cease" (p. 252). Providing hope to the client by seeing alternatives to suicide is a challenge for nurses in this context of care. Jones discusses the importance of stories as a means of helping persons who are suicidal to make meaning in their situation and to replace narratives of hopelessness with narratives of hope. Jones uses a case study to illustrate how Biblical narratives can be of assistance to a person who is suicidal. Others have written about the use of stories in the context of suicide (e.g., Kaplan & Schwartz, 2008; Schwartz & Kaplan, 2004).

Religious teachings and beliefs can be a protective factor against suicide. For example, a client may ascribe to a religious doctrine that prohibits suicide. Connection to a faith community can also provide support, which can prevent suicide (Dervic et al., 2004; van Tubergen, Grotenhuis, & Ultee, 2005). Another protective factor against suicide is connection to others (family, friends, health care professionals et al.; Oliffe, Ogrodniczuk, Bottorff, Johnson, & Hoyak, 2012).

Kalischuk and Davies (2001) focused on the healing of family members following suicide: an important aspect of family-focused care within the context of suicide. They identified several healing themes that were characteristic of the family members' "journeying toward wholeness" (p. 172), which were each, in some way, related to finding meaning and exploring spirituality:

- Cocooning (journey of descent), characterized by withdrawal for a period of time to try and make sense of what happened. At this stage, family members often asked "Why?" and were preoccupied with finding the answer(s) to this question.

- Centering (journey of growth), where family members emerged from withdrawal to commit to life and living. At this stage, various spiritual and religious strategies were used, such as prayer, rituals, meditation, and imagery.

- Connecting (journey of transcendence), involving, as one family member put it, a "different way of being in the world" (p. 177). Here, family members transcended their circumstances by being involved with others, especially those in the family unit, in more meaningful ways. They also became involved in helping others who had experiences similar to theirs—"Their purpose in life came into clearer focus as did the changes that were needed to accomplish their goals" (p. 178). The need for love and relatedness was also met through these activities.

Reflection 8.5

- Reflect on clients who were/are experiencing depression, anxiety, or who were/are suicidal. What was/is the place of spirituality/religion in terms of their experience in any of these scenarios—both in terms of impact on their illness and in terms of their illness impacting their spirituality/religion?
- What particular challenges might you encounter personally in focusing on the spiritual/religious needs of clients who are depressed, anxious, or suicidal? If you do find any of these situations to be challenging, then why might this be so and how can you address such challenges?

PSYCHOSIS

Perhaps some of the greatest challenges with respect to religion/spirituality in mental illness are presented in clients experiencing psychosis. In fact, Clarke (2010) edited a book with an overall focus on the complexities of spirituality in psychosis. Peterson and Nelson

(1987) suggest that dealing with clients who have religious delusions during psychosis is "probably the most difficult with which to deal. However, this process can be made easier if the nurse has been careful in assessing and determining whether the spiritual issues are basically healthy or unhealthy" (p. 38).

Koenig (2009) concluded from his review of the research on religion/spirituality and psychosis that generally both spirituality and religion can provide a positive force in the lives of clients experiencing psychosis. In an earlier review, Koenig and colleagues (2001) found that four of the 10 studies reviewed that focused on religion and psychosis indicated that there was less psychosis in clients who were more religiously involved. Three studies found no association between religion and psychosis, whereas two studies reported mixed results. Koenig (2009) states, "Longitudinal studies suggest that non-psychotic religious activity may actually improve long-term prognosis in patients with psychotic disorders" (p. 288). Other studies have reported religion to be important to clients experiencing schizophrenia as it instilled hope, meaning, and purpose into their lives (e.g., Huguelet, Mohr, Borras, Gillieron, & Brandt, 2006; Mohr, Gillieron, Borras, Brandt, & Huguelet, 2007). Hultsjo and Blomqvist (2013) found that meaningful work and quality relationships with family and friends were also helpful to people with psychoses, in particular in helping them remain healthy. Hutlsjo and Blomqvist also identified religious beliefs as impacting clients' health beliefs and behaviors—as well as how clients perceived and dealt with their illness.

As previously mentioned, religious delusions, some bizarre, can often accompany psychosis (Koenig, 2009; Scharf, 2007). Koenig (2009) notes that, in addition to religion, culture can also be a factor that can impact the content of psychotic delusions. An interesting study by Siddle, Haddock, Tarrier, and Faragher (2002) compared clients with religious delusions to clients with nonreligious delusions. Siddle and colleagues found that clients who had religious delusions had increased severity of symptoms (especially hallucinations and bizarre symptoms), less ability to function, longer duration of the illness, and were on higher doses of antipsychotic medication.

There are several challenges to the spiritual care of clients with psychoses. One challenge is distinguishing religious beliefs expressed during psychosis from normative religious beliefs. At times, this is obvious, as for example, when a client thinks that he or she is God. In less obvious cases, the nurse can consult with a religious leader or a spiritual care professional (Koenig, 2005; Scharf, 2007). Reference to the discussion in Chapter 2 (see section on Religion and Negative Impact on Health/Well-Being) on healthy/unhealthy religion and characteristics of healthy and unhealthy spiritual life is recommended for review.

Another challenge is with respect to distinguishing psychotic symptoms from spiritual experiences. This distinction is of particular interest when religiosity is part of the client's psychotic manifestations. Yet, as Pesut and colleagues (2011) point out:

> . . . it is not always easy to disentangle religious delusions from religious experiences common to those individuals who do not have a diagnosis of mental illness. It may actually be the level of preoccupation, conviction and extent of the thinking rather than the content that marks it as delusional (Pierre, 2001). (p. 786)

Cultural factors can also determine whether a religious/spiritual experience is to be considered normal or abnormal (Pesut et al.).

Eeles, Low, and Wellman (2003) identify subtypes of spiritual experience (as developed by Donovan, 1998) that can be helpful for consideration by nurses when attempting to distinguish spiritual experience from psychotic experience:

- Mystical experiences, characterized by heightened awareness, a sense of oneness, and transcendence beyond the physical world

- Paranormal experiences (psychic or out-of-body) that are not consistent with Western scientific knowledge

- Charismatic experiences, which are manifestations of a spirit or divinity within an individual, such as "speaking in tongues" in the Christian faith

- Regenerative experiences, which are religious enlightenment or conversion experiences, resulting in a new way of being

Eeles and colleagues make the important point that spiritual experiences can also result from seizures, drug use, or near-death experiences. Thus, there is a need for careful assessment of the client. Moreover, they acknowledge that spiritual experiences can be "simply spiritual events innovated by the divine or through an individual's own supernatural spirit" (p. 198).

Eeles and colleagues (2003) conducted a study with a sample of mental health nurses in the United Kingdom regarding the criteria that these nurses considered significant when interpreting spiritual-type experiences reported by clients. The nurses described four main domains used to evaluate spiritual-type experiences reported by clients (pp. 200–203):

- *The outcome of the spiritual experience*: It involves whether clients could generally function well; be self-disciplined; have ordered thinking; and be grounded in reality. Assessing if relational function was present was also deemed important, that is assessing any intolerance or abuse of others as a result of the experience. The clients' ability to work or study after the experience was also assessed. The risk to health was determined, for example, if clients neglected themselves or harmed themselves. Although the nurses acknowledged that clients would likely experience distress and stress related to their mental illness, they assessed for the presence of negative emotions (e.g., excessive distress) and excessive emotions (e.g., manic elation). If the clients had a measure of peace and were reassured by the spiritual experience, then the nurses generally had less concern.

- *The nature and qualities of the experience*: That is, the form, frequency, content, and duration. For example, if the spiritual experiences were continuous, similar to familiar psychotic phenomena, and put the client "in contact" with fictitious television or movie characters; caused the person to lose control; included derogatory messages (e.g., emphasizing evil), then such outcomes were not deemed to be the characteristics of spiritual experiences.

- *The context of the experience*: That is whether the experiences were normal in terms of the client's culture (including religious culture) and if they were understandable and acceptable by someone from that culture. Consistency with the client's individual beliefs was also important to determine. If bizarre behavior occurred after the experience, then the nurses viewed this as indicative of an experience that was not spiritual in nature. The history of the client was also important to context, for example, if similar experiences had occurred in the past. Moreover, the client's present situation was of interest; for example, if the client was under significant stress, had experienced loss(es), and so on, then the nurses felt that such situations might increase vulnerability to spiritual-type experiences. Other factors concerned with context included the client's use of drugs and alcohol, sleep patterns, eating habits (particularly fasting), and meditative activities.

- *Explanatory modes*: These are based on the nurse's own spiritual beliefs and their views of plausible or possible spiritual experiences—if the client's spiritual experiences lay outside of these limits, most experiences were considered pathological. Qualities such as "being with" the client, and intuition, were also deemed to be important in distinguishing spiritual experiences from mental illness. Psychological, physical, and diagnostic interpretations were considered in explaining the experience (note that these are directly related to the nurse's knowledge base). Concurrent symptomology (e.g., hearing voices) and the possibility of co-occurrence of spiritual experiences and mental illness were also considered.

These four domains provide one example of a viable framework for the assessment of spiritual experiences. It is perhaps helpful to approach these criteria as "hypotheses to be tested" as opposed to seeing the criteria as being "set in stone." Eeles and colleagues (2003) stress the importance of realizing that what is labeled as "positive" or "negative" outcomes in client experiences is essentially value laden and interpretive, based on the nurse's subjective knowledge, beliefs, and experiences: "Reduction of personal bias is desirable to ensure beneficial treatment for patients, determining that sometimes dramatic and personally significant but essentially harmless spiritual-type experiences are not mistaken for the symptoms of mental illness" (p. 205). The nurse's capability to deal with the ambiguity in evaluating spiritual experiences and mental illness is also important. If the client's experiences are indeed considered to be delusional, then the nurse can address the delusions according to common practices regarding delusional thought and behavior. The important thing is to not "dismiss" spiritual experiences as merely "part of the pathology" and therefore ignore conducting a careful assessment of such experiences. To do this is to "[specifically focus] on particular aspects of a person's *pathology*. As such . . . they [mental health professionals] are oblivious to certain other dimensions of the person's *experience*" (Swinton, 2001, p. 170).

Reflection 8.6

Reflect on the discussion about spiritual experiences and psychotic experiences. Have you witnessed both in clients with mental illness? If so, were you able to distinguish between the two? And what factors contributed positively to your competency in this regard? If you were not able to distinguish, then what steps do you need to take in order to increase your competency in this regard?

ADDICTION/SUBSTANCE ABUSE

Addiction is one mental health disorder that has long been associated with spirituality/religion. Spirituality and religion have been linked to recovery from substance abuse. The etiology of substance abuse has also been linked to spirituality, as studies indicate that lack of meaning and purpose are intricately connected to addiction (Mohr, 2006). Some authors write about addiction as a disorder with spiritual dimensions. For example, Kurtz and Ketcham (1992) maintain that such a label enables clinicians to help see the client "apart" from the disease. Caplan (1993) terms addiction as a "spiritual disease" (p. 36), characterized by "spiritual erosion" (p. 36) in terms of the client's values, relationships, and choices. Other authors, for example, Freeman (2006) and Hodge (2011), continue to write about the intricate connection between spirituality and addiction.

The connection between spirituality/religion and addiction has been well documented in the health care literature. For example, Geppert, Bogenschutz, and Miller (2007) reported on the development of a comprehensive bibliography of the literature on spirituality and addiction, covering the period from 1941 to 2004. Common findings in this body of literature included "an inverse relationship between religiosity and substance use/abuse, reduced use among those practicing meditation, and protective effects of 12-Step group involvement during recovery" (p. 389). References for this review can be found on the website of the Center on Alcoholism, Substance Abuse, and Addiction (CASAA): www.casaa.unm.edu. Arevalo, Prado, and Amaro (2008) found in their study of women receiving substance abuse treatment that there was a negative association between perceived stress and spirituality, as well as a further negative association between posttraumatic stress symptomology and spirituality. In their article, Arevalo and colleagues discuss the Mother's Hope Mind and Spiritual Study, an evaluation of an intervention that incorporated, among other components, spiritual activities. Caplan (1993) makes the following statement about depression, which is often present in addiction: "The spiritual side of depression—despair—saps faith, hope, even the energy for life itself. The patient in despair sees the past as perpetual failure, the future as hopeless" (p. 36). Loss of self is also present in addiction and, as previously identified, lack of meaning and purpose.

As previously discussed, religious beliefs and practices are known to be deterrents to substance abuse, and there is significantly less substance abuse in people who are more religious (Hodge, 2011; Koenig, 2009; Koenig et al., 2001). However, Musick, Blazer, and Hays (2000) note that, in the case of people who are from religious traditions that promote abstinence but do engage in alcohol or drug use contrary to that upbringing, then the substance abuse can become severe and intractable. Guilt and shame can be profound, which can negatively impact their mental health. Therefore, there is a need for nurses to carefully assess the religious history of those experiencing substance abuse.

As previously mentioned in this section, spirituality/religion has interconnections with the treatment of substance abuse. In fact, the Joint Commission on the Accreditation of Health Care Organizations (JCAHCO; Hodge, 2015) has mandated the assessment of spirituality in clients engaged in substance abuse treatment. In their study of clients in outpatient substance abuse treatment centers, Miller and Saunders (2011) found that spiritual and religious functioning improved over the course of the treatment of clients, in particular in terms of their existential well-being. The results from the study also suggested that if spiritual functioning improved, then there was a concurrent improvement in alcohol misuse measures, plus alcohol-related problems once the substance abuse treatment was completed. Piacentine (2013) found that spirituality, religiosity, anxiety, depression, and drug use consequences were interrelated in persons involved in methadone maintenance therapeutic treatment. For clients in treatment for opiate use who had high or increasing spiritual well-being scores, it was found that such clients had fewer days of opiate use and were more likely to have negative urine samples for opiate use (Conner, Anglin, Annon, & Longshore, 2008).

Similarly, Heinz, Epstein, and Preston (2007) found that strongly religious participants in their study had more negative urine samples for cocaine compared to nonreligious participants. Furthermore, the study revealed that time spent on religious/spiritual activities was also found to be significant in relation to the number of negative urine samples, and also with respect to treatment retention. Heinz and colleagues (2007) also noted that spirituality increased in clients who were in a methadone maintenance program. This finding was in contrast to what was seen in the case of these same clients when they were engaged in active addiction. At that time, spirituality was in many ways replaced with addiction: There was alienation from God, and struggle around defining themselves as moral beings. For the study participants connected to a religion, adherence to organized practices was also difficult for them. Participants in this study identified spirituality as facilitating recovery in that it was a source of strength, hope, and peace. Spiritual practices such as prayer were identified as being helpful. Participants generally supported the inclusion of a spiritually oriented group in the treatment plan, and they had clear ideas about how this might be organized. Hodge (2011) came to a similar conclusion in his review of the literature that many clients who have alcohol dependence want spirituality/religion to be included in their treatment plan.

There is also indication that it is not only clients but also health care professionals who want spirituality to be part of substance abuse programs. For example, Forman, Bovasso, and Woody (2001) found that 84% of the addiction treatment professionals believed that spirituality should receive greater emphasis in the treatment of clients with addiction.

There are many substance abuse treatment programs that intentionally incorporate spirituality/religion into their treatment philosophies and plans. Perhaps the best known are the 12-step programs, such as Alcoholics Anonymous (AA) and Narcotics Anonymous (NA). Spirituality is explicitly foundational to these programs, for example, in the guiding principle that encourages people with substance abuse problems to submit to a "higher power" or "God" (Ward, 2011). Furthermore, Carrico, Gifford, and Moos (2007) and Atkins and Hawdon (2007) identify that spirituality and religiosity serve to promote involvement in these programs. Noted in the research and literature is that outcomes of such programs have also been connected to a person's spirituality. Examples of such outcomes include an increase in meaning and purpose in life; the capacity to forgive; the ability to accept and love oneself; and a greater contentment with life (Ameling & Povilonis, 2001; Dadich, 2007; O'Reilly, 2004).

Chen (2006) compared two 1-year programs that were both directed at inmates who were recovering addicts. One program included both social support and spirituality (12-step), and the other program was primarily support based. Participants in the program that included both explicit spirituality and support demonstrated a higher "sense of coherence" and meaning in life, as well as a gradual decrease in the intensity of such negative emotions as anxiety, depression, and hostility. The definition of "sense of coherence" that Chen used for this study was taken from that of Antonovsky (1979), who described this concept as "a global orientation that expresses the extent to which one has a pervasive enduring though dynamic feeling of confidence that one's internal and external environments are predictable" (Antonovsky, 1979, p. 19, quoted in Chen, p. 306).

Other types of treatment programs that have incorporated spirituality have reported positive outcomes related to substance use. For example, a sample of participants in a faith-based residential rehabilitation substance abuse facility identified spirituality/religion to be useful components of the program. Spirituality was seen as helpful in diminishing cravings for a substance and also in increasing clients' self-efficacy, and also associated with a decrease in cravings (Mason, Deane, Kelly, & Crowe, 2009). Hodge (2011) describes and illustrates a three-step process to develop spiritually modified cognitive behavioral therapy (CBT) for clients with alcoholism. Instrumental in the decision to develop this program were Hodge's conclusions from the research on the incorporation of spirituality into CBT. Those conclusions were that spirituality had the potential to facilitate and speed recovery, to enhance compliance to treatment, to decrease relapse rates, and to ensure culturally relevant services. Hodge wrote the article with the intent of orienting clinicians to spiritually modified CBT, including suggestions for working with clients' spirituality in an ethical manner. Delaney, Forcehimes, Campbell, and Smith (2009) also write about how clinicians can address spirituality in addiction treatment, using a case study to illustrate this process.

Reflection 8.7

Why do you think that 12-step programs might be so helpful to those experiencing addiction and substance abuse? If you were developing a program that seeks to focus on clients' spirituality/religion and the interface with substance abuse, what aspects might you include in such a program and why?

This section of the chapter has focused on a discussion of spirituality/religion in common mental illnesses. Other mental health conditions have also been discussed in the literature with respect to their connection with spirituality/religion. Examples include borderline personality disorder (Gravitt, 2011), recovery from childhood sexual abuse (Draucker et al., 2014; Walsh, Fortier, & DiLillo, 2010), and trauma (Bidwell, 2002; Meisenhelder, 2002; Paquette, 2008; Pearson, 2009). There is also much written in the health care literature about the intersection of spirituality/religion with respect to mental health problems in children and adolescents. Reference to materials focusing on other mental health illnesses and conditions not discussed in this chapter, as well as reference to the literature on children and adolescents, is recommended.

SPIRITUAL ASSESSMENT AND SPIRITUAL CARE IN MENTAL ILLNESS

Some of the discussion in this chapter has identified some implications for spiritual assessment and spiritual care in mental health contexts, for example, the importance of including a spiritual/religious history in the assessment of clients, and the importance of including spirituality into the care of clients. This section focuses on spiritual assessment and spiritual care within the context of mental health care/mental health nursing.

There has been discussion in the health care literature about distrust and bias against religion by mental health professionals, for example, Chandler (2012). There has also been discussion about how mental illness is viewed by health professionals, and how their perceptions will then have implications for spiritual care. For example, Lakeman (2013) argues that an evidence-based scientific view has dominated perceptions of mental illness: that such illness is a biological disorder. This, in turn, impacts how mental health care is delivered. Comparisons have also been made regarding differences between a medical orientation and a spiritual orientation to clients with mental health issues (Cheney, Galanter, Dermatis, & Ross, 2009). The notion that some mental health care professionals experience discomfort in addressing spirituality/religion with clients has also been discussed (Beebe & Speraw, 2011), an assertion that is not restricted to the mental health context. There have been efforts made to educate and assist mental health professionals to intentionally incorporate spirituality/religion into the care of clients (see Clarke, 2010). Plante (2009) also wrote a book that provides practical guidance to mental health clinicians in incorporating spirituality into psychotherapy. Beebe and Speraw (2011) comment on Plante's work: "[The book is] . . . grounded in science, practical in its applications, enhanced by liberal case examples and vignettes, and targeted to mental health professionals who respect the fact that many of their clients have concerns with religious-spiritual dimensions" (p. 549). Reference to both Clarke's and Plante's books is recommended.

As in other contexts of care, sensitive and ethical spiritual assessment is important in mental health nursing. Some of the spiritual assessment models/tools discussed in Chapter 5 have been explicitly endorsed for use with clients who have mental illness. For example, Ameling and Povilonis (2001) discuss use of the FICA approach (Puchalski & Romer, 2000); Baetz and Toews (2009) identify the HOPE approach (Anandarajah & Hight, 2001) as being useful; and O'Reilly (2004) discusses the SPIRITual History Tool (Maugens, 1996). Based on a review of spiritual assessment tools, Raffay (2013) concludes that many of the existing spiritual assessment tools have not been validated on a psychiatric population, suggesting the need for further work in this regard. No matter which tool is used or what questions are asked of clients, the following are examples of important foci for assessment in clients with mental illness (Edward et al., 2004; Eeles et al., 2003; Koenig, 2009, 2005; Musick et al., 2000; Pesut et al., 2011; Scharf, 2007):

- Factors contributing to resilience, including spiritual/religious factors

- Religious/spiritual activities and rituals important to clients, including how they are helpful

- Religious/spiritual beliefs, including the assessment of distortion of beliefs

- The clients' spiritual and religious history, including history of spiritual/religious experiences and distinguishing such experiences from psychotic experiences

As in other contexts of care, the client's family may play an integral part in the client's assessment, in particular if the client is actively psychotic or delusional.

With respect to spiritual care, Baetz and Toews (2009) emphasize the importance of the clinician synthesizing research on religion/spirituality in mental illness from various orientations, such as cognitive, social, and biological orientations. In that fashion, the research is made applicable to client care. The discussion by Baetz and Toews in this regard is worth reviewing. Also important to consider are teachings common to major world religions that promote good mental health such as altruism, gratitude, love, and forgiveness. Such concepts can be incorporated into various interventions. Moreover, the importance of religion/spirituality as a positive or negative factor in coping with mental illness must be recognized and appreciated (Baetz & Toews, 2009).

Reflection 8.8

Based on the discussion so far about spirituality/religion and mental illness, develop a number of spiritual assessment questions that nurses need to ask themselves in assessing clients (if possible, discuss these with peers/colleagues and revise or modify the questions as needed. Then, develop assessment questions that you can ask clients, based on the initial set of questions developed. Pilot these questions with clients and, if necessary, revise them).

As in the case of spiritual assessment, there can be complexities associated with providing spiritual care in a mental health context, for example, incorporating spirituality/religion in a manner that takes into account the client's mental health status. The client's delusions, thought processes, suicidal tendencies, and so on impact the process of spiritual assessment and intervention, perhaps delaying it until the client's mental health improves. As purported in previous chapters in this book, being client centered, working from the client's perspective, is essential.

There are some models that can guide the process of providing spiritual care in this setting. For example, Morris (1996) discusses a spiritual well-being model that can be helpful to nurses in the spiritual assessment and treatment of women with depression. Kilmer and Lane-Tillerson (2013) describe use of the Tidal Model (Barker & Buchanan-Barker, 2005) with clients who had attempted suicide. This model is client centered and has "spiritual truths" (Kilmer & Lane-Tillerson, 2013, p. 101) embedded within it. Group-oriented strategies can also be helpful. The 12-step programs have been discussed already, but discussion groups focused on spirituality can also be helpful. For example, Moller (1999) conducted two such spirituality discussion groups with clients hospitalized on a psychiatric unit and who were admitted because of psychosis. One discussion group focused on the meaning of spirituality/religion to those participating in the group; the other group focused on what they perceived was needed from their religious leader/spiritual resource to help them spiritually while they were in hospital. From these discussions, the group leaders were able to understand psychosis from a spiritual perspective. They were also able to identify what might be helpful to clients. Although the second discussion group focused on the desired help from religious leaders/spiritual resources, the clients' responses would also be relevant for nurses; for example, clients identified being listened to, accepted, and cared for and cared about. Psychotherapy, a common approach in mental health care and mental health nursing, has also been of focus with respect to incorporating spirituality into this approach. For example, Sperry (2012) writes of spiritual-oriented psychotherapy, identifying it as an approach that attends to clients' spiritual concerns and that incorporates spiritual activities. Ameling and Povilonis (2001) identify the power of spirituality in mental health care when they state:

> [T]he language of spirituality provides a way of talking about such things as meaning and purpose. It also provides a way to talk about how the search for meaning affects the lives of the people for whom nurses care. When people are asked to talk about their spirituality, they often speak of that which enlivens, empowers, or motivates them. These are powerful and meaningful concepts in peoples' lives that can, in appropriate cases, be incorporated into mental health treatment. (p. 19)

Many of the spiritual care interventions discussed in Chapter 6 have been identified to be of assistance to clients with mental illness. For example, O'Reilly (2004) identifies generic spiritual care as being helpful to clients with mental illness. O'Reilly also stresses the importance of exploration of the content and meaning of religious delusions and hallucinations as a means of encouraging further discussion with clients. For example, if the content of a delusion or hallucination suggests a spiritual need that the client may have, then this need can be validated and addressed once the client is able to engage in such a process. The nurse can also support any spiritual or religious beliefs and interactions that are based in reality (O'Reilly). La Torre (2004) discusses the use of prayer in therapy. Luk (2011) describes the use of spiritual interventions (Christian in nature) with clients with severe mental illness. Meditation, intentional strategies to help clients develop and maintain meaning and purpose, strategies to foster hope, and the use of narratives may all be beneficial.

The use of metaphors has been identified as being of particular interest in mental health contexts as clients often interpret their spiritual needs by expressing them in metaphors. An example of such a metaphor is when a client says, "I feel very dirty," which can express a guilty feeling (Borin et al., 1983, p. 41; Koslander, da Silva, & Roxberg, 2009). The nurse can then use this metaphor to help the client explore his or her guilt.

It should be remembered that focusing on the families of clients with mental illness is imperative. Often, familial relationships are instrumental in a client's healing. Family members can also provide valuable information about the client's spiritual beliefs, needs, and practices, particularly when the client is not able to provide such information. Supporting the family throughout the client's illness is also crucial.

Spiritual assessment and interventions may be quite important in facilitating wellness in clients with mental illness. As nurses understand what is meaningful and important to clients and address it in their nursing care, the relationship between the nurse and the client can be strengthened. If the client is confused about reality or quite ill in other regards, then generic spiritual care may be the best course of action at that time. No nurse should advocate spiritual or religious practices in lieu of conventional treatments. Nor should nurses promote any personal agendas or their own spiritual values and practices upon clients. Nurses should never impose spiritual interventions when clients are in vulnerable mental states. They should keep abreast of the debates and research on useful spiritual/religious practices in mental health care, taking care not to misrepresent the state of research in this area. Religious/spiritual goals and interventions should be pursued only if clients have expressed a desire for them. Compliance with all the foregoing is essential to safeguard ethical practice (Mohr, 2006). There is ample rationale supportive of spiritual assessment and intervention being incorporated into mental health nursing practice. It is only then that the holistic care deemed to be critical to mental health care can be realized (Koslander & Arvidsson, 2007).

Reflection 8.9

From your clinical practice and experience, why is it important to have a family-oriented perspective when working with clients with mental illness? What spiritual/religious issues have you noticed within such families? Have they been addressed by health care professionals? If not, why not? How can nurses and other health care professionals adopt a family-oriented perspective in this context of care?

Taking It Further

1. Read the case studies as presented in O'Reilly (2004, pp. 49–50).

   a. What is your appraisal of the nurse's actions in each case scenario?

   b. Would you find it challenging to interact with any of these clients in terms of spiritual assessment and spiritual care? If so, why might this be so? And how can you deal with the challenge(s)?

   c. How does addressing the spiritual domain complement addressing other domains of the person in each scenario?

2. Read the case study of Trudy in La Torre (2004, pp. 39–40).

   a. How might the idea of prayer as a spiritual resource be ideally addressed in a spiritual assessment with Trudy? What specific questions might have been asked of her?

   b. How was the idea of prayer introduced by the nurse in this scenario? What is your appraisal of such an introduction?

   c. How might a discussion of the place of prayer proceed with Trudy? What aspects of prayer might be explored and how? Draft some examples of questions that would explore these aspects of prayer with Trudy.

d. Refer to guidelines for the use of prayer (see section on Prayer as Intervention in Chapter 6). As far as you can ascertain, and based on the information in the case study, which guidelines were followed by the nurse in this scenario?

e. Would you consider exploring the place of prayer in a person's life in an assessment? Why or why not?

f. Would you be comfortable in including prayer in your care of clients such as Trudy? Why or why not? If you would not be comfortable in actively participating in prayer with clients, then what appropriate action(s) might you take?

g. What specific issues or concerns does a nurse have to consider with respect to the use of prayer in a mental health nursing context?

3. Read the case studies in Morris (1996, pp. 447–450).

a. What indicators of spiritual needs are present in each case scenario? Use the model presented by Morris (p. 443) to assist you in determining these needs.

b. Compare the list of spiritual needs that you generated with those that were identified by Morris at the end of each case study.

c. How might you address each of the spiritual needs identified (those identified by yourself and/or those identified by Morris)? Compare your response with the discussion by Morris (pp. 451–453).

d. How might the model in Morris be useful in other contexts of mental health nursing practice?

4. Read the case study of Elizabeth in Delaney and colleagues (2009, pp. 193–196).

a. How did an assessment of Elizabeth's spiritual history inform the treatment plan?

b. Appraise the discussion between the therapist and Elizabeth regarding the hypothesis that spiritual practices might be of benefit to Elizabeth.

c. Would you have approached this topic with Elizabeth differently than the therapist had done? How so, and why?

d. Note the short-term and long-term outcomes of the therapist focusing on Elizabeth's spiritual resources. How do these outcomes encourage you to incorporate spiritual resources into mental health nursing practice?

5. Consider the following clients whom you might encounter in a mental health setting:

- A client who has neglected himself and abused family members because of substance abuse

- A client who is rude and demanding because of her mental illness

- A young adult who self-injures by cutting herself and has no desire to get better

- A man with schizophrenia who has used acid to scrub his body to remove perceived bugs from his skin, which is sore and rotting

- A young mother who is admitted with her newborn because of postpartum depression

- A man who is addicted to cocaine and seems to have no desire to stop using the drug

Taking and considering each of the above possible clients:

a. How might such scenarios impact you emotionally, physically, and spiritually?

b. What can be helpful to enable you to provide compassionate and holistic care in such situations?

c. How might you respond to the person in each scenario?

d. How might nursing codes of ethics be helpful in encountering such clients?

e. What personal spiritual/religious beliefs do you have that might be helpful in encountering such clients? (Adapted from Hoglund, 2013)

6. Read the case study of a client admitted to the hospital for detoxification from drugs and alcohol in Taylor (2011, pp. 200–201).

a. If you were the nurse receiving the report from the prior shift about this client (paragraph 1), then what thoughts, feelings, and concerns might you have about meeting him?

b. What do you think was the rationale for the nurse taking the blood pressure equipment to the room rather than the usual practice of having the client come outside of the room to have his blood pressure checked (paragraph 2)?

c. What is your appraisal of how the nurse handled the issue of giving the client medication (paragraph 3)?

d. What actions/words of the nurse caused the client to say, "You're the first person who seems to give a damn" (paragraph 4)?

e. How did the nurse facilitate disclosure from the client? What did she say or do that encouraged the client to talk to the nurse (consider the entire case study in your reflection on these questions)?

f. How did the nurse broach the topic of faith/spirituality with the client? Was it appropriate? Why or why not?

g. How did the nurse facilitate conversation about spiritual matters? Was it appropriate? Why or why not?

h. What were the indications of spiritual distress in the client?

i. What is your appraisal of the appropriateness of the nurse's self-disclosure regarding her personal faith perspective?

j. In your opinion, was it an appropriate action for the nurse to offer to get a Bible and to pray for/with the client? Why or why not?

k. This entire scenario took place within one evening shift. What does this suggest to you about spiritual care?

l. How might the nurse's perspective and beliefs about nursing impact how she approaches and relates to clients (last paragraph)?

m. How are the ethical guidelines in Taylor (pp. 197–198) illustrated throughout this case study? Give specific examples.

n. What insights have you gained from reflecting on this case study that can be of help to you in your clinical practice with clients with mental health problems?

7. Read the two case studies in Cox (2003) of J (p. 32) and S (pp. 32–33).

a. What information in each case study would support a diagnosis of spiritual distress?

b. How did the assessment of each client incorporate aspects of spirituality?

c. What spiritual needs can you identify in each client?

d. Appraise the nursing interventions directed at meeting the clients' spiritual needs. Would you have added other interventions? If so, then what would they be? And why would you incorporate these into the care of each client?

e. What client outcomes support the efficacy of the spiritually based interventions?

f. What part did culture play with respect to possible interventions in each of the case studies?

g. What aspects of Roger's nursing theory are evident in each case study?

8. Read the case study of Iona in Dombeck (1996, pp. 69–70).

a. What spiritual needs are evident in this scenario? What information is given to support each need?

b. What signs of spiritual disequilibrium are evident?

c. How might you address Iona's spiritual issues? Compare your ideas for intervention with Dombeck's ideas (p. 70; pp. 72–73).

9. Read the case study of Debbie in Agrimson and Taft (2008, pp. 457–458).

a. Imagine that you were a nurse who encounters Debbie at the point where Debbie is realizing that her marriage is not happy but that she is choosing to stay in the marriage for the reasons given. How might you work with Debbie at that point in her life to impact positively on her mental health?

b. Imagine that you are a nurse who encounters Debbie shortly after her son's death. How might you work with her at this point to deal with her depression and suicidal thoughts?

c. Use the information in Table 1 (p. 458) on the antecedents and defining attributes of spiritual crisis to identify any spiritual crisis that you might have experienced (or are currently experiencing) in your own life. How did you (or can you) deal with such a crisis?

d. Appraise the potential for the discussion on the concept of spiritual crisis in this article to inform your clinical practice with respect to assessing for spiritual crisis.

10. In Shelly and John (1983) read the scenarios of Linda (pp. 56—just the conversation between the nurse and Linda), Donna (p. 57—just the first two paragraphs of the case scenario, ending your reading at the end of Donna's statement), and Mike (pp. 58–59—just to the end of Mike's statement on p. 59).

   a. From the information that you read about each of these persons, what spiritual needs are suggested? What information supports the identification of those needs? Compare your needs appraisal with the commentary by the authors in each scenario.

   b. In the case of Linda, what is your appraisal of the nurse's comment: "Do you ever think about the fact that God loves you and accepts you just the way you are?" (p. 56) What would the nurse need to know about Linda in order for this comment to be appropriate?

   c. How might you respond to Donna's statement? To what aspect(s) in the statement would you respond first; and why? Formulate a number of responses (in actual words) that you could make to Donna, and choose the one that you think is the best. Are there other aspects that you would want to explore, perhaps further in the conversation? If so, then what would these be?

   d. How might you respond to Mike's last statement? Formulate a number of responses (in actual words) and choose the one that you think is the best.

   e. In each of these scenarios, how might the information presented assist the nurse in formulating interventions for each client?

11. Read the case study of Mrs. Thomas in Shelly and John (1983, pp. 88–92).

   a. What do you know about Mrs. Thomas's religious tradition (Pentecostalism)? If you need to, then it would be advisable to research the main tenets of this religious tradition.

   b. Comments about Janet's (the nurse) assessment of Mrs. Thomas are provided in the case study. What questions do you think that Janet may have asked Mrs. Thomas in order to obtain this information? What were the foci of the assessment?

   c. Appraise the care plan that Janet and the team developed for Mrs. Thomas. Does it appear that this plan was well individualized to this particular client? What is the rationale for your response?

   d. Read the principles of spiritual care planning and intervention provided by Shelly and John (pp. 85–86). Identify how the case study of Mrs. Thomas illustrates these principles.

   e. If you were a nurse caring for Mrs. Thomas, what personal or professional challenges might you face? How would you address these challenges?

12. Read the following vignettes in Shelly and John (1983): (a) Larry, Donald, and Gail (p. 63); (b) Rosa, Judy, Jeff, and Andy (pp. 66–67; (c) Bruce (p. 68); and (d) Fred, Trish, Tim, and Cindy (pp. 68–69).

   a. These clients are all connected in some way to the Christian faith but in each, there is evidence of distorted or unhealthy religious beliefs. Research information about the concepts described in relation to each of these clients from the Christian worldview—for example, sin, guilt, forgiveness, view of God's control in one's life, view of self as a person, and concept of suffering.

   b. How might you respond to each of these clients? What might you say to them to address the issue of distorted or unhealthy beliefs?

   c. What challenges might each of these clients pose for you personally and professionally? How might you deal with such challenges?

REFERENCES

Agrimson, L. B., & Taft, L. B. (2008). Spiritual crisis: A concept analysis. *Journal of Advanced Nursing, 65*(2), 454–461. doi:10.1111/j.1365-2648.2008.04869.x

Aldwin, C. M. (2007). *Stress, coping, and development* (2nd ed.). New York, NY: Guilford Press.

Ameling, A., & Povilonis, M. (2001). Spirituality: Meaning, mental health and nursing. *Journal of Psychosocial Nursing and Mental Health Services, 39*(4), 15–20. doi:10.3928/0279-3695-20010401-08

Anandarajah, G., & Hight, E. (2001). Spirituality and medical practice: Using the HOPE questions as a practical tool for spiritual assessment. *American Family Physician, 63*(1), 81–89.

Antonovsky, A. (1979). *Health, stress, and coping: New perspectives on mental and physical well-being*. San Francisco, CA: Jossey-Bass.

Arevalo, S., Prado, G., & Amaro, H. (2008). Spirituality, sense of coherence, and coping responses in women receiving treatment for alcohol and drug addiction. *Evaluation and Program Planning, 31*(1), 113–123. doi:10.1016/j.evalprogplan.2007.05.009

Atkins, R. G., & Hawdon, J. E. (2007). Religiosity and participation in mutual-aid support groups for addiction. *Journal of Substance Abuse Treatment, 33*(3), 321–331. doi:10.1016/j.jsat2007.07.001

Baetz, M., & Toews, J. (2009). Clinical implications of research on religion, spirituality, and mental health. *Canadian Journal of Psychiatry, 54*(5), 292–301.

Barker, P., & Buchanan-Barker, P. (2005). *The Tidal Model: A guide for mental health professionals*. East Sussex, England: Brunner-Routledge.

Beebe, L. H., & Speraw, S. (2011). Book review: Spiritual practices in psychotherapy: Thirteen tools for enhancing psychological health. *Issues in Mental Health Nursing, 32*(8), 549. doi:10.3109/0161 2840.2011.587939

Bidwell, D. R. (2002). Developing an adequate "pneumatraumatology": Understanding the spiritual impacts of traumatic injury. *The Journal of Pastoral Care and Counseling, 56*(2), 135–143. doi:10.1177/ 154230500205600204

Bowen, R., Baetz, M., & D'Arcy, C. (2006). Self-rated importance of religion predicts one year outcome of patients with panic disorder. *Depression & Anxiety, 23*(5), 266–273. doi:10.1002/da .20157

Buswell, J., Clegg, A., Grant, F., Grout, G., Minardi, H. A., & Morgan, A. (2006). Ask the experts: Spirituality in care. *Nursing Older People, 18*(1), 14–15. doi:10.7748/nop2006.02.18.1.14.c2408

Caplan, P. S. (1993). Addiction as a spiritual disease. *Addict Recovery, 13*(6), 36–37.

Carrico, A. W., Gifford, E. V., & Moos, R. H. (2007). Spirituality/religiosity promotes acceptance-based responding and 12-step involvement. *Drug and Alcohol Dependence, 89*(1), 66–73. doi:10.1016/j .drugalcdep.2006.12.004

Chandler, E. (2012). Religious and spiritual issues in DSM-5: Matters of the mind and searching of the soul. *Issues in Mental Health Nursing, 33*(9), 577–582. doi:10.3109/01612840.2012.704130

Chen, G. (2006). Social support, spiritual program, and addiction. *International Journal of Offender Therapy and Comparative Criminology, 50*(3), 306–323. doi:10.1177/0306624X05279038

Cheney, B., Galanter, M., Dermatis, H., & Ross, S. (2009). Medical versus spiritual orientations: Differential patient views toward recovery. *The American Journal of Drug and Alcohol Abuse, 35*(5), 301–304. doi:10.1080/00952990903060119

Clarke, I. (2010). *Psychosis and spirituality: Consolidating the new paradigm* (2nd ed.). Chichester, England: Wiley-Blackwell.

Conner, B. T., Anglin, M. D., Annon, J., & Longshore, D. (2008). Effect of religiosity and spirituality on drug treatment outcomes. *Journal of Behavioral Health Services & Research, 36*(2), 189–198. doi:10.1007/s11414-008-9145-z

Cox, T. (2003). Theory and exemplars of advanced practice spiritual intervention. *Complementary Therapies in Nursing and Midwifery, 9*(1), 30–34. doi:10.1016/S1353-6117(02)00103-8

Dadich, A. (2007). Is spirituality important to young people in recovery? Insights from participants of self-help support groups. *Southern Medical Journal, 100*(4), 422–425. doi:10.1097/SMJ.0b013e318031611a

Delaney, H. D., Forcehimes, A. A., Campbell, W. P., & Smith, B. W. (2009). Integrating spirituality into alcohol treatment. *Journal of Clinical Psychology, 65*(2), 185–198. doi:10.1002/jclp.20566

Dervic, K., Oquendo, M. A., Grunebaum, M. F., Ellis, S., Burke, A. K., & Mann, J. J. (2004). Religious affiliation and suicide attempt. *American Journal of Psychiatry, 161*(12), 2303–2308. doi:10.1176/appi.ajp.161.12.2303

Dombeck, M. B. (1996). Chaos and self-organization as a consequence of spiritual disequilibrium. *Clinical Nurse Specialist, 10*(2), 69–73.

Donovan, P. (1998). *Interpreting religious experience.* Oxford, England: Religious Experience Research Centre.

Draucker, C. B., Martsolf, D. S., Roller, C., Knapik, G., Ross, R., & Stidham, A. W. (2014). Healing from childhood sexual abuse: A theoretical model. *Journal of Child Sexual Abuse, 20*(4), 435–466. doi:10.1080/10538712.2001.588188

Edward, K., Welch, A., & Chater, K. (2009). The phenomenon of resilience as described by adults who have experienced mental illness. *Journal of Advanced Nursing, 65*(3), 587–595. doi:10.1111/j.1365-2648.2008.04912.x

Eeles, J., Lowe, T., & Wellman, N. (2003). Spirituality or psychosis? An exploration of the criteria that nurses use to evaluate spiritual-type experiences reported by patients. *International Journal of Nursing Studies, 40*(2), 197–206. doi:10.1016/S0020-7489(02)00061-5

Folkman, S. (2008). The case for positive emotions in the stress process. *Anxiety, Stress, & Coping, 21*(1), 3–14. doi:10.1080/10615800701740457

Forman, R. E., Bovasso, G., & Woody, G. (2001). Staff beliefs about addiction treatment. *Journal of Substance Abuse Treatment, 21*(1), 1–9. doi:10.1016/S0740-5472(01)00173-8

Freeman, D. R. (2006). Spirituality in violent and substance-abusing African American men: An untapped resource for healing. *Journal of Religion and Spirituality in Social Work, 25*(1), 3–22. doi:10.1300/J377v25n01_02

Geppert, C., Bogenschutz, M. P., & Miller, W. R. (2007). Development of a bibliography on religion, spirituality and addictions. *Drug and Alcohol Review, 26*(4), 389–395. doi:10.1080/09595230701373826

Gravitt, W. J. (2011). God's ruthless embrace: Religious belief in three women with borderline personality disorder. *Issues in Mental Health Care, 32*(5), 301–317. doi:10.3109/01612840.2010.558234

Heinz, A., Epstein, D. H., & Preston, K. L. (2007). Spiritual/religious experiences and in-treatment outcome in an inner-city program for heroin and cocaine dependence. *Journal of Psychoactive Drugs, 39*(1), 41–49. doi:10.1080/02791072.2007.10399863

Hodge, D. R. (2011). Alcohol treatment and cognitive–behavioral therapy: Enhancing effectiveness by incorporating spirituality and religion. *Social Work, 56*(1), 21–31. Retrieved from http://sw.oxfordjournals.org/content/56/1/21.full.pdf

Hodge, D. R. (2015). *Spiritual assessment in social work and mental health practice.* New York, NY: Columbia University Press.

Hoglund, B. A. (2013). Practicing the code of ethics, finding the image of God. *Journal of Christian Nursing, 30*(4), 228–233. doi:10.1097/CNJ.0b013e3182a18d40

Huguelet, P., Borras, L., Gillieron, C., Brandt, P. Y., & Mohr, S. (2009). Influence of spirituality and religiousness on substance misuse in patients with schizophrenia and schizo-affective disorder. *Substance Use and Misuse, 44*(4), 502–513. doi:10.1080/10826080802344872

Huguelet, P., Mohr, S., Borras, L., Gillieron, C., & Brandt, P. (2006). Spirituality and religious practices among outpatients with schizophrenia and their clinicians. *Psychiatric Services, 57*(3), 366–372. doi:10.1176/appi.ps.57.3.366

Hultsjo, S., & Blomqvist, K. B. (2013). Health behaviors as conceptualized by individuals diagnosed with a psychotic disorder. *Issues in Mental Health Nursing, 34*(9), 665–672. doi:10.3109/01612840.2013.794178

John, S. D. (1983). Healthy and unhealthy religious beliefs. In J. A. Shelly & S. D. John (Eds.), *Spiritual dimensions of mental health* (pp. 61–71). Downers Grove, IL: InterVarsity Press

Jones, E. (2010). Suicide prevention through stories of hope. *Journal of Christian Nursing, 27*(3), 252–257. doi:10.1097/CNJ.0b013e3181df8012

Kalischuk, R. G., & Davies, B. (2001). A theory of healing in the aftermath of youth suicide. *Journal of Holistic Nursing, 19*(2), 163–186. doi:10.1177/089801010101900206

Kaplan, K., & Schwartz, M. (2008). *A psychology of hope: A biblical response to tragedy and suicide* (Rev. and expanded ed.). Grand Rapids, MI: Eerdmans.

Keltner, N. L. (2005). Whatever became of sin? Revisiting Menninger's question. *Perspectives in Psychiatric Care, 41*(3), 142–145. doi:10.1111/j.1744-6163.2005.00027.x

Kilmer, D. L., & Lane-Tillerson, C. (2013). When still waters become a soul tsunami: Using the Tidal Model to recover from shipwreck. *Journal of Christian Nursing, 30*(2), 100–104. doi:10.1097/CNJ.0b013e31825b8d73

Koenig, H. G. (1997). *Is religion good for your health? The effects of religion on physical and mental health.* London, England: Routledge.

Koenig, H. G. (2005). *Faith and mental health: Religious resources for healing.* West Conshohocken, PA: Templeton Foundation Press.

Koenig, H. G. (2007). Religion and depression in older medical inpatients. *American Journal of Geriatric Psychiatry, 15*(4), 282–291.

Koenig, H. G. (2009). Research on religion, spirituality and mental health: A review. *Canadian Journal of Psychiatry, 54*(5), 283–291.

Koenig, H. G., McCullough, M. E., & Larson, D. B. (2001). *Handbook of religion and health.* New York, NY: Oxford University Press.

Koslander, T., & Arvidsson, B. (2007). Patients' conceptions of how the spiritual dimension is addressed in mental health care: A qualitative study. *Journal of Advanced Nursing, 57*(6), 597–604. doi:10.1111/j.1365-2648.2006.04190.x

Koslander, T., da Silva, A. B., & Roxberg, A. (2009). Existential and spiritual needs in mental health care: An ethical and holistic perspective. *Journal of Holistic Nursing, 27*(1), 34–42. doi:10.1177/0898010108323302

Kurtz, E., & Ketcham, K. (1992). *The spirituality of imperfection.* New York, NY: Bantum Books.

Lakeman, R. (2013). Talking science and wishing for miracles: Understanding cultures of mental health practice. *International Journal of Mental Health Nursing, 22*(2), 106–115. doi:10.1111/j.1447-0349.2012.00847.x

Landeen, J., Pawlick, J., Woodside, H., Kirkpatrick, H., & Byrne, C. C. (2000). Hope, quality of life, and symptom severity in individuals with schizophrenia. *Psychiatric Rehabilitation Journal, 23*(4), 364–369. doi:10.1037/h0095142

La Torre, M. A. (2004). Prayer in psychotherapy: An important consideration. *Perspectives in Psychiatric Care, 40*(1), 2–40. doi:10.1111/j.1744-6163.2004.00002.x

Luk, A. L. (2011). Investigating the long-term effects of a psychiatric rehabilitation programme for persons with serious mental illness in the community: A follow-up study. *Journal of Clinical Nursing, 20*(19–20), 2712–2720. doi:10.1111/j.1365-2702.2010.03622.x

Mason, S. J., Deane, F. P., Kelly, P., & Crowe, T. P. (2009). Do spirituality and religiosity help in the management of cravings in substance abuse treatment? *Substance Use & Misuse, 44*(13), 1926–1940. doi:10.3109/10826080802486723

Maugens, T. A. (1996). The SPIRITual history. *Archives of Family Medicine, 5*(1), 11–16. doi:10.1001/archfami.5.1.11

Meisenhelder, J. B. (2002). Terrorism, posttraumatic stress, and religious coping. *Issues in Mental Health Nursing, 23*(8), 771–782. doi:10.1080/01612840260433659

Mental Health Foundation. (1999). *The courage to bare our souls: A collection of pieces written out of mental distress.* London, England: Mental Health Foundation.

Michalak, E. E., Yatham, L. N., Kolesar, S., & Lam, R. W. (2006). Bipolar disorder and quality of life: A patient-centered perspective. *Quality of Life Research: An International Journal of Quality of Life Aspects of Treatment, Care and Rehabilitation, 15*(1), 25–37. doi:10.1007/s11136-005-0376-7

Miller, M. L., & Saunders, S. M. (2011). A naturalistic study of the associations between changes in alcohol problems, spiritual functioning, and psychiatric symptoms. *Psychology of Addictive Behaviors, 25*(3), 455–461. doi:10.1037/a0022224

Mohr, S., Gillieron, C., Borras, L., Brandt, P., & Huguelet, P. (2007). The assessment of spirituality and religiousness in schizophrenia. *Journal of Nervous & Mental Disease, 195*(3), 247–253. doi:10.1097/01.nmd.0000258230.94304.6b

Mohr, W. K. (2006). Spiritual issues in psychiatric care. *Perspectives in Psychiatric Care, 43*(3), 174–183. doi:10.1111/j.1744-6163.2006.00076.x

Moller, M. D. (1999). Meeting spiritual needs on an inpatient unit: Patients and family members speak out. *Journal of Psychosocial Nursing, 37*(11), 5–10. doi:10.3928/0279-3695-19991101-04

Morris, E. H. (1996). A spiritual well-being model: Use with older women who experience depression. *Issues in Mental Health Nursing, 17*(5), 439–455. doi:10.3109/01612849609009412

Musick, M. A., Blazer, D. G., & Hays, J. C. (2000). Religious activity, alcohol use and depression in a sample of elderly Baptists. *Research on Aging, 22*(2), 91–116. doi:10.1177/0164027500222001

Narayanasamy, A. (1991). *Spiritual care: A resource guide.* London, England: Central Health Studies, BKT Information Services & Quay.

Narayanasamy, A. (1999). ASSET: A model for actioning spirituality and spiritual care training in nursing. *Nurse Education Today, 19*(4), 274–285. doi:10.1054/nedt.1999.0637

Oliffe, J. L., Ogrodniczuk, J. S., Bottorff, J. L., Johnson, J. L., & Hoyak, K. (2012). "You feel like you can't live anymore": Suicide from the perspectives of Canadian men who experience depression. *Social Science & Medicine, 74*(4), 506–514. doi:10.1016/j.socscimed.2010.03.057

O'Reilly, M. l. (2004). Spirituality and mental health clients. *Journal of Psychosocial Nursing, 42*(7), 44–53.

Paquette, M. (2008). The aftermath of war: Spiritual distress. *Perspectives in Psychiatric Care, 44*(3), 143–145. doi:10.1111/j.1744-6163.2008.00168.x

Park, C. L., & Folkman, S. (1997). Meaning in the context of stress and coping. *Review of General Psychology, 1*(2), 115–144. doi:10.1037/1089-2680.1.2.115

Pearson, G. S. (2009). When to forgive. *Perspectives in Psychiatric Care, 45*(3), 159–160. doi:10.1111/j.1744-6163.2009.00217.x

Pesut, B., Clark, N., Maxwell, V., & Michalak, E. E. (2011). Religion and spirituality in the context of bipolar disorder: A literature review. *Mental Health, Religion & Culture, 14*(8), 785–796. doi:10.1080/13674676.2010.523890

Peterson, E. A., & Nelson, K. (1987). How to meet your client's spiritual needs. *Journal of Psychosocial Nursing, 25*(5), 34–39.

Phillips, R. E., & Stein, C. H. (2007). God's will, God's punishment, or God's limitations: Religious coping strategies reported by young adults living with serious mental illness. *Journal of Clinical Psychology, 63*(6), 529–540. doi:10.1002/jclp20364

Piacentine, L. B. (2013). Spirituality, religiosity, depression, anxiety, and drug-use consequences during methadone maintenance therapy. *Western Journal of Nursing Research, 35*(6), 795–814. doi:10.1177/0193945913479452

Pieper, J. Z., & van Uden, M. H. (2012). *"Whenever God shines His light on me . . ."* Religious coping in clinical healthcare institutions. *Mental Health, Religion & Culture, 15*(4), 403–416. doi:10.108 0/13674676.2011.579456

Plante, T. G. (2009). *Spiritual practices in psychotherapy: Thirteen tools for enhancing psychological health.* Washington, DC: American Psychological Association.

Puchalski, C., & Romer, A. L. (2000). Taking a spiritual history allows clinicians to understand patients more fully. *Journal of Palliative Medicine, 3*(1), 129–137. doi:10.1089/jpm.2000.3.129

Raffay, J. (2013). How staff and patient experience shapes our perception of spiritual care in a psychiatric setting. *Journal of Nursing Management, 22*(7), 940–950. doi:10.1111/jonm.12056

Rew, L., & Wong, J. Y. (2006). A systematic review of associations among religiosity/spirituality and adolescent health attitudes and behaviors. *Journal of Adolescent Health, 38*(4), 433–442. doi:10.1016/j .jadohealth.2005.02.004

Sawatzky, R., Ratner, P., & Chiu, L. (2005). A meta-analysis of the relationship between spirituality and quality of life. *Social Indicators Research, 72*(2), 153–188. doi:10.1007/s11205-004-5577-x

Scharf, A. (2007). Religion and mental illness: Safe spirituality or risky religious intervention? *Journal of Christian Nursing, 24*(2), 71–75. doi:10.1097/01.CNJ.0000265568.04964.45

Schwartz, M., & Kaplan, K. (2004). *Biblical stories for psychotherapy and counseling.* Binghamton, NY: Haworth Pastoral Press.

Shelly, J. A. (1983). What are spiritual needs? In J. A. Shelly & S. D. John (Eds.), *Spiritual dimensions of mental health* (pp. 55–60). Downers Grove, IL: InterVarsity Press.

Shelly, J. A., & John, S. D. (1983). *Spiritual dimensions of mental health.* Downer's Grove, IL: Intervarsity Press.

Siddle, R., Haddock, G., Tarrier, N., & Faragher, E. B. (2002). Religious delusions in patients admitted to hospital with schizophrenia. *Social Psychiatry and Psychiatric Epidemiology, 37*(3), 130–138. doi:10.1007/s001270200005

Sperry, L. (2012). *Spirituality in clinical practice: Theory and practice of spiritually oriented psychotherapy* (2nd ed.). New York, NY: Routledge.

Swinton, J. (2001). *Spirituality and mental health care: Rediscovering a "forgotten" dimension.* London, England: Jessica Kingsley.

Taylor, E. J. (2011). Spiritual care: Evangelism at the bedside? *Journal of Christian Nursing, 28*(4), 194–202. doi:10.1097/CNJ.0b013e31822b494d

Thompson, I. (2002). Mental health and spiritual care. *Nursing Standard, 17*(9), 33–38. doi:10.7748/ ns2002.11.17.9.33.c3296

Van Tubergen, F., Grotenhuis, M., & Ultee, W. (2005). Denomination, religious context, and suicide: Neo-Durkheimian multilevel explanations tested with individual and contextual data. *American Journal of Sociology, 111*(3), 797–823. doi:10.1086/497307

Walsh, K., Fortier, M. A., & DiLillo, D. (2010). Adult coping with childhood sexual abuse: A theoretical and empirical review. *Aggression and Violent Behavior, 15*(1), 1–13. doi:10.1016/j.avb.2009.06.009

Ward, T. D. (2011). The lived experience of adults with bipolar disorder and comorbid substance use disorder. *Issues in Mental Health Nursing, 32*(1), 20–27. doi:10.3109/01612840.2010.521620

World Health Organization Quality of Life-Spirituality, Religiousness and Personal Beliefs Group. (2006). A cross-cultural study of spirituality, religion, and personal beliefs as components of quality of life. *Social Science & Medicine, 62*(6), 1486–1497. doi:10.1016/j.socscimed.2005.08.001

9

Spirituality and the Older Adult

Worldwide, there is an increase in the number of people older than 65. In fact, the most rapidly growing population demographic in the near future will be people who are older than 80 years (Baltes & Smith, 2003; Colby & Ortman, 2015; Haugen & Innstrand, 2012). Because of the increasing number of people older than 80 years of age, the concept of the "young old" and the "old old" has arisen (Borella et al., 2013). As greater focus is placed on the older adult, many aspects of aging may be better understood, for example, the many physical, psychosocial, spiritual, and environmental changes that occur with increasing age, as well as the lifestyle practices of this age group.

Increasing frailty and its impact will continue to challenge not only older adults but also the health care system (MacKinlay & Hudson, 2008). As people live longer, they will likely experience chronic diseases and other health care issues. Nursing care for the aging population will be needed and spiritual care must be an integral part of such nursing care (Choi, Tirrito, & Mills, 2008; Chow, 2005; Haugen, Rannestad, Hammervold, Garasen, & Espres, 2014; MacKinlay, 2006; MacKinlay & Hudson, 2008).

THE AGING PROCESS AND SPIRITUALITY

Foundational to any discussion pertaining to spirituality in older adults is an understanding of its developmental characteristics. Erikson (1963) identifies the developmental task of the last stage of the life cycle is to achieve integrity over despair. In this stage of life, it is normal for an elderly person to revisit earlier life stages (reminiscence). Sometimes, a reframing of life events occurs in this process. If the developmental tasks accompanying this life stage are successfully achieved, then the outcome is integrity, which, in turn, leads to wisdom. Acknowledging that one's life span is approaching its end is also part of achieving integrity. If this developmental task is not successfully achieved, then the person may enter despair (Erikson, 1963; MacKinlay, 2001a).

MacKinlay (2001a) discusses three stages of the aging process, drawing on the foundational work of Peck (1968):

- "Ego differentiation versus work-role preoccupation" (MacKinlay, 2001a, p. 114): In this stage, a person deals with the role changes that occur with the onset of retirement. The work-role identity is lost and the person's value system shifts in an attempt to redefine one's self worth. Loss of meaning and purpose may be an important issue at this stage.

- "Body transcendence versus body preoccupation" (MacKinlay, 2001a, p. 114): In this stage, a person needs to accept an aging body, with all its issues and limitations, and possibly pain and chronic illness. Transcending the physical decline of the body is an important task at this stage. If transcendence is not attained, then the person may become preoccupied with physical decline.

- "Ego transcendence versus ego preoccupation" (MacKinlay, 2001a, p. 114): In this stage, as a person grows older, he or she comes to realize that death is more imminent and that reality must be accepted. The task is to let go of self-centeredness and transcend the self. If not attained, then the person may become preoccupied with the self.

Although these stages are psychosocial in intent, note that they are also connected intricately to spirituality, as meaning, transcendence, and a sense of the self may all be operational in these stages.

With respect to spiritual development, older adults can be in various stages of faith or spiritual development. Fowler's stages of faith (Fowler, 1981) are prominent in terms of examining spiritual development, as his use of the term "faith" is similar to the more generic use of the term "spirituality." A review of Fowler's stages is recommended (see section on Spiritual Development in Chapter 1). Older adults can have any one of the Fowler's stages as their terminal stage, although most older adults are likely to be between stage three and stage six as their terminal stage. Fowler's final stage of faith development is closely related to wisdom, an outcome of Erikson's developmental stage of ego integrity (Erikson, 1963; MacKinlay, 2001a).

Reflection 9.1

- Reflect on the stages of the aging process. Can you identify older adults who display the characteristics described in this aging process? Talk with these adults about how they are experiencing the aging process.
- Reflect on Fowler's stages of faith development. Can you identify older adults who have reached particular stages? Talk to these adults about their spiritual development.
- What insights did you gain from your conversations that can impact your nursing practice with older adults?

Aging itself has been described as a spiritual, as opposed to a biological, process (Lee-tun, 1996). From a physiological perspective, growing older means physical decline as the body grows older and begins to wear out. Loss of family and friends through death, loss of physical abilities, loss of independence, and other detriments often accompany aging (Emery, 2006). One's perceived identity may also be threatened or lost. Connection to other people may diminish due to physical decline, thus diminishing social support sources. Financial resources may lessen. When any of these losses occur, not only can depression, loneliness, and alienation result, but also loss of the spirit may occur and spiritual distress can be the result (Blazer, 1991; Dunn, 2008; Emery & Pargament, 2004; Heriot, 1992). However, unlike physiological growth, spiritual growth can continue until the point of death. As Leetun (1996) states, "Spiritual awakening and development help older adults recognize how aging can be both a time for growth and letting go" (p. 60). In fact, Sorajjakool (1998) maintains that the best time of life to reflect on spirituality may be the later stages of life. Spirituality can take on new meaning in light of the many issues that the older adult must embrace. Previously held coping strategies may no longer be adequate for coping with life circumstances, and a search for new meaning may commence (Ark, Hull, Husaini, & Craun, 2006; Bondevik & Skogstad, 2000; MacKinlay, 2001a). As MacKinlay (2001a) states, "As individuals become more conscious of the approaching end of their lives the search for final meaning of life gains greater urgency. Questions such as 'Why was I here?' 'Has my life been worthwhile?' gain a new importance" (p. 120). Transcendence, a concept integral to many conceptualizations of spirituality, has been identified as contributing to successful aging (McCarthy & Bockweg, 2012). Based on a concept analysis of transcendence, McCarthy and Bockweg developed a conceptual model of transcendence in order to identify activities that might promote transcendence in aging. Reference to this model (p. 89) and the ensuing discussion is recommended.

As can be seen, older adults can choose to be spiritually healthy despite the decline that occurs with aging. They can draw on spiritual resources to counter or buffer the stressors of aging. Religiosity (subjective or intrinsic), organizational religious behavior (e.g., attending religious services), and nonorganizational religious behavior (e.g., prayer) are examples of resources that older adults can access (Ark et al., 2006; Levin, Chatters, & Taylor, 1995; Levin, Markides, & Ray, 1996; Levin, Taylor, & Chatters, 1994). Leetun (1996) has developed a "Wellness Spirituality Protocol," which presents the possible responses of older adults to life conditions/illnesses. The protocol identifies how to diagnose and evaluate wellness spirituality, and provides management strategies to facilitate spiritual well-being. This protocol can be quite helpful as a practical model to assist and manage the wellness spirituality of older adults. Leetun's protocol is further discussed later in this chapter (see section on Spiritual Assessment of the Older Adult).

MacKinlay (2001a) illustrates the concept of spiritual wellness in the older years in the profile of an 80-year-old woman whom she calls "Eva." Eva claimed that she was not religious as she had not attended church for many years. But she had developed a deep sense of spirituality:

> She had not attended church for many years; she lived alone, in fairly fragile
> health, surrounded by her cats, her garden and lots of interesting books. She went
> to a contact centre for older people each week. Eva had a sense of peace and joy in

her life. Eva had grappled with loss and adversity in her long life. She had been both mother and father to her children, as her husband had died while she was pregnant. Eva had never remarried. She had grown spiritually through all of this and continued to question life. Eva described herself as a first World War baby boomer. She said experience had made her question life and its meaning. She was a real survivor and displayed a deep wisdom in the way she spoke of the important things of life. (p. 112) Eva [had] a sense of spiritual integrity. (p. 113)

The spiritual integrity that Eva seemed to have has been described as: "A state where an individual shows by their life example and attitudes, a sense of peace with themselves and others, and development of wholeness of being. The search for meaning and a degree of transcendence is evident" (MacKinlay, 1998, quoted in MacKinlay, 2001a, p. 113).

It is important to remember that an older adult's behavior and beliefs can be culturally determined, including his or her beliefs and behavior about health and spirituality (Chow & Nelson-Becker, 2010; Rawlings-Anderson, 2004). Not only should one consider culture based on ethnicity or geographic origin, but culture can also be considered in terms of various subcultures within the broader culture, such as various religious groups. It is also important to be aware of how older people are viewed in the predominant culture (and in various subcultures). For example, are they viewed as wise and cherished; or as a burden to others?

MacKinlay (2001a) identifies the spiritual needs of older adults to include the need for worship; the need to find ultimate meaning in life; the need to reminisce, focusing from the time lived; the need to cope with various losses; the need to cope with an aging body with its implications for a sense of self; and the need to have forgiveness and reconciliation. MacKinlay more fully describes in her article the changes that occur in the spiritual dimension as a person ages. For example, the death of loved ones may raise new questions about meaning and purpose. Chronic illness(es) and/or disability may cause a person to shift from a position of "doing" to "being," or create struggle and tension as the person tries to hold on to previously held roles and activities. MacKinlay states:

> In a sense, there is an inextricable connection between physical decline and spiritual development . . . . Transcendence and growing into a sense of integrity, as well as coming to final meanings of life can be seen as critical tasks of ageing . . . . [Even] the process of dying itself is part of the spiritual journey. (MacKinlay, 2001a, p. 120)

Specifically with respect to religion and the older adult, Killick (2000) raises an important point to consider. Killick stresses that older people today may have grown up and been socialized in an era where traditional religion systems had greater power and influence. For many, their spirituality may have been rooted in the traditions of these more influential systems. In Western society today, religious systems have lost power, and many nurses and other health care professionals who are caregivers for older adults have grown up in a more secular society with less emphasis on religion. Even with the increase in spirituality in the recent years, the focus of this increase is quite different from that of the past years. Thus, the nurse and older adult may be coming from two very distinct worldviews, an important point in terms of the potential impact on care.

The aforementioned discussion has provided many facts about aging. Facts and statistics, however, are not enough to obtain a full understanding of older adults because they provide only a limited insight into the needs of this population. To best assist the older adult to deal with the issues accompanying aging, it is necessary to see the world from the perspective of the older adult. For example, research indicates that older adults are interested in spirituality, including spiritual growth (Lucas, Orshan, & Cook, 2000). MacKinlay and Hudson (2008) make an excellent point when they argue for evidence-based practice to include the perceptions of older adults themselves.

AGING, SPIRITUALITY, AND HEALTH

Many of the research findings with respect to religion/spirituality and health discussed earlier in this book are also relevant and applicable in the context of the older adult population. A few examples are provided to illustrate such findings.

From a review of the literature, Kim, Reed, Haywood, Kang, and Koenig (2011) identify spirituality as a resource for older adults globally. Spirituality assists them to not only deal with the challenges of aging, but also enhance their physical and psychological well-being, their life satisfaction, their social support, and their ability to cope with dying. Fry (2000) found that significant predictors of well-being for older adults in the community, as well as in institutions, included having personal meaning, engaging in spiritual practices, and placing importance on being involved with religion. Religious involvement has also been noted to contribute to lower levels of anxiety and depression in older adults, as well as increase their ability to cope with the health concerns that are common in this age group (Huang, Hsu, & Chen, 2011). In a study of older adult women living in the community, Maddox (2000) found that spirituality/faith was important in contributing to their sense of wellness, and in bringing them through hardship and crises. Involvement in a faith community provided "a spiritual lifting" (Maddox, 2000, p. 28) for them, a connection with others, and strength to meet life's challenges. Personal spiritual practices were also important to them, as were visits from religious leaders. Dobbs, Emmett, Hammarth, and Daaleman (2012) found that chronically ill older adults living in the community identified that closeness to God was a particularly significant factor that contributed to their ability to discuss advanced care planning with health care professionals. Collins and Bowland (2012) comment on the critical place of spirituality in terms of effecting health and well-being:

> In many ways, spirituality is the precious oil that graces our endeavors to maintain connection, remember the good times, live in the moment, bear suffering, and maintain balance in the face of uncertainty and decline. (p. 246)

SPIRITUAL ASSESSMENT OF THE OLDER ADULT

Given the importance of spirituality/religion to older adults and the aging process, spiritual assessment is an important nursing activity for this age group. Thompson and colleagues (2011) advocate for a holistic and longitudinal assessment of older adults because of the complex and distinctive needs of this age group. In such an assessment, various parameters of wellness should be explored in order to examine older adults' well-being and also any barriers to wellness (e.g., physical, cognitive, social, spiritual, and functional parameters). Thompson and colleagues describe the use of e-health tools to facilitate such an assessment. They conclude that there is potential for this method of assessment to impact public health policy, identify targeted populations for intervention, and also indicate interventions that can promote and maintain wellness in older adults. Rawlings-Anderson (2004) discusses the use of assessment frameworks to ascertain older adults' cultural and religious needs. Rawlings-Anderson maintains that spiritual assessment of this population needs to acknowledge their life experiences and the impact of the same on their health, cultural, and religious beliefs. Specific questions for health care professionals to ask themselves are provided by Rawlings-Anderson. Examples provided include: "Is the person likely to be traumatized or depressed due to life events?" "Are there religious commendations or restrictions?" and "Does impaired mobility affect activities such as personal prayer, ritual washing or attendance at worship?" (p. 31). Reference to the article by Rawlings-Anderson is recommended to consider additional questions relative to religion (p. 31) and culture (p. 32).

Leetun's Wellness Spirituality Protocol (Leetun, 1996), found in Appendix B, is focused not only on assessment but also on caring for the spiritual needs and concerns of older adults. This protocol incorporates:

- Clinical presentation of possible responses to the life conditions and illness that impact or challenge older adults' wellness spirituality. Leetun quotes Pilch's definition of "wellness spirituality" (Pilch, 1988) as:

  > A way of living, a lifestyle that views and lives life as purposeful and pleasurable, that seeks out life-sustaining and life-enriching options to be chosen freely at every opportunity, and that sinks its roots deeply into spiritual values or specific religion beliefs. (Leetun, 1996, p. 60)

- Diagnosis and evaluation of older adults' wellness spiritual activities

- Management approaches available to support or restore the client's ability to perform activities that may reflect his or her spiritual well-being

---

Reflection 9.2

Review Leetun's protocol in Appendix B. Complete the assessment component of the protocol by considering your own life. What insights did you gain from this exercise with respect to your own spiritual well-being? What did you learn about the utility and functionality of the protocol? Appraise the protocol for its potential in the assessment and care of older adults. Pilot the use of this protocol in the nursing care of older adults in your practice for even more evaluation.

In reviewing Leetun's (1996) protocol, it can be seen that she provides a focus for assessment based on four aspects of spirituality. Other authors also describe foci for the spiritual assessment of older adults. For example, Ark and colleagues (2006) identify religiosity and religious coping styles as important to assess. Touhy (2001) specifically identifies the assessment of hope and spirituality as important to include in the spiritual assessment of older adults. Bondevik and Skogstad (2000) identify existential values, experience of loneliness, and a sense of purpose in life as important assessment foci. Ark and colleagues (2006) describe the religious coping styles typical of older adults that should be assessed:

- Coping styles that arise out of religious beliefs and practices, for example, attending a place of worship, belonging to a faith community, prayer, reading religious materials, and feeling close to God

- Self-directed religious coping, where the person relies more on self than on a higher power

- Deferring religious coping, for example "giving" problems to God so that He can solve them

- Collaborative religious coping, for example, seeing both self and God as active partners in the coping process

Various spiritual assessment tools have been specifically developed to explore aspects of religion and spirituality in older adults. For example, the Herth Hope Index (Herth, 1992) is a 12-item abbreviation of the Herth Hope Scale (Herth, 1990). The Herth Hope Scale is developed by Meraviglia, Sutter, and Gaskamp (2008) as: "The tool most appropriate for assessing terminally ill older adults" (p. 10). Kerrigan and Harkulich (1993) developed an assessment tool adapted from Stoll's (1979) Guidelines for Spiritual Assessment for use with residents in nursing homes. The tool consists of open-ended questions, but it also has a checklist of common answers to these questions that can be used to facilitate documentation of the client's responses. Review of this tool is recommended (pp. 48–49) for its potential in long-term care contexts. The Geriatric Spiritual Well-Being Scale (GSWS) developed by Dunn (2008) determines the level of spiritual well-being in older adults who may or may not have internalized religious beliefs. Reed (1991) developed the Self-Transcendence Scale (STS) for older adults. Hungelmann, Kenkel-Rossi, Klassen, and Stollenwerk (1996) developed the JAREL Spiritual Well-Being Scale (JAREL SWBS), a 21-item scale developed for older adults. Their scale incorporates the broad dimensions of spiritual well-being. Of course, other spiritual assessment tools and scales discussed in Chapter 5 (see section on Spiritual Assessment Tools/Models) may also be used with older adults with or without adaptation.

With respect to spiritual needs, older adults have spiritual needs similar to those discussed in Chapter 5 (see section on Spiritual Needs). Lloyd (2003a) includes a hierarchy of spiritual needs of older adults, cast in the familiar triangle that Maslow used in identifying his hierarchy of human needs (Maslow, 1968). Lloyd's adapted triangle is found in Figure 9.1.

Lloyd (2003a) advocates for supporters of older adults to be spiritual companions to them so as to assist the older adults to meet their spiritual needs. This is accomplished, in part, by using "spiritually-enhanced active listening" (p. 1). Lloyd describes an important part of this type of listening to be distinguishing between a client's basic feelings (deeper

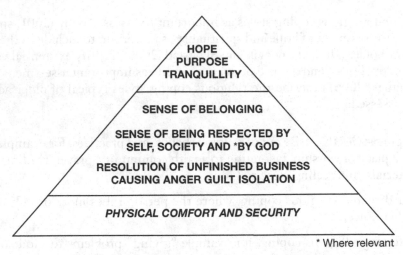

Figure 9.1 Hierarchy of spiritual needs.

feelings) and his or her reactive feelings (what is expressed). For example, an older adult client may express anger (reactive feeling) that his son is not visiting him, but the deeper feeling may actually be a feeling of abandonment.

An important point with respect to the spiritual assessment of older adults (stressed throughout this book) is to obtain *their* perspectives on their own spirituality. This is important for effective holistic care to be given. As MacKinlay (2008) states, "To neglect to understand the patients' view is to miss important information and perspectives" (p. 152). To stress this point, MacKinlay refers to a finding from her research, indicating that use of a professionally designed spiritual assessment tool alone (without in-depth interviewing of the older adults) "failed to account for the importance of family and relationships for the older adult" (p. 152).

SPIRITUALITY AND HEALTH CONDITIONS IN OLDER ADULTS

Spirituality and its implications have been the focus of study in relation to various health conditions commonly encountered by older adults. One such health condition common in older adults that has received attention is myocardial infarction (MI; Bartels, 2003), which is often accompanied by depression and anxiety (Branco, 2000; Haugen & Innstrand, 2012). Spirituality/religion can be of assistance in dealing with these issues. Stroke is also common in older adults and is one of the leading causes of death and disability in this age group. The Joanna Briggs Institute (2010) completed a review of 165 studies on the psychosocial and spiritual experience of older adults recovering from stroke. Findings from this review (with italics to highlight words that connect to spirituality) that have implications for spiritual care include:

- *Connectedness* to others is impacted by stroke, including spiritual connectedness. Being connected was important to recovery, for example, connecting with family, friends, other victims, and health professionals. Such connectedness instilled *hope*, provided encouragement, comfort, and confidence. *Prayer* was seen as an important connection to a higher power and prayer provided strength. Facilitating such connections is important to the spiritual care of stroke victims.

- Not only is stroke an unexpected event that results in confusion and fear, but also there is an experience of a body–mind split. Recovery from a stroke involves reconstructing one's life theme in terms of attitude, especially having an attitude of *hope* and drawing on *inner strengths* and other positive attributes of the person. This reconstruction involved not only coping with a physical disability but also reconstructing *the self*—in general, adjusting to the reality of this new self. An integral part of spiritual care with stroke victims, then, is to facilitate the development of a new *meaning* of the self as well as to develop and foster *hope* within the person in that context.

- Stoke was perceived as having life-altering consequences in multiple areas of the person's life, for example, as just discussed, a change in one's *sense of self.* Assessing such consequences and helping clients deal with them are important aspects of spiritual care in this context.

Nurses should give attention to spiritual needs in older adults with chronic illness as it may be the case in such instances that the spiritual reserves of the client would be depleted. Also, as discussed in Chapter 7 (see the section on Spirituality and Chronic Illness), spirituality and religion are known resources for those dealing with chronic health problems. Spirituality can enable the older adult to adapt to the chronic condition, as well as have a healthy response to stressful events (Landis, 1996; Loeb, Penrod, Falkenstern, Gueldner, & Poon, 2003; Maddox, 2000). Dossey (1997) found that chronic illness and resulting quality of life issues often result in anxiety, ineffective coping, sleep disturbance, isolation, and emotional issues. Spirituality/religion can be effective in dealing with such issues.

MacKinlay (2003) has edited a book composed of a collection of papers presented at a conference on mental health and pastoral care in later life. This book provides a wide range of perspectives on mental health and spirituality in older adults, for example, theological and cultural aspects of mental health as a focus, as well as the implications for spiritual care in mental health contexts. Qualitative research and case studies are included relative to mental health and spirituality for this age group. Specific issues related to mental health in older adults are discussed, for example, depression, suicide, and dementia. Spirituality as a protective factor for good mental health in older adults is also considered. Lloyd (2003b) also writes about spirituality and mental illness in older adults. He illustrates the use of a holistic model that incorporates spirituality into the care of older adults with depression. Lloyd also gives examples of secular and spiritual/faith-based programs that focus on the mental health of older adults. Reference to both of these resources is recommended for an in-depth discussion on spirituality and mental health in older adults.

As older adults are nearing the end of their lives, terminal illness is characteristic of this age group. Much has been written about spirituality and terminally ill older adults. For example, Moberg (2005), in addressing end-of-life contexts, writes about the sense of belonging and support provided through connection with self, others, and God or a higher power. Such connections often counteract the loneliness and despair that often accompany terminal illness. Moberg also identifies the spiritual awareness that often accompanies old age as providing hope and support in cases of terminal illness. Meraviglia and colleagues (2008) also discuss spirituality and terminal illness in older adults; in particular, the connection between terminal illness and risk for spiritual distress. They stress the importance of assessing for signs of spiritual distress—for example, loneliness, isolation, hopelessness, anxiety, and depression. Examples of effective interventions discussed by Meraviglia and colleagues to address spiritual distress include facilitating connectedness and encouraging hope. Monitoring outcomes of interventions for spiritual distress are also important, for example, signs of hopefulness and the level of connection with others. Reference to their article is recommended to review evidence-based guidelines for providing spiritual care to terminally ill older adults at risk for spiritual distress. Lowis, Jewell, Jackson, and Merchant (2011) found that religious/spiritual beliefs and faith in God were used by older adults not only to cope with life in general, but also to actively influence their thoughts and feelings about death. Literature and music were particularly important to these adults. Faith in God, intrinsic religiosity, a belief in life after death, and a sense of purpose in life have all been shown to be predictive of fear and lower death anxiety (Ardelt & Koenig, 2006; Fortner, Neimeyer, & Rybarczyk, 2000).

Reflection 9.3

Reflect on the findings regarding spirituality and the various health problems that older adults can encounter. Do these findings "ring true" for you in terms of your own experience with older adults? How can you use these findings to inform your nursing care of older adults who may be experiencing such health problems?

SPIRITUALITY/SPIRITUAL CARE AND DEMENTIA

Spirituality is of relevance to older adults who are cognitively impaired (Collins & Bowland, 2012; Kumar, Tims, Cruess, & Mintzer, 1999). MacKinlay (2008) maintains that nurses need to have enhanced awareness about spirituality and dementia so that more effective ways of providing spiritual care can be developed.

Richards (1990) warns against an attitude of dismissal in terms of how spirituality may be relevant in the context of dementia. Such an attitude can be expressed in the following manner: "Spiritual aspects of a confused person's life don't matter—he wouldn't understand" (p. 63). Attitudes of that nature can lead to the neglect of a person's spiritual needs. Rather, when a person's response, or ability to respond, is limited, the attitude should be that even in those circumstances, some things still get through to the person. In fact, it is suggested that dementia itself can stimulate people to explore meaning and purpose in their lives—especially in the early stages of dementia (Carr, Hicks-Moore, & Montgomery, 2011; Dunn, 2004). Bryden (2005) and Davis (1989) each provide first-person accounts of themselves as older adults dealing with dementia, and they bear witness to the importance of spirituality/religion in dementia.

Buckwater (2003) presents a vignette of an older adult with end-stage dementia. This vignette demonstrates that older adults in such a context can have a "wide awake" (p. 21) soul and be able to communicate:

> My roommate was dying. The lady in black with the funny white collar had just done something with oil and prayers. No family was present. She then sat down beside my friend and began to quietly sing old-time hymns. Something within me began to stir. Before I knew it, though I was curled up in a fetal position and hadn't spoken a word in 3 years, I began to match her pitches when she got to "Amazing Grace." From somewhere down deep and ancient the tones came. And as my vocal cords vibrated, so did my soul. The lady with the collar came over and thanked me for helping her to lullaby Mary into Eternity. Then she moved our beds closer together and sat between us. How warm her hand felt in mine. The cross around her neck glowed. I never took my eyes off it. Together we sang "Blessed Assurance" and "Love Lifted Me." That is, she sang and I hummed snatches now and then. After—I don't know how long—she kissed Mary on the forehead and gently wiped away the tears that were running down my face, thanked me once again, and left. I fell into the deepest, most peaceful sleep. (pp. 20–21)

Buckwater points out that the loss of self, which may be characteristic of older adults with profound memory impairment, does not necessarily mean loss of the soul. Buckwater suggests that caregivers of such older adults need to intervene and assist the older adult whose memory loss causes a disturbance in his or her soul. As was seen in the vignette, love and acceptance, touch, presence, and human-to-human connection are important to offer. Connection can be made through religious/spiritual rituals, activities, visual symbols, smells, and sounds, which can cue the older adult. For example, it was music, deemed by Buckwater as "the strongest bridge to the soul over the tangles of the mind of the patient with AD [Alzheimer's disease]" (p. 21), that was very effective in establishing connection and positive emotions within the older adult in the vignette. The family of an older adult with dementia can also provide valuable information about the spirituality of the older adult. They could relate, for example, what provided meaning for the person in the past. As Buckwater states: "Our souls . . . retain body-memories [related to religious/spiritual practices] even when we've lost almost everything else" (p. 23).

A critical point to make with respect to older adults with dementia is that they are first and foremost *persons*; and as it has been referred to many times in this book, spirituality is part of personhood. As McFadden, Ingram, and Baldauf (2000) state: "When persons cannot comprehend language nor think in any way usually conceptualized as cognitive activity, still they retain personhood" (p. 71). McFadden and colleagues also comment on the need to "see" the personhood of the person with dementia: "The person with dementia retains emotional responsiveness and ways of connecting with other persons, although sometimes these forms of connection are very subtle and can only be perceived by those who 'have eyes to see'" (p. 70). Page (2005) is in agreement with this statement in that she indicates that the remnant identity that survives in dementia clients can be strengthened, thus improving the older adult's quality of life. Page calls for nurses to look beyond the physical and mental states of persons with dementia and see the whole person. She identifies three areas to focus on when providing spiritual care to older adults with dementia:

- The need for meaning (family members can help identify what was meaningful to the person): What provided meaning for the person can then be "woven" into conversations with that person.

- The need for love and relatedness, which can be met through relationships. Caring and loving others help to instill self-worth and provide meaning and purpose to life. For the older adult with dementia, as mentioned previously, touch can communicate caring (i.e., love and relatedness). Photographic records of the person's life, family, and friends can also trigger memories and assist the person to connect to the past in a meaningful way.

- Creating an environment in which the older adult feels valued, and where his or her spiritual needs, beliefs, and values are considered: This is imperative to good nursing care. Nurses can create such environments by the tone of their voice, their body language, the use of touch, and/or eye contact—all of which affirm the worth of the person.

Killick (2000) maintains that even people with dementia deserve to have an "audience" as they relate their stories. Such stories may not make any sense at first glance, but they can be extremely meaningful to the client. Through stories, nurses can obtain information about what was meaningful to the client (Page, 2005). They also help nurses more clearly understand the value of spiritual practices and resources to the person with dementia (Collins & Bowland, 2012). Thus, these stories can provide valuable information to nurses in terms of providing spiritual care to the client.

People with dementia can respond to faith symbols, rituals, and practices that are familiar to them and that can bring them great comfort (Higgins, 2013; Richards, 1990). Mooney (2006) wrote about the place of rituals in helping to orient clients with Alzheimer's disease to reality, calming them and lowering their excessive emotional responses and agitated physical behavior. Mooney maintains that such rituals do not need to be intellectually focused because that may pose problems for those with Alzheimer's disease manifesting a decline in intellectual functioning. Rather, the rituals can be at an experiential level. They can also be mediated through other people on behalf of the client. For example, a nurse might read a familiar prayer to the client, or arrange for familiar songs to be sung to him or her. Such rituals can be comforting and decrease anxiety and fear. They can also promote communication with God or the Divine. As Ellor (1997) says:

> If an older adult needs an amputation of the leg, the world knows how to respond.
> We help replace the lost mobility with crutches, an artificial leg or other
> alternative ambulatory devices. When a person is losing memory and cognition,
> we need to do similar things: find ways to use alternatives to memory and rational
> thinking. These people continue to be persons with souls . . . . They call us to be
> creative . . . . This is an important challenge [for the nurse], not a burden. (p. 20)

From a review of recent literature, Higgins (2013) identifies faith, faith communities, and practicing one's faith or religion as all being important to people with dementia. Even for those living in long-term care facilities, these things are important. Higgins suggests a number of activities that health care professionals can employ to meet the religious needs of older adults with dementia who are living in long-term care facilities:

- A number of practical aspects including ensuring access to worship services in the long-term care facility, perhaps by fostering linkages with local faith communities; being present at such services to assist with any behavioral issues that may arise during the service; providing space for worship services; ensuring that the resident does not have conflicting appointments during the time of the service; and determining the length of the service and the environmental ambiance of the service

- If possible, facilitating residents to attend faith communities external to the long-term care facility

- Supporting residents' participation in private prayer as well as employing ethical guidelines for the use of prayer with clients

- Providing and facilitating the reading of meaningful spiritual literature to the client

- Meeting religious needs in end-of-life care

- Discussing faith issues and practices with the resident and his or her family

Any and all of these activities should be tailored to address the specific needs and circumstances of clients, which stresses the importance of assessing the spiritual history and spiritual preferences of clients.

Carr and colleagues (2011) explored the meaning of spiritual care from the perspective of older adults with moderate–severe dementia, as well as from the perspectives of their families and care providers. For the older adults with dementia, an important aspect of spiritual care for them was that care providers respect their religious background, beliefs, and practices. With respect to the care providers in this study, Carr et al. noted:

> "Their sense of the spiritual, of God, of relationships, and of interdependence of life, was often infused in their everyday encounters and served at times to energize and sustain them in their lives and work." (p. 410)

Carr and colleagues conclude:

> . . . the essence of spiritual care in dementia, as described by participants in this study, is rooted in the promotion of personhood through intentional caring attitudes and actions. In this sense, spiritual care is not something reserved for someone or something that is done in isolation of other aspects of care. (p. 409)

In this study, spiritual care was seen as mutually beneficial to both the person being cared for and the caregiver. Some perceived challenges to spiritual care were similar to those discussed earlier in this book (see the section on Challenges to Incorporating Spiritual Care Into Nursing Practice, Education, and Research in Chapter 3). However, the presumptive perception that people with dementia cannot focus or understand was also determined to be a barrier. Referring to the challenges associated with providing spiritual care to those with dementia, Carr and colleagues state:

> [There was] disconnection from the person on the part of the one caring and a failure to understand the meaning of spiritual care in its broadest sense . . . even

when a person with dementia cannot connect with the nurses, chaplains, and other direct care providers, these caregivers can still make an effort to connect with that person . . . there is an essential sacredness to genuinely caring for the personhood of another. This is perhaps especially true when that person is living with severe dementia and cognitive impairment. (p. 409)

Reflection 9.4

In reflecting on the comments made and the case scenario presented by Buckwater (2003), how can these better prepare you to focus on spirituality in clients with dementia?

SPIRITUAL CARE AND LONG-TERM CARE FACILITIES

For many in the "old old" age category of life, it is common for them to experience physical disability, illness, loss of function, and loss of social connection. Such conditions may require the older adult to reside in a nursing home or another long-term care facility (Haugen et al., 2014; MacKinlay, 2001b). In long-term care facilities, the purpose of life can be impacted as the older adult is removed from many activities, tasks, and routines that provide meaning (Bondevik & Skogstad, 2000; Branco, 2000). Depression is common. Many of the frail elderly as well as those older adults who have dementia and delirium may have a condition labeled "failure to thrive" (MacKinlay, 2001b, p. 29). MacKinlay (2001b) connects failure to thrive to spirituality: " . . . how much of this concept may be related to lack of nourishment for the soul, or perhaps this failure to thrive syndrome is really a loss of meaning in life" (p. 30).

Sources of meaning identified by Seeber (2000) in a mixed population of residents in nursing homes included relationships with other people outside of the nursing home; control of daily routine; privacy; intimacy/sexual expression; intellectual stimulation; support for self-identity; ethnic-cultural habits; a sense of security regarding health and well-being; optimism; quality of their environment; and rituals/religious observance (p. 147). Reference to Seeber for an in-depth discussion of each of these sources of meaning is recommended.

MacKinlay (2001b) interviewed frail elderly in nursing homes, and found that the spiritual needs for these people included the need to find meaning, the need to find hope, the need for relationships, and the need for God. MacKinlay points out the vital role that nurses can have in helping the frail elderly meet such needs, noting that achieving them on their own is often too hard, if not impossible. Many of the participants in the study verbalized their desire to talk with someone about their spiritual needs. MacKinlay concludes:

[A] frail bed bound person is not really cared for simply because they are fed, washed, turned, and kept pain free, and given the right medications, important as these things are. No, that person's spirit must be fed too, each person is still a human being, no matter what his or her cognitive status and/or ability to communicate. Each person has a soul that needs recognizing and connecting with, at the deepest level. (p. 29)

Spirituality is known to be a beneficial resource for older adults who are residing in nursing homes. For example, Wallace and O'Shea (2007) found that residents in nursing homes supported spirituality as a framework for living life, for choosing between right and wrong, and for fostering a sense of peace. Patterson, King, Ball, Whittington, and Perkins (2003) found that residents in assisted living facilities used religious practices to cope with the challenges that they faced. Such practices provided continuity with their earlier lives; gave relief from pain; provided the opportunity for socialization; gave them courage, meaning, and purpose; and prepared them for impending death. The core theme in this study was continuity, or maintaining a sense of self. Spirituality was identified as the only significant predictor of hope in a study of institutionalized older adults (Touhy, 2001). Touhy identified intrapersonal connectedness and connection to a higher power or some purpose greater than themselves to be particularly important to older adults in terms of maintaining hope.

CAREGIVERS OF OLDER ADULTS

No discussion about the care of older adults would be complete without reference to their caregivers, and, in particular, those who look after older adults who live at home. Choi and colleagues (2008) studied the role that religious beliefs and practices, as well as faith-based organizations, play in the lives of caregivers of elderly and disabled long-term care recipients of community health agencies. Religious coping practices were found to have positive impact on the caregivers, for example, enabling them to cope with stress. There was less role overload and role preoccupation, and less depression than in the case of caregivers who did not engage in such practices. Religious beliefs and practices were also operant in the caregivers' decisions to care for the family member at home. Morano and King (2005) also found that religion/spirituality mediated the caregivers' perception of stress and their reaction to it. Berg-Weger, Rubio, and Tebb (2001) note that religion/spirituality has also been noted to contribute to caregivers' overall sense of well-being. Thus, it is important for nurses to facilitate use of appropriate religious/spiritual resources for caregivers. Also important is facilitating conversations between older adults and their caregivers about spirituality. Paying attention to the caregivers' spirituality is critical because of the high degree of influence that caregivers' spirituality can have on the well-being of older adults (Kim et al., 2011).

Paun (2004) conducted a qualitative study of persons who were spousal caregivers of older adults with Alzheimer's disease. Paun found that the religious/spiritual beliefs and practices of these caregivers were reflected in four major themes:

- Taking charge (while still preserving normalcy and dignity for their spouses): Caregivers strived to maintain their spouses' engagement in religious practices.

- Adjusting and coping: Religious practices and beliefs helped caregivers cope with the caregiving situation.

- Making sense of the situation: Caregivers deliberately focused on the positive aspects of their lives. Many saw caregiving as their "mission," with God supporting them. They also spoke of the subjective importance of the values of altruism and caring in their lives. Their religious/spiritual beliefs enabled them to see caregiving as part of a larger plan for their own lives.

- Looking into the future: Although these caregivers did not have much hope in terms of the caregiving situation improving, they did verbalize hope and trust in God.

Paun's work has implications for how nurses should respond to the caregivers of older adults: the caregivers' spiritual needs must be assessed; they must be encouraged to continue with religious/spiritual practices that are helpful to the caregivers; they must be given emotional support; and if necessary, they should be referred to religious or spiritual leaders who can also support their religious/spiritual practices. Encouraging the use of respite care is also important.

Similar to the comments of Paun (2004), other authors have suggested activities in which nurses should engage with caregivers of older adults. For example, based on professional knowledge and personal experience with caregiving, Collins and Bowland (2012) suggest that nurses be open to older adults and their caregivers in terms of talking about religious/spiritual practices and beliefs; identify and address the spiritual needs of caregivers; explore religious/spiritual practices and beliefs as sources of support; encourage the use of music as a therapeutic intervention; identify sources of support in faith communities; and encourage and support the spiritual growth of caregivers.

Reflection 9.5

In thinking about various caregivers of older adults, what factors have contributed to their decision to take care of their loved one? What factors have helped them cope with caregiving and which of these are related to spirituality/religion? If possible, talk with caregivers, asking them specifically about spiritual or religious resources that they use.

SPIRITUAL CARE OF OLDER ADULTS

Generic spiritual care, as well as many of the spiritual care interventions discussed in Chapter 6 (see the section on Spiritual Care Interventions), can be utilized in the care of older adults, whether they are in long-term care facilities or not (Sullivan & Asselin, 2013; Wallace & O'Shea, 2007; Wilkes, Cioffi, Fleming, & LeMiere, 2011). For example, the arts (music, literature) are noted to improve older adults' health (Bungay, Clift, & Skingley, 2010; Cohen, Peristein, Chapline, Firth, & Simmens, 2006). Support and encouragement of older adults' religious beliefs, practices, and involvement have also been identified as an appropriate and helpful spiritual intervention (Huang et al., 2011; Theis, Biordi, Coeling, Nalepka, & Miller, 2003). Spiritual resources important to older adults, such as prayer, are seen as important within the context of the dying process (Doorenbos, Wilson, & Coenen, 2006). In fact, prayer is a common spiritual coping practice for older adults (Dunn & Horgas, 2000). A more specific finding was made by Musgrave, Allen, and Allen (2002) in that religion provided comfort during stressful times for African American older adults.

Narayanasamy and colleagues (2004) identified a variety of spiritual interventions noted by nurses to be important in the care of older adults: respect for privacy; helping clients connect; helping them address unfinished business; listening to their concerns; comforting and reassuring them; and assisting them to engage in various religious practices. Bush (2001) explored the research and the theoretical foundations of the use of touch in older adults. Bush maintains that older adults are particularly receptive to touch and asserts that the use of touch should be integral to the care of the older adult, improving their functional capacity and orientation (particularly true for the cognitively impaired). Bush concludes from her review of the literature with older adults that there are a number of benefits to the use of touch:

- It enhances comfort for not only older adults but also their caregivers—especially during the dying process.

- It improves symptoms of confusion and agitation in cognitively impaired older adults.

- It improves the sensory stimulation levels for older adults (thereby promoting relationships and interrelationships with the environment).

- It ameliorates the impact of long-term institutionalization as well as short-term hospitalization.

Of course, in considering the use of touch, nurses need to consider aspects related to its use, as outlined in Chapter 4 (see the section on Communication). Bush calls for more rigorous research on this viable, cost-effective, and nonintrusive nursing intervention.

Storytelling as a spiritual intervention was discussed in Chapter 6 (see the section on Stories and Intervention). Killick (2000) discusses how dementia affects storytelling, including the importance of having someone listen and pay attention to the person's stories. Killick uses the example of a woman with dementia (Lily) to show the power of story as an intervention in the context of dementia. He analyzes her story concluding that: "Such a window into another's world is worth a dozen correct chronologies" (p. 10). Reference to Killick's article is recommended for the review and discussion of Lily's story (pp. 8–10).

Reflection 9.6

If you are working with older adults in your nursing practice, or have a family member who is an older adult, reflect on a view that their stories are a window on their spirituality, and how stories can open up possibilities for you to relate to them in a more significant manner.

The manner in which spiritual care interventions are applied to older adults has been studied and certain guidelines have been established. For example, Meraviglia and colleagues (2008) provide an evidence-based guideline for promoting the spirituality of older adults who are terminally ill. Emblen (2006) notes that spiritual growth can occur in older adults if they are "action-oriented" (p. 57): if their desires, attitudes, and behaviors change to suit their present context of life. The resulting implication is that nurses may be able to assist clients to be action oriented. Emblen developed guidelines, known as GRACE (p. 57), to assist nurses in this process. Although Emblen writes from a Christian worldview, many of the guidelines can be applied to older adults with other worldviews:

- G—Goals. Facilitating specific short-term and long-term goals for general growth and spiritual growth is important. Such goals can be incorporated into the older adult's care plan.

- R—Robust health. Planning for good biological health, including a healthy lifestyle, is important. Examples include planning times of activity and rest, and planning activities to maintain an active mind.

- A—Acknowledgment of this stage of growth and development. Older persons need to be assisted to see that their current stage of life can be seen in positive terms; and that energy needs to be directed at the positive "fruits" of this stage (such as wisdom).

- C—Christian fruits. Older adults should be assisted to develop the Christian "fruits" of calmness, humility, gentleness, compassion, joy, and patience. These are in contrast to stress, a critical spirit, impatience, sadness, and hatefulness. If the person is not Christian, an adaptation is that the nurse can ask what "healthy fruits" are desired by the person at this stage of life and then assist him or her to attain them.

- E—Enabling stories to be told that provide positive spiritual experiences. An example is encouraging stories that demonstrate hope, courage, God's goodness, and so on.

Spiritual interventions have been identified for older adults who live in long-term care facilities. For example, Touhy (2001) suggests the following interventions: helping residents attend and participate in worship services in the long-term care facility if they so wish; having spiritual readings in large print and in audio formats so that visually and hearing-impaired residents can have access to them; praying with and for residents; conducting life review, wisdom circles, and spiritual groups; and creating opportunities to care for others. Other spiritual care interventions noted to be useful with older adults in long-term care facilities include the following:

- Having discussion groups about spirituality; encouraging resident leadership in religious activities in the institution; encouraging external faith communities to participate in the life of the institution (Patterson et al., 2003)

- Strengthening intrapersonal transcendence by encouraging personal interests and learning; interpersonal transcendence can be achieved by involvement with others, sharing wisdom, and helping others. Interpersonal transcendence should also be strengthened by facilitating acceptance of aging (including the changes accompanying aging), and also by finding meaning in past experiences (Haugen & Innstrand, 2012; Wang, 2011)

- Assisting older adults in long-term care facilities to develop meaning (Seeber, 2000)

- Advocating for and facilitating an environment that facilitates spiritual well-being and spiritual growth. Examples include providing religious resources in institutions, and making them more homelike (Emery, 2006; Patterson et al., 2003)

- Referring residents to a religious leader or spiritual care professional (Wallace & O'Shea, 2007)

THE PERSON OF THE NURSE IN CARING FOR OLDER ADULTS

As in any setting or context of care, the person of the nurse is important in providing spiritual care. This is particularly true in long-term care facilities, as nurses will generally have a long-term relationship with residents (Haugen et al., 2014). MacKinlay (2001a) developed a project to increase nurses' awareness of their own spirituality (as well as increasing awareness of nursing home residents' spirituality). Outcomes of the project included an increased sensitivity by the nurses to the spiritual needs of residents, and an increase in the nurses' ability to identify spiritual behaviors.

Overvold, Flannelly, Weaver, and Koenig (2005) conducted a study of staff in a large nursing home in the United States and found that many of the staff members relied on religious faith to decrease the stress of care giving and to provide meaning and purpose in their role. These authors postulated that finding meaning and purpose in providing care to residents in a nursing home can act as a protective factor against job dissatisfaction and burnout.

Dick (2014) also identified that nursing staff in long-term care settings personally availed of spiritual resources. In particular, such resources helped the nurses deal with the death of residents, "an inevitable part of aged care" (p. 168). Specific resources used by the nurses included connecting with nature; having a sense of meaning and purpose in their work; seeking comfort in relationships (e.g., with colleagues, family, and friends); and having hope that the resident would have a good death and go to a better place. These nurses also hoped that they had made a difference.

Reflection 9.7

- Reflect on factors that have contributed to your own view of older adults, for example, societal views of this age group, your personal/professional experience with older adults, and any other perceived factors. How do your views of older adults inform your nursing practice—positively or negatively?
- What strengths do you bring to the spiritual care of the older adult? What is challenging for you in this regard?

Throughout the discussion in this chapter, spirituality as it relates to older adults has been explored, as well as spiritual care in a variety of contexts relative to older adults. Overriding all spiritual care with this age group is the importance of treating the older adult with dignity and respect. It is also critical that one be aware of personal and subjective biases about aging and older adults. Finally, a willingness to "be with" the older adult will go a long way to the provision of quality care!

Taking It Further

1. Read the case study of Mrs. Smith, an older adult who has had a hip fracture repair, in Kim-Godwin (2013, p. 212).

   a. Answer the questions at the end of the case study.

   b. How would you facilitate discussion of Mrs. Smith's perception of God? What might be challenging for you in conducting such a conversation?

2. Re-read the case study of Eva as presented by MacKinlay (2001a) in this chapter (see the section on Aging, Spirituality, and Health).

   a. What foundational spiritual needs are being met in the case of Eva? What evidence is presented to support your answer?

   b. What spiritual needs might still be present in Eva? How might you address them? What specific interventions might you use?

   c. What feelings are you aware of within yourself as you read the case study of Eva? What is the origin of such feelings? Might they be conducive to your nursing care of Eva; or not?

3. Read the case study of Mrs. James, an older adult with Alzheimer's disease, in Collins and Bowland (2012, pp. 239–240).

   a. If you were caring for Mrs. James, how would you address her religious needs? Who else might be involved and why?

   b. What specific challenges might you personally face in caring for Mrs. James's religious needs? How might you address such challenges?

4. Read the stories in Mooney (2006) of Sarah, an 82-year-old woman who resides in a long-term care facility (pp. 6–8), and also of Helen, another woman who resides in a long-term care facility on a special care unit (pp. 8–9).

   a. What is your response to the actions of the nurse with each of these clients?

   b. Why do you think that the outcome was so positive in each of these case scenarios?

   c. What is the potential of the nurses' actions (or modifications of same) for the nursing care of older adults with dementia?

   d. What rituals have you observed to be meaningful for older adults with dementia? What has been the outcome when older adults with dementia have participated in such rituals?

5. Read the case study of Helen, an older adult with Stage IV chronic obstructive lung disease in Chrash, Mulich, and Patton (2011, pp. 533–535).

   a. Read the additional questions related to the HOPE spiritual assessment tool that were not used in this case study. Then appraise the use of the HOPE spiritual assessment tool in this case study in terms of its success in assessing Helen's spirituality/spiritual needs.

   b. What actions did the nurse employ after the assessment was completed? And what was the outcome of the actions?

   c. What is your appraisal of the potential of the HOPE spiritual assessment tool for your own nursing care of older adults?

6. Read the case study of Sam, a man who is caring for his invalid wife at home, in Burkhardt (1989, pp. 72–73).

   a. How might Sam describe his spirituality?

   b. What evidence is there in the case study that Sam's spiritual needs are being met?

   c. What is the role of the nurse with respect to Sam's spiritual well-being?

7. Read the case study of Mr. Huff, a man who resides in a nursing home, in Crain (1994, pp. 4–8).

   a. What words and actions of the student nurse illustrate a caring attitude?

   b. How did aspects of Mr. Huff's story or his physical condition impact on the student nurse's care of Mr. Huff?

   c. What nonverbal cues impacted the care of Mr. Huff; and how?

   d. What part did observation and listening play in the care of Mr. Huff?

   e. What educational concepts did the student nurse use as a foundation for her care of Mr. Huff?

   f. How did the student nurse incorporate the family into Mr. Huff's care? Why was this important?

   g. How does the student nurse answer the question: "Why am I doing this nursing?" Does her answer resonate with how you might answer this same question? If not, what would your answer be to this question?

   h. Answer the Discussion Questions in Crain (1994) pertaining to the case of Mr. Huff (p. 8).

8. Read the case study of Mrs. Adams, and the description of the same, in McSherry (1996, pp. 48–49).

   a. If you had been assigned to care for Mrs. Adams during the first few days of her admission, how would you respond to her withdrawal and lack of communication?

   b. How would you respond to Mrs. Adams's anger and frustration toward God and also her guilt? How might you introduce these topics to Mrs. Adams? What aspects would you want to explore regarding each?

  c. How might you have helped Mrs. Adams find meaning in her grief and also in the midst of her illness?

  d. How are environmental and behavioral cues related to spiritual needs? How can observations about Mrs. Adams's environment open up possibilities for her spiritual care?

9. Read the 12 case scenarios in O'Brien (2011, pp. 268–270; p. 271).

  a. For each of these clients, summarize the impact of religious beliefs and practices on his or her health and well-being.

  b. For each of these clients, how would you proceed to explore in more depth how his or her spiritual and religious beliefs and practices are strengths? What aspects would you focus on? How might you explain the rationale for your inquiry? How can your reflection and/or discussion in this regard inform your nursing practice with older adults?

10. Read the case study of Loretta in Deloughry (2008, pp. 239–240).

  a. What spiritual/religious practices were instigated by Loretta's family during her hospitalization? What actions did Loretta take after her discharge from the hospital that nurtured and expressed her spirituality?

  b. What made Loretta well (in your reflection on this question, please note Figure 9.1 in Deloughry, p. 241)?

  c. How does Loretta's example illustrate the fact that spiritual growth can occur as one ages, even in the midst of physical decline?

  d. How can Loretta's example inform your practice with older adults who are in declining health?

11. Read case study 4 (Mr. Robert Smith) in Narayanasamy (1991, p. 52).

  a. What information is given in the case study to support the two spiritual needs identified in the nursing care plan (p. 52)?

  b. Several activities are identified in the care plan to address the two spiritual needs exhibited by Mr. Smith. For each activity, outline how you would achieve that activity. For example, what might you say? What strategies might you employ to achieve the activity given?

  c. What particular challenges might Mr. Smith's situation pose for you personally? If any, how might you deal with these challenges?

12. Read the case study of Mrs. Murphy in Narayanasamy (1991, pp. 55–56).

  a. What information is given in the case study to support the three spiritual needs/issues identified in the nursing care plan (p. 56)?

  b. Several activities are identified in the care plan to address the spiritual needs/issues exhibited by Mrs. Murphy. For each activity, outline how you would achieve that activity. For example, what might you say? What strategies might you employ to achieve the activity given?

c. What particular challenges might Mrs. Murphy's situation pose for you personally? If any, how might you deal with these challenges?

REFERENCES

Ardelt, M., & Koenig, C. S. (2006). The role of religion for hospice patients and for relatively healthy older adults. *Research on Aging, 28*(2), 184–215. doi:10.1177/0164027505284165

Ark, P. D., Hull, P. C., Husaini, B. A., & Craun, C. (2006). Religiosity, religious coping styles, and health service use: Racial differences among elderly women. *Journal of Gerontological Nursing, 32*(8), 20–29.

Baltes, P. B., & Smith, J. (2003). New frontiers in the future of aging: From successful aging of the young old to dilemmas of the fourth age. *Gerontology, 49*(2), 123–135. doi:10.1159/000067946

Bartels, S. J. (2003). Improving the system of care for older adults with mental illness in the United States: Findings and recommendations for the President's New Freedom Commission on Mental Health. *American Journal of Geriatric Psychiatry, 11*(5), 486–497. doi:10.1097/00019442-200309000-00003

Berg-Weger, M., Rubio, D. M., & Tebb, S. S. (2001). Strengths-based practice with family caregivers of the chronically ill: Qualitative insights. *Families in Society: Journal of Contemporary Human Services, 82*(3), 263–272. doi:10.1606/1044-3894.191

Blazer, D. (1991). Spirituality and aging well. *Generations: Journal of the American Society on Aging, 15*(1), 61–65.

Bondevik, M., & Skogstad, A. (2000). Loneliness, religiousness, and purpose in life in the oldest old. *Journal of Religious Gerontology, 11*(1), 5–21. doi:10.1300/J078v11n01:_03

Borella, E., Carretti, B., Cantarella, A., Riboldi, F., Zavagnin, M., & DeBeni, R. D. (2013). Benefits of training visuospatial working memory in young-old and old-old. *Developmental Psychology, 50*(3), 714–727. doi:10.1037/a0034293

Branco, K. J. (2000). Religiosity and depression among nursing home residents: Results of a survey of ten states. *Journal of Religious Gerontology, 12*(1), 43–61. doi:10.1300/J078v12n01_05

Bryden, C. (2005). *Dancing with dementia*. London, England: Jessica Kingsley.

Buckwater, G. L. (2003). Addressing the spiritual and religious needs of persons with profound memory loss. *Home Healthcare Nurse, 21*(1), 20–24.

Bungay, H., Clift, S., & Skingley, A. (2010). The Silver Song Club Project: A sense of well-being through participatory singing. *Journal of Applied Arts & Health, 1*(2), 165–178. doi:10.1386/jaah.1.2.165_1

Burkhardt, M. A. (1989). Spirituality: An analysis of the concept. *Holistic Nursing Practice, 3*(3), 69–77.

Bush, E. (2001). The use of human touch to improve the well-being of older adults. *Journal of Holistic Nursing, 19*(3), 256–270. doi:10.1177/089801010101900306

Carr, T. J., Hicks-Moore, S., & Montgomery, P. (2011). What's so big about the "little things": A phenomenological inquiry into the meaning of spiritual care in dementia. *Dementia, 10*(3), 399–414. doi:10.1177/1471301211408122

Choi, G., Tirrito, T., & Mills, F. (2008). Caregiver's spirituality and its influence on maintaining the elderly and disabled in a home environment. *Journal of Gerontological Social Work, 51*(3–4), 247–259. doi:10.1080/01634370802039528

Chow, E. O. W., & Nelson-Becker, H. (2010). Spiritual distress to spiritual transformation: Stroke survivor narratives from Hong Kong. *Journal of Aging Studies, 24*(4), 313–324. doi:10.1016/j.jaging.2010.06.001

Chow, R. K. (2005). Life's quest for spiritual well-being: A holistic and gerontological nurse perspective. *NSNA Imprint, 52*(4), 80–83.

Chrash, M., Mulich, B., & Patton, C. M. (2011). The APN role in holistic assessment and integration of spiritual assessment for advance care planning. *Journal of the American Academy of Nurse Practitioners, 23*(10), 530–536. doi:10.1111/j.1745-7599.2011.00644.x

Cohen, G. D., Peristein, S., Chapline, J. J., Firth, K. M., & Simmens, S. (2006). The impact of professionally conducted cultural programs on the physical health, mental health, and social functioning of older adults. *The Gerontologist, 46*(6), 726–734. doi:10.1093/geront/46.6.726

Colby, S. L., & Ortman, J. M. (2015). Projections of the size and composition of the US population 2014-2060. Retrieved from http://www.census.gov

Collins, W. L., & Bowland, S. (2012). Spiritual practices for caregivers and care receivers. *Journal of Religion, Spirituality & Aging, 24*(3), 235–248. doi:10.1080/15528030.2012.648585

Crain, A. (1994). Why are you doing this for me? A student nurse cares enough to help a patient regain self-respect. *Journal of Christian Nursing, 11*(2), 4–8.

Davis, R. (1989). *My journey into Alzheimer's disease*. Wheaton, IL: Tyndale House Publishers.

Deloughry, T. E. (2008). Spirituality and elder care. In V. B. Carson & H. G. Koenig (Eds.), *Spiritual dimensions of nursing practice* (Rev. ed., pp. 236–278). West Conshohocken, PA: Templeton Foundation.

Dick, H. V. (2014). "Knowing the person is happy that you were there": The spiritual resources staff in a residential aged care facility use to cope with resident deaths. *Journal of Religion, Spirituality & Aging, 24*(1–2), 164–176. doi:10.1080/15528030.2012.633056

Dobbs, D., Emmett, C. P., Hammarth, A., & Daaleman, T. P. (2012). Religiosity and death attitudes and engagement of advance care planning among chronically ill older adults. *Research on Aging, 34*(2), 113–130. doi:10.1177/0164027511423259

Doorenbos, A. Z., Wilson, S. A., & Coenen, A. (2006). A cross-cultural analysis of dignified dying. *Journal of Nursing Scholarship, 38*(4), 352–357. doi:10.1111/j.1547-5069.2006.00126.x

Dossey, B. M. (1997). Complementary and alternative therapies for our aging society. *Journal of Gerontological Nursing, 23*(9), 45–51. doi:10.3928/0098-9134-19970901-11

Dunn, D. (2004). Hearing the story: Spiritual challenges for the ageing in an acute mental health unit. In Jewell Albert (Ed.), *Ageing, spirituality and well-being* (pp. 153–160). London, England: Jessica Kingsley.

Dunn, K. S. (2008). Development and psychometric testing of a new geriatric spiritual well-being scale. *International Journal of Older People Nursing, 3*(3), 161–169. doi:10.1111/j.1748-3743.2007.00107.x

Dunn, K. S., & Horgas, A. L. (2000). The prevalence of prayer of a spiritual self-care modality in elders. *Journal of Holistic Nursing, 18*(4), 337–352. doi:10.1177/089801010001800405

Ellor, J. W. (1997). Celebrating the human spirit. In D. K. McKim (Ed.). *God never forgets: Faith, hope, and Alzheimer's disease* (pp. 1–20). Louisville, KY: Westminster John Knox Press.

Emblen, J. (2006). How can we help elders finish strong? *Journal of Christian Nursing, 31*(1), 57. doi:10.1097/CNJ.0000000000000041

Emery, E. E., & Pargament, K. I. (2004). The many faces of religious coping in late life: Conceptualization, measurement and links to well-being. *Ageing International, 29*(1), 3–27. doi:10.1007/s12126-004-1007-2

Emery, P. (2006). Building a new culture of aging: Revolutionizing long-term care. *Journal of Christian Nursing, 23*(1), 16–23. doi:10.1097/01.CNJ.0000262347.97634.8f

Erikson, E. H. (1963). *Childhood and society*. New York, NY: W. W. Norton.

Fortner, B. V., Neimeyer, R. A., & Rybarczyk, B. (2000). Correlates of death anxiety in older adults: A comprehensive review. In A. Tomer (Ed.), *Death attitudes and the older adult: Theories, concepts, and applications* (pp. 95–108). Philadelphia, PA: Brunner-Routledge.

Fowler, J. (1981). *Stages of faith: The psychology of human development and the quest for meaning*. San Francisco, CA: Harper & Row.

Fry, P. S. (2000). Religious involvement, spirituality and personal meaning for life: Existential predictors of psychological well-being in community-residing and institutional care elders. *Aging & Mental Health, 4*(4), 375–387. doi:10.1080/713649965

Haugen, G., & Innstrand, S. T. (2012). The effect of transcendence on depression in cognitively intact nursing home patients. *International Scholarly Research Notices: Psychiatry*, Volume 2012. doi:10.5402/2012/301325

Haugen, G., Rannestad, T., Hammervold, R., Garasen, H., & Espnes, G. A. (2014). The relationships between self-transcendence and spiritual well-being in cognitively intact nursing home patients. *International Journal of Older People Nursing, 9*(1), 65–78. doi:10.1111/opn.12018

Heriot, C. S. (1992). Spirituality and aging. *Holistic Nursing Practice, 7*(1), 22–31.

Herth, K. (1990). Fostering hope in terminally ill people. *Journal of Advanced Nursing, 15*(11), 1250–1259. doi:10.1111/j.1365-2648.1990.tb01740.x

Herth, K. (1992). Abbreviated instrument to measure hope: Development and psychometric evaluation. *Journal of Advanced Nursing, 17*(10), 1251–1259. doi:10.1111/j.1365-2648.1992.tb01843.x

Higgins, P. (2013). Meeting the religious needs of residents with dementia. *Nursing Older People, 25*(9), 25–29. doi:10.7748/nop2013.11.25.9.25.e501

Huang, C., Hsu, M., & Chen, T. (2011). An exploratory study of religious involvement as a moderator between anxiety, depressive symptoms and quality of life outcomes of older adults. *Journal of Clinical Nursing, 21*(5–6), 609–619. doi:10.1111/j.1365-2702.2010.03412.x

Hungelmann, J., Kenkel-Rossi, E., Klassen, L., & Stollenwerk, R. (1996). Focus on spiritual well-being: Harmonious interconnectedness of mind–body–spirit-use of the JAREL spiritual well-being scale. *Geriatric Nursing, 17*(6), 262–266.

Kerrigan, R., & Harkulich, J. T. (1993). A spiritual tool: An assessment tool helps nursing homes meet residents' spiritual needs. *Health Progress, 74*(4), 46–49.

Killick, J. (2000). Storytelling and dementia. *Elderly Care, 12*(2), 8–10.

Kim, S., Reed, P., Hayward, R. D., Kang, Y., & Koenig, H. G. (2011). Spirituality and psychological well-being: Testing a theory of family interdependence among family caregivers and their elders. *Research in Nursing & Health, 34*(2), 103–115. doi:10.1002/nur.20422

Kim-Godwin, Y. (2013). Prayer in clinical practice: What does evidence support? *Journal of Christian Nursing, 30*(4), 208–215. doi:10.1097/CNJ.0b013e31826c2219

Kumar, A. M., Tims, F., Cruess, D. G., & Mintzer, M. J. (1999). Music therapy increases serum melatonin levels in patients with Alzheimer's disease. *Alternative Therapies in Health and Medicine, 5*(6), 49–56.

Landis, B. J. (1996). Uncertainty, spiritual well-being and psychosocial adjustment to chronic illness. *Issues in Mental Health Nursing, 17*(3), 217–231. doi:10.3109/01612849609049916

Leetun, M. C. (1996). Wellness spirituality in the older adult: Assessment and intervention protocol. *Nurse Practitioner, 21*(8), 60, 65–70. doi:10.1097/00006205-199608000-00006

Levin, J., Chatters, L., & Taylor, R. (1995). Religious effects on health status and life satisfaction among Black Americans. *Journal of Gerontology, Series B: Psychological Sciences and Social Sciences, 50*(3), 154–163. doi:10.1093/geronb/50B.3.S154

Levin, J., Markides, K., & Ray, L. (1996). Religious attendance and psychological well-being in Mexican Americans: A panel analysis of three-generation data. *The Gerontologist, 36*(4), 454–463. doi:10.1093/geront/36.4.454

Levin, J., Taylor, R., & Chatters, L. (1994). Race and gender differences in religiosity among older adults: Findings from four national surveys. *Journal of Gerontology, 49*(3), S137–S145. doi:10.1093/geronj.49.3.S137

Lloyd, M. (2003a, November). *Spiritual nurturing as a technique: Advancing the search for meaning.* Paper presented at the NSW Elderly Suicide Prevention Network Conference, Sydney, Australia.

Lloyd, M. (2003b). Challenging depression: Taking a spiritually enhanced approach. *Geriaction, 21*(4), 26–29.

Loeb, S. J., Penrod, J., Falkenstern, S., Gueldner, S. H., & Poon, L. W. (2003). Supporting older adults living with multiple chronic conditions. *Western Journal of Nursing Research, 25*(1), 8–29. doi:10.1177/0193945902223883

Lowis, M. J., Jewell, A. J., Jackson, M. I., & Merchant, R. (2011). Religious and secular coping methods used by older adults: An empirical investigation. *Journal of Religion, Spirituality & Aging, 23*(4), 279–303. doi:10.1080/15528030.2011.566543

Lucas, J. A., Orshan, F., & Cook, F. (2000). Determinants of health-promoting behavior among women ages 65 and above living in the community. *Scholarly Inquiry for Nursing Practice: An International Journal, 14*(1), 77–100.

MacKinlay, E. (2003). *Mental health and spirituality in later life.* Binghamton, NY: Haworth Pastoral Press.

MacKinlay, E. (2008). Practice development in aged care nursing of older people: The perspective of ageing and spiritual care. *International Journal of Older People Nursing, 3*(2), 151–158.

MacKinlay, E., & Hudson, R. (2008). A review of literature in 2006. *International Journal of Older People Nursing, 3*(2), 139–144. doi:10.1111/j.1748-3743.2008.00117.x

MacKinlay, E. B. (1998). *The spiritual dimension of ageing: Meaning in life, response to meaning, and well-being in ageing* (Unpublished doctoral dissertation). LaTrobe University, Melbourne, Australia.

MacKinlay, E. B. (2001a). Understanding the ageing process: A developmental perspective of the psychosocial and spiritual dimensions. In E. MacKinlay, J. W. Ellor, & S. Pickard (Eds.), *Aging, spirituality, and pastoral care: A multi-national perspective* (pp. 111–122). Binghamton, NY: Haworth Pastoral Press.

MacKinlay, E. B. (2001b). Health, healing and wholeness in frail elderly people. *Journal of Religious Gerontology, 13*(2), 25–34. doi:10.1300/J078v13n02_03

MacKinlay, E. B. (2006). *Spiritual growth and care in the fourth age of life.* London, England: Jessica Kingsley.

Maddox, M. (2000). Spiritual wellness in older women. *Journal of Christian Nursing, 17*(1), 27–29. doi:10.1097/00005217-200017010-00013

Maslow, A. H. (1968). *Toward a psychology of being.* New York, NY: Van Nostrand.

McCarthy, V. L., & Bockweg, A. (2012). The role of transcendence in a holistic view of successful aging: A concept analysis and model of transcendence in maturation and aging. *Journal of Holistic Nursing, 31*(2), 84–92. doi:10.1177/0898010112463492

McFadden, S., Ingram, M., & Baldauf, C. (2000). Actions, feelings and values: Foundations of meaning and personhood in dementia. *Journal of Religious Gerontology, 11*(3–4), 67–86. doi:10.1300/j078v11n03_07

McSherry, W. (1996). Raising the spirits. *Nursing Times, 92*(3), 48–49.

Meraviglia, M., Sutter, R., & Gaskamp, C. D. (2008). Providing spiritual care to terminally ill older adults. *Journal of Gerontological Nursing, 34*(7), 8–14. doi:10.3928/00989134-20080701-08

Moberg, D. O. (2005). Research in spirituality, religion and aging. *Journal of Gerontological Social Work, 45*(1–2), 11–40. doi:10.1300/J083v45n01_02

Mooney, S. F. (2006). When memory fails: Helping dementia patients remember God. *Journal of Christian Nursing, 23*(1), 6–14. doi:10.1097/01.cnj.0000262345.07937.33

Morano, C. L., & King, D. (2005). Religiosity as a mediator of caregiver well-being: Does ethnicity make a difference? *Journal of Gerontological Social Work, 45*(1–2), 69–84. doi:10.1300/J083v45n01_05

Musgrave, C., Allen, C., & Allen, G. (2002). Spirituality and health for women of color. *American Journal of Public Health, 92*(4), 557–560. doi:10.2105/AJPH.92.4.557

Narayanasamy, A. (1991). *Spiritual care: A resource guide.* Lancaster, England: Quay Books.

Narayanasamy, A., Clisset, P., Parumal, L., Thompson, D., Annasamy, S., & Edge, R., (2004). A qualitative study of nurses' responses to the spiritual needs of older people. *Journal of Advanced Nursing, 48*(1), 6–16. doi:10.1111/j.1365-2648.2004.03163.x

O'Brien, M. E. (2011). *Spirituality in nursing: Standing on holy ground* (4th ed.). Sudbury, MA: Jones & Bartlett.

Overvold, J. A., Flannelly, K. J., Weaver, A. J., & Koenig, H. G. (2005). A study of religion, ministry, and meaning in caregiving among health professionals in an institutional setting in New York City. *The Journal of Pastoral Care & Counseling, 59*(3), 225–235. doi:10.1177/154230500505900305

Page, M. (2005). How well do we care for people's spiritual needs? *Kai Tiaki Nursing New Zealand, 11*(10), 18–19.

Patterson, V. L., King, S. V., Ball, M. M., Whittington, F. J., & Perkins, M. M. (2003). Coping with change: Religious activities and beliefs of residents in assisted living facilities. *Journal of Religious Gerontology, 14*(4), 79–93. doi:10.1300/J078v14n04_05

Paun, O. (2004). Female Alzheimer's patient caregivers share their strength. *Holistic Nursing Practice, 18*(1), 11–17.

Peck, R. C. (1968). Psychological development in the second half of life. In B. L. Neugarten (Ed.), *Middle age and aging: A reader in social psychology* (pp. 88–92). Chicago, IL: University of Chicago Press.

Pilch, J. J. (1988). Wellness spirituality. *Health Values, 12*(3), 28–31.

Rawlings-Anderson, K. (2004). Assessing the cultural and religious needs of older people. *Nursing Older People, 16*(8), 29–33. doi:10.7748/nop2004.11.16.8.29.c2343

Reed, P. G. (1991). Self-transcendence and mental health in oldest-old adults. *Nursing Research, 40*(1), 5–11. doi:10.1097/00006199-199101000-00002

Richards, M. (1990). Meeting the spiritual needs of the cognitively impaired. *Generation: Aging and the Human Experience, 14*(4), 63–64.

Seeber, J. J. (2000). Meaning in long-term care settings: Viktor Frankl's contribution to gerontology. *Journal of Religious Gerontology, 11*(3–4), 141–157. doi:10.1300/J078v11n03_11

Sorajjakool, S. (1998). Gerontology, spirituality, and religion. *Journal of Pastoral Care & Counseling, 52*(2), 147–156. doi:10.1177/002234099805200204

Stoll, R. I. (1979). Guidelines for spiritual assessment. *American Journal of Nursing, 79*(9), 1574–1577. doi:10.1097/00000446-197909000-00041

Sullivan, L. J., & Asselin, M. E. (2013). Revisiting quality of life for elders in long-term care: An integrative review. *Nursing Forum, 48*(3), 191–204. doi:10.1111/nuf.12030

Theis, S. L., Biordi, D. L., Coeling, H., Nalepka, C., & Miller, B. (2003). Spirituality in caregiving and care receiving. *Holistic Nursing Practice, 17*(1), 48–55. doi:10.1097/00004650-200301000-00010

The Joanna Briggs Institute. (2010). The Joanna Briggs Institute Best Practice Information Sheet: The psychosocial and spiritual experiences of elderly individuals recovering from a stroke. *Nursing & Health Sciences, 12*(4), 515–518.

Thompson, H. J., Demiris, G., Rue, T., Shatil, E., Wilamowska, K., Zaslavsky, O., & Reeder, B. (2011). A holistic approach to assess older adults' wellness using e-health technologies. *Telemedicine and e-Health, 17*(10), 794–800. doi:10.1089/tmj.2011.0059

Touhy, T. A. (2001). Nurturing hope and spirituality in the nursing home. *Holistic Nursing Practice, 15*(4), 45–56. doi:10.1097/00004650-200107000-00008

Wallace, M., & O'Shea, E. (2007). Perceptions of spirituality and spiritual care among older nursing home residents at the end of life. *Holistic Nursing Practice, 21*(6), 285–289. doi:10.1097/01.HNP.0000298611.02352.46

Wang, J. (2011). A structural model of the bio-psycho-socio-spiritual factors influencing the development towards gerotranscendence in a sample of institutionalized elders. *Journal of Advanced Nursing, 67*(12), 2628–2636. doi:10.1111/j.1365-2648.2011.05705.x

Wilkes, L., Cioffi, J. M., Fleming, A., & LeMiere, J. (2011). Defining pastoral care for older people in residential care. *Contemporary Nurse, 37*(2), 213–221. doi:10.5172/conu.2011.37.2.213

10

Spirituality in Palliative Care

Palliative care is a growing area of nursing practice. As the number of older adults increases, clinical specialties such as palliative and hospice care continue to expand. This chapter focuses on spirituality in palliative and hospice care as well as the role of a nurse in providing spiritual care within that context of practice.

The World Health Organization (WHO) defines palliative care as

> an approach that improves the quality of life of patients and their families facing the problems associated with life-threatening illness, through the prevention and relief of suffering by means of early identification and impeccable assessment and treatment of pain and other problems, physical, psychosocial and spiritual. (WHO, 2007, para. 1)

Hospice care has a similar aim in being described as care that is

> toward a different goal: maintaining or improving quality of life for someone whose illness, disease or condition is unlikely to be cured. Each patient's individualized care plan is updated as needed to address the physical, emotional and spiritual pain that often accompanies terminal illness. Hospice care also provides practical support for the caregiver(s) during the illness and grief support after the death. (Hospice Foundation of America, 2014, para. 1)

In this chapter, the terms "palliative care" and "hospice care" are used interchangeably.

DEATH AND DYING

Wynne (2013) states that "death and dying are frightening and isolating concepts that people may have difficulty in understanding" (p. 41). In addition to fear and isolation, when faced with impending death, individuals may also experience an overwhelming sense of loss, that is, an awareness of the inevitable impending loss of life (Carr, 2008; Meraviglia, Sutter, & Gaskamp, 2008). The person's sense of security as he or she knew it is shattered (Milligan, 2011).

As a person approaches death, his or her awareness of existential aspects of himself or herself may be heightened. Spiritual issues and concerns may come to the forefront and be of prime importance to the person (Steinhauser et al., 2000; Taylor, 2000; Van Dover & Bacon, 2001). Spiritual/existential suffering, struggle, and distress may result. Characteristics of these states of being may include loss of meaning in life, disappointment, regret, anxiety, and identity crisis (Kissane, 2000). Issues of faith may be important to healing (Steinhauser et al., 2000). As Satterly (2001) states, "Dying is first and foremost a spiritual experience" (p. 30). And MacKinlay (2001) adds that "the process of dying itself is part of the spiritual journey" (p. 120).

What are some of the tasks associated with dying? Death can occur at any stage of human development, which means that a person can be working through tasks of a particular life stage and the situation of death is juxtaposed upon normative developmental tasks. Two tasks that have been identified to be associated with the dying process include the acknowledgment and expression of feelings of guilt, anger, and fear; and the accommodation and/or reshaping of one's spirituality to encompass the concepts of finality and death. Accomplishing these tasks can make the death experience be one of acceptance, and even fulfillment (West, 1996). West makes three important points with respect to the "working through" of these tasks:

- This process is not necessarily done on a conscious level.

- The tasks can be met satisfactorily only if the dying person is comfortable, that is, if pain and other symptoms are well controlled.

- To engage in these tasks, the person must feel valued and safe emotionally, physically, and spiritually.

Therefore, nurses need to respond with respect, caring, compassion, and empathy in order to best help the dying person achieve these tasks.

Spirituality (including meaningfulness) has been identified as essential to a "good death"—a peaceful death—by both health care professionals and clients alike (Kruse, Ruder, & Martin, 2007; Steinhauser et al. 2000). As palliative care is a model and philosophy of care that is based on a holistic approach, therefore, spiritual care is essential to palliative care (Hayden, 2011).

Reflection 10.1

Itemize the feelings as well as the tasks that can accompany death and dying. Have you witnessed such feelings and tasks in terminally ill clients you have encountered in your nursing practice? How did you address such feelings and tasks with the client(s)?

SPIRITUALITY AND PALLIATIVE CARE

Palliative and hospice care are well recognized as settings particularly important for a focus on the spiritual beliefs, values, attitudes, and practices of clients, as well as a focus on providing spiritual care (Gijsberts, 2015; Iversen & Sessanna, 2012; Pitroff, 2013; Ruder, 2013; Tiew, Kwee, Creedy, & Chan, 2013). In a review of original research on spiritual care, Cockell and McSherry (2012) found that there was "a preponderance of research within the fields of palliative care and oncology . . . . Spiritual care is more likely to be discussed by health-care practitioners within the contexts of palliative care or on-cology care" (p. 965). In fact, Cockell and McSherry note that one-third of the studies focused on these two areas. They postulate that the tendency for spirituality to be of an intensified focus in these two areas of clinical practice is due to the fact that when cure is no longer possible, then other types of care—in particular spiritual care—emerge. Cockell and McSherry also argue that the research on spirituality in palliative care and oncology can also be relevant to practice in other areas.

DeLima and colleagues (2012) report on the essential components/practices for op-timal care as set out by the International Association for Hospice and Palliative Care (IAHPC). Practices intended to meet clients' spiritual needs necessarily focus on as-sessment and intervention related to the spiritual needs and any existential stress of cli-ents and families. Grief and bereavement needs and the spiritual support of health care workers are also a focus of the established practices. The complete document outlining the methodology and results of the process of developing the essential practices can be viewed on the IAHPC website: www.hospicecare.com.

In the literature, there is discussion of the importance of education for palliative care professionals to better prepare them for holistic practice. For example, Iversen and Sessanna (2012) describe the use of the Theory of Caring (Watson, 2012) and Emanci-patory Pedagogy (Hills & Watson, 2011) as frameworks for such education. Iversen and Sessanna outline the focus, topics, carative factors/processes, and content of their pro-gram of education. Refer to this article for further details.

It is clear from the definitions of palliative care and hospice care, and from the re-search on spirituality in palliative and hospice care, that spirituality is a key component of such care. It is appropriate to examine some of the findings related to the place of spirituality/religion at the end of life. The following discussion is only a sample of the vast literature on this topic.

SPIRITUALITY/RELIGION AT THE END OF LIFE

Gijsberts (2015) states that "the concept of spirituality at the end of life is complex and culturally sensitive" (p. 175). From a review of instruments measuring spirituality in the health care literature (1980–2009), Gijsberts and colleagues (2011) identified the fol-lowing dimensions of spirituality as important at the end of life:

- Spiritual well-being (peace, harmony, trust, hope, acceptance, meaning and pur-pose, connectedness, completion, fulfillment, positive affect, and comfort)

- Spiritual cognitions and behavior (spiritual beliefs, spiritual activities, and spiri-tual relationships)

- Spiritual coping (all behaviors and cognitions used to decrease distress and in-crease spiritual well-being)

By including these three dimensions, Gijsberts and colleagues constructed a model that depicted a conceptualization of spirituality at the end of life (p. 857). An impressive list of instruments used to measure spirituality at the end of life is also provided, along with the content validity of each instrument (pp. 855–856). Reference to this article is recommended. Other authors have also identified dimensions of spirituality important at the end of life, for example, Vachon, Fillion, and Achille (2009) identified and discussed 11 dimensions: "(1) meaning and purpose in life, (2) self-transcendence, (3) transcendence with a higher being, (4) feelings of communion and mutuality, (5) beliefs and faith, (6) hope, (7) attitude toward death, (8) appreciation of life, (9) reflection upon fundamental values, (10) the developmental nature of spirituality, and (11) its conscious aspect" (p. 53).

The assertion that spirituality and religion have an impact on clients' decisions and behavior has been mentioned in earlier chapters. That reality is also true at the end of life. The religious or spiritual beliefs of clients may impact their decision about prolonging life, or decisions as to how end-of-life care is provided. Although some clients may be explicit about their spiritual or religious issues with health care professionals, Mitchell (2011) makes the point that such issues "often present as distress or agitation in the patient" and that "spiritual, religious, and cultural issues are not difficult to understand; although they can be complex, they often come down to humanity" (pp. 678–679). Mitchell stresses the importance of identifying spiritual and religious issues on an ad hoc basis for every individual client due to the diversity of religious, spiritual, and cultural beliefs and practices. Clients themselves have also identified spiritual issues to be important at the end of life (Hills, Paice, Cameron, & Shott, 2005; Steinhauser et al., 2000).

Penman, Oliver, and Harrington (2013) examined the essence of spiritual engagement from the lived experiences of palliative clients and caregivers. Salient findings included the following:

- Such engagement reflected personal transformation where a change in direction in terms of the purpose (and of life itself) occurred: " . . . a new way of thinking" (p. 42). This change occurred in both clients and caregivers.

- Engagement in spiritual matters involved the emotions of love, compassion, and altruism, especially for caregivers.

- Engagement in spiritual matters was manifested through maintaining relationships. Intrapersonal and transpersonal relationships were also part of this theme.

- Religious practices, especially prayer, were important ways to engage in spiritual matters.

- Cultural influences impacted engagement in spiritual practices.

As an outcome of the study, Penmen and colleagues developed a conceptual model, The Relational Model of Spiritual Engagement. This model is useful not only to explain spiritual engagement but also to increase understanding of spirituality at the end of life, including the concerns, decisions, and actions of clients and their caregivers. Reference to this model (p. 44) and the discussion of the same (pp. 44–45) provide further details. Penman and colleagues maintain that the primacy of relationships and social networks for clients and caregivers should lead to nurses valuing, supporting, and nourishing such relationships. Facilitating spiritual engagement for both clients and caregivers is also an important role for nurses.

Reflection 10.2

Think about some time or event in your own life when you "engaged in spiritual matters." Review the findings by Penman and colleagues. Did you experience any such findings in your own life in engaging with spiritual matters? For example: Did spiritual transformation occur? What emotions did you experience? What place, if any, did relationships have in your engagement? What religious or spiritual practices enabled you to engage? What cultural influences impacted your engagement?

Boston, Bruce, and Schreiber (2011) identify that existential suffering and spiritual concerns are frequently encountered by terminally ill clients. They label this suffering and these concerns as being "among the most debilitating conditions in dying patients and yet are a neglected area of palliative care" (p. 605). Boston and colleagues reviewed the literature on existential suffering in palliative care (1970–2009). This review identified themes related to existential suffering, for example, the lack of consistency in definitions and conceptual understandings of existential suffering and the significance of existential suffering in palliative care. The review continued with a critical commentary of the themes identified, current gaps in the research literature on the topic, and recommendations for future research to bridge these gaps. For an in-depth discussion of these findings, reference to Boston and colleagues is recommended.

Bolmsjo (2000) identified that existential issues in palliative care clients are related to

- Dignity (being treated like a person, begin respected, and having a dignified death)

- Autonomy (loss of autonomy and impact of same in the dying process)

- Guilt (rational and irrational thoughts that produce guilt, including self-blame for illness)

- Relationships (unresolved conflicts with people, concern about those being left behind, isolation, and loneliness)

- Communication (being told information about their situation, receiving mixed messages from the palliative care team, how their diagnosis was communicated)

Satterly (2001) identifies that it is sometimes the case that religious or spiritual pain is present in those who are dying, adding to the struggles that they face. He separates these two types of pain for clarity purposes. Religious pain, a highly subjective and personal pain, is described as "a condition in which a patient in feeling guilty over the violation of the moral codes and values of his or her religious tradition" (p. 32). In this type of pain, the client's subjective interpretation of religious beliefs is operant. Satterly identifies fear as the primary emotion for people experiencing religious pain. Anxiety is also present due to anticipation of punishment—perhaps in the hereafter. Because guilt is a key feature of religious pain, it is important to determine how forgiveness fits with the client's religious tradition; as well as how the client views guilt and forgiveness.

Satterly suggests that the process of forgiveness is key in relieving religious pain. He further identifies childhood religious legacies as a primary source of religious pain, pointing to the need for assessment of the same.

With respect to spiritual pain, Satterly (2001) identifies this type of pain as being "about the business of a person's relationship with the source (God) of his or her life" (p. 34). He further describes this pain as "the felt absence of the ever-present God" (p. 37). Thus, while religious pain focuses on morals, values, behavior, and religious codes, spiritual pain is about a relationship that is "damaged or suspect" (p. 34). At the root of spiritual pain, he identifies shame, which he describes as people viewing themselves as being unworthy or damaged; resulting in them recoiling from attempts to love: "People in spiritual pain are those who have concluded, through their own self-judgment, that there is something wrong with them at their core" (p. 35). He makes the following statement about how the process of approaching death connects to shame and relationships: "Patients in spiritual pain now approaching death and a possible day of reckoning find themselves terrified of divine exposure. The fear is that God will see what has been so successfully hidden from all other relationships over decades [referring here to the hiding of the true self to receive approval and love from others]" (p. 35). Satterly suggests that spiritual pain may be relieved through an exploration of the nature of the person's relationship to his or her perceived source of life. The concept of love is operant in this examination, as is the exploration of shame. He believes that, when persons can love themselves unconditionally, seeing themselves as lovable persons, then spiritual pain can be relieved. Nurses, and other professionals on the palliative care team, can show unconditional love and acceptance to clients in spiritual pain, thus modeling love to the client. Although Satterly's discussion may be more relevant to clients who are religious, it is also relevant to many clients who may not be currently religious but still have a residual background in some religion. Such clients may similarly be prone to experiencing these types of pain as their religious background may surface at the end of their lives.

Others have identified the importance of managing spiritual/religious issues, distress, and pain at the end of life. In fact, Dobratz (2005) found that hospice clients identified that the management of spiritual distress was as vital as controlling physical pain.

Reflection 10.3

- Reflect on the concept of religious pain. Have you experienced such pain in your own life? What helped to relieve it? Have you seen religious pain in clients, even in those who are not "religious" but who have an ethical/moral code that guides their lives? How have you responded to such pain?
- Reflect on the concept of spiritual pain. Have you ever experienced such pain? What helped to relieve it? Have you seen spiritual pain in clients? How have you responded to such pain?
- What do you think of Satterly's notion that the best response to a client's spiritual pain is to show the client unconditional love? Can you think of any clinical situations that would support or disprove this assertion?

In an earlier section in this chapter, the statement was made that spirituality can contribute to a "good death" (see the section on Death and Dying). Spirituality can be beneficial in many other and related ways. A high level of spiritual well-being can generate a sense of peace and serenity for the dying client (Kruse et al., 2007). Spirituality can bring comfort to clients and families and be a source of hope for them (Doorenbos, Wilson, & Coenen, 2006; Kruse et al., 2007). Spiritual coping can assist them in dealing with existential concerns related to death and dying (Milligan, 2011). Spirituality can also enhance and improve the quality of life in clients and their families (Iversen & Sessanna, 2012). It can also relieve physical pain. For example, in the study by Dobratz (2004), quoted in Dobratz (2005), greater pain was experienced by clients when spiritual expressions were absent in their lives. A client's spiritual life (and that of their families) can also be strengthened through spiritual/religious practices (Kruse et al., 2007).

Bereaved family members have also identified what is important to a positive end of life. In a study by Steinhauser and colleagues (2000), bereaved persons identified peacefulness as the most frequently sought attribute. In this study, peace was connected to religion/God for some people, but for others, it was related to a sense of tranquility.

SPIRITUAL NEEDS AT THE END OF LIFE

Milligan (2011) states death and dying are times when "at least some patients will experience spiritual distress that may contribute to suffering and spiritual work—such as resolving spiritual issues and coming to terms with the personal reality of death. These will manifest as spiritual care needs" (p. 50). Spiritual needs, such as the need for meaning and purpose and the need for forgiveness, have already been alluded to in the discussion in this chapter. These needs can be especially acute and important at the end of life. For example, Milligan (2011) identifies questions that dying clients may ask health care professionals, questions that are related to meaning and purpose: "Why me?"; "Is there an afterlife or heaven or god?"; and "What has been the point of my life?" (p. 50). The spiritual needs of love and belonging and meaning and purpose are identified as prominent in a palliative care context, as suggested by Boston and colleagues (2011).

The need to prepare for death has also been identified as a spiritual need at the end of life. This need includes addressing unmet issues before death; addressing concerns about the afterlife; having a deeper understanding of death and dying; forgiving oneself and others; reviewing one's life; and being forgiven by others and perhaps God (Galek, Flannelly, Vane, & Galek, 2005).

In a study by Ross and Austin (2015), palliative care clients who were experiencing end-stage heart failure identified the following spiritual needs to be important:

- The need for love and belonging (these clients experienced isolation and loneliness)

- The need for hope and coping (hope-enhancing strategies were used by the clients, for example, keeping their dreams alive and maintaining a fighting spirit)

- The need for meaning and purpose (making sense of the illness, asking "Why?" and feeling useless)

- The need for faith and belief (especially related to the dying process)

- The need for religious faith and/or transcendence as a resource for coping

Vassallo (2001) applied the list of spiritual needs of terminally ill clients (as identified by Highfield & Carson, 1983) to describe how these needs were operant in clients dying at home—although their discussion may be equally relevant for clients in palliative and hospice settings. Vassallo discusses the fact that dying people often struggle with *meaning and purpose* in life, especially in terms of past life lived and life as it is in the midst of dying. These clients often look inward for answers to those existential questions of life that frequently emerge as part of the dying process. Meaning and purpose is also sought for the remaining time that they have to live. Examples of sources of meaning for this end time of life are family, suffering, and religious beliefs. Clients may identify the *need for forgiveness and reconciliation* with those for whom they may have had conflict or from whom they had been estranged in the past. This need can arise upon review of one's life. The *need to give love* is also discussed by Vassallo: a need that may be expressed through words and/or actions. In fact, the dying process can open up possibilities for this need to be more explicitly experienced in the client's life than was the case before the client became ill. Mending broken relationships through forgiveness and reconciliation is also a form of giving love. The *need for hope* can express itself in dying as a hope for inner peace, and a desire for less physical and emotional difficulties. It can also be expressed in hoping for repair of broken relationships from the past. Hope for something better in an afterlife can also be expressed. Finally, the *need for creativity* can be expressed in the legacy left, and also in the possibility of growth experiences in the midst of the dying process.

Using a list of spiritual needs identified in her Spiritual Needs Inventory (SNI; Hermann, 2001), Hermann (2007) determined clients' perceptions of the degree to which their spiritual needs were met as they neared the end of their lives. Salient findings from Hermann's study include the following:

- The need to pray was perceived to be met by 96% of the clients.

- The need to sing, listen to music, use inspirational materials, talk about day-to-day things, see the smiles of others, and use phrases from a religious text was perceived to be met by 80% to 89% of the clients.

- The need to talk with someone about spiritual issues, have information about family and friends, be around children, be with people who share spiritual beliefs, and think about happy thoughts was perceived to be met by 70% to 79% of the clients.

- The need to laugh, read a religious text, be with family and friends, and read inspirational materials was perceived to be met by 60% to 68% of the clients.

- The need to go to religious services was perceived to be met by only 30% of the clients.

The list of spiritual needs is fairly broad in the SNI, as can be seen in the aforementioned findings. However, on further examination, it is found that most of these spiritual needs are related to the need for love and relatedness, and the need for spiritual/religious activities. Diversity in spiritual needs has important implications for nurses in terms of nurses appreciating the broad nature of what is considered to be spiritual. Some of the spiritual needs that clients perceived to be met are related to their living in the midst of dying. This is an important point. As Hermann (2001) phrases it, nurses need to recognize clients in palliative care as "living, not merely dying" (p. 71). In a more recent study, Buck and McMillan (2012) tested the SNI on a sample of informal care-givers of terminally ill clients in a hospice context. They concluded that there was "early evidence for the validity and reliability of the SNI" (p. E332) to meet the spiritual needs of caregivers as well as clients.

The need for hope has some interesting dimensions in a palliative care context. Hope takes on a different perspective when death is imminent. Puchalski (2004) comments on this when she states:

> Early on, the person may hope for a cure; later, when a cure becomes unlikely, the person may hope for time to finish important projects or goals, travel, make peace with loved ones or with God, and have a peaceful death. This can result in healing, which can be manifested as a restoration of one's relationships or sense of self. (p. 495)

The spiritual beliefs of clients and families can provide a means for attaining hope. Through a case study, Pattison and Lee (2011) examine the Christian view of hope. As movement to end of life occurs, the reframing of hope is discussed by these authors. They also discuss practical aspects of caring for clients in the face of changing hope. Refer to the case study of Emma at the end of this chapter in this regard (see Case Studies, number 2). Not only is hoping a focus in dying, but it also functions as a mechanism connected to spirituality that can help people cope with dying (Puchalski, 2004).

As can be determined from this discussion, any of the foundational spiritual needs discussed in Chapter 5 (see the section on Spiritual Needs) are relevant in the context of palliative care. Such needs include, for example, the need for love and relatedness; the need for meaning and purpose; the need for forgiveness; and the need for hope. However, as can also be seen, death and dying bring added dimensions to these needs. Moreover, because of the context of dying, additional spiritual needs present themselves, such as the need to prepare for death. It is critical for nurses in a palliative care context to not only possess knowledge of foundational spiritual needs and how the process of death and dying impacts such needs but also be cognizant and alert to the specific spiritual needs related to death and dying.

Reflection 10.4

From the aforementioned discussion, itemize a list of possible spiritual needs of those who are dying. Have such needs been evident in terminally ill clients for whom you provided nursing care? How did these needs manifest themselves? How did you respond to such needs? Was it adequate in terms of helping clients meet their spiritual needs? If not, what else might you have done?

SPIRITUAL ASSESSMENT IN PALLIATIVE CARE

As identified in the definition of palliative care earlier in this chapter (see section on Spirituality and Palliative Care), the relief of suffering in a palliative care context is assisted by an "impeccable assessment" (WHO, 2007, para 1). Because of the importance of spirituality in palliative care, spiritual assessment is imperative. There is also indication that clients in palliative care want to be asked questions about spirituality/religion, and this is especially true for those clients who identify as being religious or spiritual (Taylor & Brander, 2013).

Taylor (2013) identified two foci for spiritual assessment in palliative care: indications and manifestations of spiritual needs, and the efficacy of spiritual practices. Taylor appropriately points out that a spiritual assessment can reveal whether a client's spiritual needs *are* being met. She identifies guidelines for the assessment of terminally ill clients, similar to the principles for spiritual assessment identified in Chapter 5 (see the section on Principles of Spiritual Assessment). An important point that Taylor stresses is that nurses must "match" the language of the client. Another legitimate observation related to clients who are dying is that some may be too ill to speak, hear, or understand a verbal assessment. In such cases, the family may be called upon as a resource. Nonverbal means of communication may also be instigated.

Taylor and Brander (2013) suggest that, in a spiritual assessment in palliative care, nurses should focus on what is positive, primary, and most pertinent, such as spiritual/religious beliefs and practices and how they impact the person's life:

> Ask only questions that are relevant to the health care challenge and care anticipated. Do not veer off course out of curiosity or because of an evangelical desire to delve more deeply. Indeed, one way to show respect is to not tread where one does not belong. (p. 354)

Puchalski and colleagues (2009) reported on a census conference, which was held on palliative care, in particular, recommendations related to the spiritual assessment and care as a dimension of palliative care. Key criteria for spiritual assessment and care included the following:

- Using a standardized spiritual assessment tool where possible

- Reevaluating the impact of spiritual interventions and client/family preferences

- Ensuring that clients/families have access to appropriate spiritual care professionals/religious leaders

- Being sensitive in the use of religious/spiritual symbols due to cultural and religious diversity

- Encouraging clients/families to display their own religious symbols

- Documenting clients'/families' spiritual and existential concerns

Some of the spiritual tools discussed in Chapter 5 (see section on Spiritual Assessment Tools/Models) and elsewhere in this book have also been identified as being relevant in the context of palliative care. For example, Brown, Whitney, and Duffy (2006) and

Milligan (2011) discuss use of the FICA approach (Puchalski & Romer, 2000). Milligan also discusses use of the HOPE approach to spiritual assessment (Anandarajah & Hight, 2001), whereas Taylor (2001) illustrates the use of Fitchett's 7×7 Model for Spiritual Assessment (Fitchett, 1993). Earlier in this chapter (see section on Spirituality/Religion at the End of Life) reference was made to a list of spiritual assessment tools used in palliative care contexts (Gijsberts et al., 2011). Additionally, although it is somewhat dated, it is still worth reviewing a synthesis of the content of spiritual assessment forms from 53 hospices provided by Dudley, Smith, and Millison (1995). However, relying on empirical research studies and expert opinions, the Department of Health (2011) in the United Kingdom put forth the proposition that a formal spiritual assessment in palliative care may not be the best approach. In the alternative, narrative methods and generic questions have been emerging as legitimate means of assessment in palliative care.

Several authors have developed questions designed for spiritual assessment in palliative care. As Milligan (2011) asserts, sometimes simple questions are all that is needed to initiate and continue discussion on spiritual matters. Steed (2012) suggests six questions that nurses can ask of themselves concerning the general assessment of clients in palliative care. Such questions focus on characteristic indicators of quality palliative care. One question in particular is an explicit focus on spiritual needs: "Are the patient's spiritual needs addressed?" (p. 60). In discussing this question, Steed acknowledges the impact that spirituality can have on clients' values, preferences, and goals—especially as they relate to end-of-life care and the decisions that clients may have to make at this time. Another example of questions developed for spiritual assessment of the terminally ill clients is provided by van der Poel (1998), quoted in Prebendary and Speck (1999), who identified five questions dealing with the following:

- The place of God in the patient's life
- The patient's attitude toward himself or herself
- The patient's relationship with family and friends
- The patient's understanding of and interest in prayer
- The patient's attitude toward his or her religious denomination or church (Prebendary & Speck, p. 286)

Further, van der Poel identifies a number of substatements under each of the aforementioned questions, formed within a Likert-type scale to assist nurses with the assessment.

Taylor and Brander (2013) itemized a list of 21 questions for use in the spiritual assessment of clients in hospice care. They included a quantification of the mean level of comfort that nurses had in their study when the nurses asked each question of clients (Table 2, p. 182). Examples of questions provided by Taylor and Brander include the following:

- Would you like to explore religious matters with someone?
- If you would like to continue to practice or explore your spirituality or religion, what would help?
- When life is hard, how have you kept going? Is there anyone or anything that has helped you? How helpful are these supports? (p. 351)

In another article, Taylor (2013) offers additional information (pp. 183–184):

- A focus for indirect spiritual assessment (e.g., what to observe and listen for)

- Guidelines for direct assessment methods (e.g., using prompts and "entering wedges," p. 183), which are statements to open up discussion about spirituality/religion with clients

- A list of topics for spiritual assessment (e.g., spiritual support and the importance of spirituality and/or religion to clients)

- Cautionary comments about spiritual assessment (e.g., to respect that some clients are private and may consider a spiritual assessment as intrusive as well as not pushing religion upon clients)

Reference to Taylor and Bender (2013) as well as Taylor (2013) is recommended for further details.

A taxonomy of the spiritual needs of clients in palliative care (and the needs of their families) can provide a framework for spiritual assessment and also for developing spiritual assessment questions. One such taxonomy has already been alluded to in this chapter (see the section on Spiritual Needs at the End of Life), and that of the SNI, developed by Hermann (2001). This tool was developed from clients' perspectives of their spiritual needs. Dimensions of spirituality important at the end of life can also provide an organizing framework from which to develop questions for spiritual assessment. Examples of such dimensions have been discussed previously in this chapter (see the section on Spirituality/Religion at the End of Life). The dimensions developed by Gijsberts and colleagues (2011) and by Vachon and colleagues (2009) are also relevant.

It is appropriate for nurses to complete an initial screening assessment in a palliative/hospice care context (Taylor & Brander, 2013). Jackson (2004) gives some examples of initial questions that nurses can ask of clients. One sample line of questioning is: "When you were admitted to the hospice, you gave us a lot of information. One of the questions you were asked was about your mood at that time. How are you feeling now?" (p. 25). Depending on the client's answer, further questions can then be asked to explore not only the client's feelings, but also other aspects that could be important in a spiritual assessment, for example, the extent to which the person is experiencing hope and peace. The first question is usually a "bridge" to talk about spirituality. In this manner, questions are not designed or sequenced for use as a script or an interview format, but, rather, the questions are used in a process as prompts for the nurse to be able to engage in ongoing discussion with the client about spirituality.

Nurses can also proceed with spiritual assessment from unprompted statements that clients may make to the nurse. For example, Taylor (2001) presents a number of client statements for each of seven dimensions of spirituality (based on the work of Kloss, 1988; Maloney, 1993; Pruyser, 1976). Taylor identifies statements that could be considered negative or less healthy utterances; and also statements that would be considered positive or healthier. For example, for the spirituality dimension "involvement in spiritual/religious community, and experience of communion" (p. 399), an example of a negative, less healthy statement by a client might be: "Why should I have to ask for help from my church? They don't bother to call me!" (p. 399). A more positive, healthy response might be: "I still feel connected to my church because I know that they are praying for me" (p. 399). Taylor also provides an interesting case study of a terminally ill client that serves to show how Fitchett's 7×7 Model for Spiritual Assessment (Fitchett, 1993) is applied. Although the dimensions of spirituality and also Taylor's statements are underpinned by a Christian worldview, it remains the case that dimensions of spirituality from a variety of worldviews can be used as a framework for assessment.

Reflection 10.5

Using the questions given in this section, or by composing your own questions, develop an interview guide for use in the spiritual assessment of terminally ill clients in the setting in which you work. Share these with peers/colleagues for feedback; and revise if necessary. Pilot the questions in your clinical practice, noting the outcomes of such questions for the client, for yourself, and for the relationship between you and the client. Continue to revise the questions if necessary.

The same principles of spiritual assessment discussed in Chapter 5 that are of general application apply also to palliative care (see the section on Principles of Spiritual Assessment). Examples of such principles are the inclusion of religious assessment if religion is important to a client, and the use of observation skills in the assessment process. In a palliative care setting, the client's family may also be more involved in the spiritual assessment because of the acuity of the client who is dying. Family members may also be the target for spiritual assessment because of the intensity of this experience for family members themselves.

SPIRITUAL CARE/INTERVENTIONS IN PALLIATIVE CARE

Based on the nature of death and dying, and also from the research on how spirituality impacts aspects of the dying process, Wynne (2013) maintains that it is imperative that spiritual care and support be offered in end-of-life care. Others who concur with this opinion are Puchalski and Ferrell (2010), Ruder (2008), and Taylor and Brander (2013). In fact, spiritual support has been identified as one domain essential for the quality of care in end-of-life care in critical care contexts (Clarke et al., 2003).

Given the importance of spiritual care in palliative contexts, much activity has occurred relative to the inclusion of spiritual care. For example, clinical practice guidelines related to spirituality/religion and existential aspects of care have been developed (National Consensus Project for Quality Palliative Care, 2009). Projects demonstrating the integration of spiritual care in palliative care have been reported, for example, Otis-Green and colleagues (2012). Website resources to help improve spiritual care in palliative care have also been identified (Otis-Green et al.). Models of care have been described for use with terminally ill clients, for example, a holistic model in Kendall (1999) and the use of a humanistic model (developed by Paterson & Zderad, 1988) in the care of terminally ill clients living at home (Vassalo, 2001). Reference to these resources is recommended for further details.

Price, Stevens, and LaBarre (1995) identify three areas of focus for the spiritual care of clients who are dying: relationships (for love and belonging, for forgiveness); meaning (in life and in illness); and self-worth (in the midst of illness). In a hospice context, Yardley, Walshe, and Parr's (2009) study identified clients' feelings as an important focus for the provision of spiritual care. These clients also thought with respect to the training of professionals who work in palliative care contexts that the most important area for such training needed to be with respect to attitudes; and, in particular, attitudes focused on empathy, genuineness, caring, being nonjudgmental, sensitivity, and willingness to engage with clients.

Generic spiritual care (presence, listening, etc.) characterizes the nature of spiritual care at the end of life and can contribute to a "good death" (Hayden, 2011; Saunders, 2000). In fact, Milligan (2011) identifies presence not only as very important in spiritual care at the end of life, but goes further to suggest that it may be all that is required. This importance of presence is in keeping with the idea of spiritual care in end-of-life care akin to the nurse accompanying clients and their families on their journey through the dying process (Hayden, 2011; Milligan, 2011; Vassalo, 2001). As Vassalo states, "Hospice nurses and the dying persons become the 'we' in the nursing situation by sharing lived experiences" (p. 23). Another metaphor used to describe spiritual care in palliative care is that of a "spiritual tapestry" (Bailey, Moran, & Graham, 2009). Each nurse contributes to the tapestry, adding color and texture through the connections between him- or herself and clients; and weaving his or her knowledge and skills regarding spirituality into the tapestry.

Puchalski, Lumford, Harris, and Miller (2006) identify six roles of the nurse in palliative care: building a trusting relationship with the client that includes conveying dignity and respect; providing an environment that is peaceful and supportive; acknowledging his or her role has changed with respect to the goals of care; actively listening, being present, and attending to the client/family; conducting a spiritual assessment; and collaborating with the palliative care team.

Although generic spiritual care is foundational in palliative care, there have been specific interventions noted to be especially effective in this setting. Examples are presented in Table 10.1.

Some of these interventions have been identified to be more common than others. For example, Kisvetrova and colleagues' (2013) study identified spiritual support to be the most frequent intervention by palliative care nurses (spiritual support included such actions as treating clients with dignity and respect, listening, and being present). Such support was seen to help protect clients against death anxiety. Palliative care clients have also identified spiritual help and support to be important to them (Ross & Austin, 2015). Clients in Ross and Austin's study described such support as linking them to chaplains/spiritual care professionals; helping them keep hope alive; and having an affirming attitude. Ross and Austin advocate for a spiritual support home-visiting service for clients who are dying at home, identifying nurses as one of the key professionals who might offer such a service. Some of the interventions in Table 10.1 have also been discussed using case examples to illustrate the process and outcome of the intervention. For example, Jenko, Gonzalez, and Alley (2010) and Jenko, Gonzalez, and Seymour (2007) provide clinical examples and techniques to help nurses conduct a life review in a palliative care context.

Table 10.1 **Nursing Interventions for Palliative Care**
Respecting/facilitating spiritual/religious rituals
Creating an environment conducive to spiritual care
Consulting/referring to a chaplain/spiritual care professional
Using prayer
Providing spiritual support
Assisting with life review
Encouraging connection with others

Sources: Holloway (2006), Jenko, Gonzalez, and Alley (2010), Jenko et al. (2007), Kisvetrova, Klugar, and Kabelka (2013), Kuuppelomaki (2001), Milligan (2011), Ross and Austin (2015), and Tiew et al. (2013).

In the course of implementing spiritual care at the end of life, conversations about death and dying will likely occur. Such conversations are noted to be different from most conversations in life: "Interactions at the end of life are often reported to have a depth of meaning and connection that is unusual in everyday life" (Planalp, Trost, & Berry, 2011, p. 483). On what should such conversations focus? In a study exploring conversations between hospice volunteers and clients, Planalp and colleagues (2011) found that the volunteers identified the most common meaningful conversations to focus on meaning, religion and prayer, and death and the hereafter. Other meaningful conversations occurred around family situations and relationships, spiritual issues, unfinished business, loss of capacities, and shared common interests. Planalp and colleagues note that such conversations "should and do arise from patients' concerns and the rapport they have established with volunteers. Sometimes, all that is needed is for the volunteer to listen" (p. 486). Although this study focused on volunteers, implications for nurses conversing with clients in palliative care can also be drawn from this study.

Others have identified meaning and purpose to be a key focus for discussion and interventions in palliative care. For example, Morita and colleagues (2007) reported the impact of a workshop that was designed to help nurses deal with meaninglessness in terminally ill clients. The workshop was deemed to be beneficial in improving the nurses' clinical skills in this regard.

Nurses should strive to create an environment conducive to communicating with clients in end-of-life care. For example, they should give full attention to clients, ask openended questions, actively listen and reflect emotions, give information, acknowledge uncertainty, consider the cultural, religious, and/or spiritual as a context for discussion, and identify the clients' beliefs about death/dying. Such actions will ascertain client priorities for conversation (Griffie, Nelson-Marten, & Muchka, 2004).

Nurses sometimes avoid discussing death and dying in the face of client comments that suggest such conversation is important. Griffie and colleagues (2004) attribute this avoidance to the idea that death can be "the elephant in the room—something unavoidable and yet taboo . . . . The elephant's presence is undeniable in hospital corridors, in waiting rooms, and at bedsides, but few acknowledge it" (p. 49). Griffie and colleagues maintain that explicitly addressing death/dying with clients can relieve their anxiety, enable them to think more clearly, help them face their fears, and help them make decisions. Griffie and colleagues label such discussion as "essential to good nursing care at the end of life" (p. 50). One area that Milligan (2011) identified as being appropriate for nurses to discuss relative to death and dying was assisting clients with planning for death or a funeral—if the client wishes such help.

A final point with respect to spiritual care in palliative care is really a reminder: Always consider culture in the practice of spiritual caregiving. Although death is a constant for all humanity, the range of approaches to death represented in society today is quite broad. As such, within the commonality of death it is important for nurses to pay particular attention to the complexity of particular spiritual/religious needs of people from various cultures (Holloway, 2006). Mazanec and Tyler (2003) identify three key components of culture relevant to end-of-life care:

- *Ethnicity*, including the role ethnicity plays in communication, values, beliefs, and practices regarding illness and death

- *Age*, including developmental stage, generational differences in views of illness, death, and dying and how to deal with same

- *Spirituality*, including religious affiliation, spiritual/religious practices, rituals, and beliefs regarding illness, death, and dying, and the hereafter

---

Reflection 10.6

Review the nature of spiritual care and identified interventions pertinent to end-of-life care. Which do you include in your care of terminally ill clients and what has been the outcome? Are there others not mentioned that you have used with positive impact on clients? Are there interventions that you might like to employ based on what you have read in this section?

Spirituality and spiritual/religious care have been the topic of research and discussion with respect to various cultures and from the perspectives of both clients and nurses. Examples include the following:

- The meaning of spirituality and spiritual care to terminally ill clients who are Chinese (Mok, Wong, & Wong, 2010)

- The impact of a training program for Japanese nurses to address meaninglessness in terminally ill clients (Morita et al., 2007)

- Cultural influences in end-of-life care among Jewish clients (Bonura, Fender, Roesler, & Pacquiao, 2001)

- Spiritual aspects of palliative care for Muslim clients (Cheraghi, Payne, & Salsali, 2005)

Reference to these and other resources on culture and end-of-life care is recommended.

There are many contexts in which palliative care is offered that have not been specifically addressed, but which have important implications for nursing in those contexts of care. One example is the spiritual care of dying children and care of their families. Much has been written about spiritual care in the palliative care of children. Topics explored include spirituality and spiritual support in neonatal end-of-life care (Rosenbaum, Smith, & Zollfrank, 2011) and spiritual care as it pertains to children in palliative care (Davies, Brenner, Orloff, Sumner, & Worden, 2002; Foster, Bell, & Gilmer, 2012; Heilferty, 2004; O'Shea & Kanarek, 2013; Peterson, 2014; Tamburro, Shaffer, Hahnlen, Felker, & Ceneviva, 2011; Weidner et al., 2011). Researching spirituality in end-of-life care in specific contexts of nursing ensures that quality care will be tailored to the particular clinical practice setting.

SPIRITUAL CARE OF THE BEREAVED

No discussion of spirituality in end-of-life care would be complete without paying attention to the bereaved. The bereaved person's experience can be influenced by a number of factors: the type of death that his or her loved one experienced; if the death was anticipated or sudden; the age of the deceased; the nature and intensity of the relationship of the bereaved to the deceased person; personality characteristics of the bereaved person; and others. For example, it has been noted that those who mourn a sudden death are more likely to experience abnormal or pathological grief, extended grief, and a grief more difficult to resolve. They are also more likely to feel overwhelmed and their ability to function will be impacted. Also characteristic of such mourners is helplessness, a sense of unreality and guilt, a need to blame, and a strong need to make sense of the loss (Fast, 2003). However, bereaved persons can also experience growth and development in the grieving process, including spiritual growth and development (Hogan, Greenfield, & Schmidt, 2001).

Often, bereaved persons are family members of the deceased. Conversing with and focusing on the family's spirituality has been a point stressed in this chapter. Focusing on families is important not only in terms of the outcomes with those families, but also in terms of the client outcomes (Kissane, 2000; Waldrop, Milch, & Skretny, 2005). The suffering of both may be alleviated. One example of an intervention directed at families is provided by Tan, Wilson, Olver, and Barton (2011). Using Murphy's family meeting model (Murphy, 1999), a family meeting was instigated with the intention and design, in part, to address spiritual and psychosocial needs. Participants in the family meeting identified the spiritual impact of the meeting primarily in terms of relationships, new understandings of themselves, and also in terms of finding meaning and purpose. Tan and colleagues conclude that the family meeting contributed to the enrichment of participants' spirituality. Griffie and colleagues (2004) also discuss meeting with families of terminally ill clients in the form of a family conference. An outline of the process and focus of such a conference is provided (p. 54) along with discussion of the same (pp. 54–56). Reference to these two resources is recommended.

A key issue discussed by Cutcliffe (2006) with respect to nurses assisting the bereaved is that of hope. He maintains that when nurses help the bereaved engage in cathartic release of painful emotions, hope is inspired. He sees this cathartic release as enabling the bereaved to see the future in a more hopeful manner. Cutcliffe discusses strategies that nurses can use to facilitate such release, for example, providing the opportunity for clients to reflect, purposefully utilizing silence, and providing unconditional and continual support. An earlier article by Cutcliffe (1995) describes the concept of hope as well as a theoretical framework that nurses can use to instill and inspire hope in terminally ill clients who have HIV infection. Reference to both of these articles will provide additional details.

Reflection 10.7

Reflecting on times of loss and grief, and the spiritual issues inherent in these, is key to understanding and responding to clients/families who are experiencing loss and grief (the following exercise is adapted from Beckman, Boxley-Harges, Bruick-Sorge, & Salmon, 2007).

- Reflect on a loss experience in your own life (death, divorce, abandonment, etc.).
- What feelings did you experience at the time of the loss?
- What spiritual issues and concerns, if any, arose during this experience?
- What or who provided comfort at this time? How did they help?
- What coping strategies did you engage in at the time? Were any of these spiritual or religious strategies? Which were helpful, and why were they helpful? Which were not helpful, and why not?

THE PERSON OF THE NURSE IN PALLIATIVE CARE

If you peruse the health care literature on the topic of palliative care, it is clear that such care is often offered by way of a team approach, with nurses being an integral part of such a palliative care team. In fact, a team approach may be a preferred method of care in this setting. The efficacy of the team approach in palliative care has been studied (e.g., Kao, Hu, Chiu, & Chen, 2014). All clients received the usual care, but some received additional visits from the hospital-based palliative care team (intervention group). Those who received the extra visits from the palliative care team had significant improvement in their spiritual well-being; whereas for the group of clients who received only the usual care, there was no significant improvement in spiritual well-being. There was also a positive impact in the intervention team with respect to symptom management.

How is the person of the nurse impacted by working with terminally ill clients and their families? Working in such a setting can be stressful as nurses constantly witness suffering and death. In fact, caring for clients who are dying has been identified as one of the most difficult, stressful, and challenging aspects of nurses' work (Holland & Neimeyer, 2005; Vachon, Fillion, Achille, Duval, & Leung, 2011). However, such work can stimulate the nurses' own subjective evaluation of the meaning of life and their own sense of mortality (Wasner, Longaker, Fegg, & Borasio, 2005).

The spiritual/religious background of a nurse has been determined to impact his or her experience in working with terminally ill clients. For example, Bjarnason (2010) found that nurses with religious backgrounds were generally more confident using questions/discussion with clients about advance directives and educating them about same. Nurses with high religiosity also had more difficulty with decisions to withdraw/withhold treatment at the end of life and allow clients to die. There was no significant relationship discovered between the nurses' religiosity and their ability to discuss end-of-life care, including discussing death and dying with clients. In their study, Ekedahl and Wengstrom (2010) found that the religious orientation of the nurses (who worked with terminally ill clients) impacted how they viewed their work (e.g., setting boundaries between work and personal life so as to promote their own health). Their religiosity also provided personal protection in that it facilitated their ability to cope with working with the terminally ill clients. Prayer was a common coping strategy for these nurses. Christopher (2010) also studied the impact of nurses' religiosity, identifying it as a factor that made the nurses more willing to advocate for clients receiving treatment in line with the clients' religious beliefs. Their religiosity also enabled them to be more willing to relinquish relationship control in end-of-life care so that clients control conversations about such care. This was especially true if the religiosity was intrinsic.

Ronaldson, Hayes, Aggar, Green, and Carey (2102) found that nurses working in palliative care had a higher level of spiritual perspectives and a more advanced practice of spiritual care than the acute care nurses in their study. Although the characteristics of the nurses in both settings might explain this finding (e.g., age and advanced experience), the setting of palliative care was itself seen as more conducive to a focus on spirituality.

A number of studies have explored nurses' experiences of working in palliative care. For example, Pittroff (2013) conducted a study of inpatient palliative care nurse consultants who were experienced in this area of care. Although the term "palliative care nurse consultant" might evoke an image of a highly specialized nurse, the nurses in Pittroff's study had not had formal education in spiritual care other than through conferences or personal study. However, their personal life experiences (especially with loss), participation in a faith community, and their evolving nursing practice all contributed to their expertise. These nurses described attending to clients' spiritual needs as reinforcing their own spirituality. They described experiencing the "mystery of human existence" (p. 166) and described providing care at the end of life "as a 'gift'" (p. 166). They also saw "the role of providing presence, support, and spiritual advocacy as 'honor and privilege'. . . . The experience of being with people undergoing loss and death creates a context of hospitality, invitation, and mutuality of care" (p. 166). These characteristics were identified by Pittroff as "the etiquette these nurses embody in providing spiritual care . . . . The manners and humbled relational stances of the nurses engage and permit actualization of spirituality and transcendent meanings and concerns" (p. 166). Pittroff identified these and other aspects of their work, as well as their spiritual care practices, as representing "humbled experts" (p. 164).

Another example of a focus on nurses' experiences in working with dying clients is that of Vachon, Fillion, and Achille (2012). These authors explored three aspects of the nurses' experiences: death confrontation, spiritual-existential experience, and caring attitudes. With respect to death confrontation, many nurses saw death as having meaning and purpose, not only in terms of death itself, but also in terms of their own lives. Some viewed death as "transition to another state of being" (p. 156). Some nurses also found that working with dying clients created personal awareness of their own death. With respect to the second theme of spiritual-existential experience, this experience was individualistic but a common theme was that nurses described the experience as providing "a sense of coherence between their values and actions" (p. 158)—although some nurses did experience distress when there was a sense of incoherence between the two. The spiritual-existential experience was also described as "a search for meaning and purpose" (p. 159). The experience also provided a sense of connection in relationships with friends/family/clients; but also a sense of isolation. In essence, the spiritual-existential experience was described as a state of being that was characterized by mindfulness. The third theme of caring attitudes referred not only to orientation toward suffering but also to how a response to suffering was handled by the nurses (e.g., if they engaged in self-care activities to promote their health). Vachon and colleagues (2012) developed a typology of the nurses' experiences in palliative care based on the three themes (Table 3, p. 164). Reference to this typology and the illuminative comments of the nurses illustrating aspects of the typology is recommended. Also for review is an earlier article by Vachon and colleagues (2011), which describes the spiritual and existential experience of palliative care nurses with respect to a meaning-centered intervention (Fillion, Dupuis, Tremblay, De Grace, & Breitbart, 2006; Greenstein & Breitbart, 2000). The intervention was directed at these nurses and the impact of this intervention on the nurses' spiritual and existential awareness is described.

From this discussion, it can be surmised that it is imperative that nurses focus on themselves when working with terminally ill clients. They must especially be aware of their own spirituality and their views on death and dying. They must also take care of themselves so that they can better care for clients and families in palliative care.

Reflection 10.8

Reflect on the following comments in an article by Conrad (1985):

> … a nurse who is uncomfortable discussing spiritual matters with another should honestly examine herself to determine if she is qualified to care for the dying since spiritual support is such an important part of nursing care of the dying. (p. 420)

(continued)

Reflection 10.8 (continued)

…the more a nurse has struggled on her own spiritual journey, including dealing with the thought of her own death, the better she is able to help another on his spiritual pilgrimage. (p. 419)

- What is your perspective on each of these statements? Do you agree or disagree and why?
- How does working with terminally ill clients and their families impact you personally? Can you relate to some of the nurses' comments in the study by Vachon and collegues (2012) and also the study by Pittroff (2013)?

This chapter has provided a mere introduction to spirituality and spiritual issues in palliative care. Accessing the literature resources mentioned in the chapter further contributes to knowledge acquisition. There are many other resources that can be accessed to improve knowledge and clinical skills in palliative care. There are also specific organizations that exist to increase knowledge about death, dying, and bereavement: in the United States, there is the Association for Death Education and Counseling (www.adec.org); and in Canada, there is the King's University College Centre for Education about Grief and Bereavement (www.kings.uwo.ca/thanatology).

Taking It Further

1. Read the case study of Jamilla in Hendriks and colleagues (2102, pp. 1053–1054).

    a. What aspects of the case study had implications for the religious care of Jamilla? Itemize these and research them in sources about the Muslim religion.

    b. Reflect on the impact on the nurse of caring for Jamilla. To what aspects of the nurse's experience can you relate in terms of caring for clients who are dying?

    c. What are your reactions to the Islamic beliefs about life and death as presented in the article? How do these beliefs compare with your own spiritual/religious beliefs?

    d. Would you face any personal challenges in caring for Jamilla? If so, what would these be and why would they be challenging? How might you deal with such challenges?

    e. In the article, the question is posed: "How should the medical team deal with this dilemma?" (p. 1054, referring to Jamilla's Islamic beliefs and faith creating a desire within her to do everything possible to prolong her life, along with her awareness that, from a medical viewpoint, all options had been exhausted and prolonging life would mean more suffering). Have you encountered such dilemmas in your own clinical practice, perhaps not related to Islamic beliefs but to other spiritual/religious beliefs of clients/families? How might you answer the question posed?

f. What dilemmas did the nurses caring for Jamilla encounter with respect to pain control? How might such a situation impact you?

g. What further assessment would you have completed with respect to Jamilla's spiritual/religious needs and why?

h. A comment made toward the end of the article is:

> It seemed . . . a miracle had happened to all of us [referring to the both Jamilla and the medical/nursing professionals]. Outside the medical paradigm, we encountered transcultural differences regarding religion and faith that were strongly influencing our understanding and policy of palliative care. Accepting the paradigm of religion and the related vision of life turned out to be an eye opener and changed our frame of reference. It also focused us to practice an even more patient-centered way of communication between the medical team, the patient, and her family. (pp. 1054–1055)

Can you relate to this statement from your own nursing experience? What are your reflections on the implications for practice of such a statement for the care of clients in palliative care?

2. Read the case study of Emma in Pattison and Lee (2011, pp. 733–739).

a. What are *your* sources of hope? How do they compare/contrast with Emma's? How do they compare/contrast with her family's sources of hope? What are the implications of your own sources of hope in terms of any spiritual care that you might provide for Emma and her family?

b. What manifestations of hope can be identified in this case study? How did these change over the course of Emma's illness?

c. What challenges to nursing care were presented relative to Emma's physical condition? How might such concerns impact spiritual care?

d. What comments are made about the family's hope? How might the nurse support the family in this regard?

e. What do you learn about the Christian view of hope from the article? Research this further in literature resources about the Christian faith. How was the Christian view of hope manifested in Emma's dying and also after her death?

f. What personal challenges would caring for Emma and her family pose for you? How might you deal with such challenges?

3. Read the case study of Anne (p. 160) and Maryann (pp. 161–163) in Ruder (2008).

Anne:

a. What cues did Anne provide that might lead the nurse to identify or hypothesize spiritual needs?

b. Can you relate to the nurse's lack of comfort in probing about death and also about spiritual needs?

c. How might the nurse have probed further to open up a discussion about death and spirituality? What might be said (in actual words)? What might the focus be for such probing?

d. How might the nurse have better dealt with the situation?

Maryann:

a. What information is given about Maryann's spirituality in the case study?

b. How would the information about Maryann's spirituality impact the spiritual care provided?

c. In the discussion about Maryann's care, a comment is made: "It was very important to Maryann that her health clinicians prayed with her and listened as she discussed her spiritual beliefs" (p. 162). If you were caring for Maryann, how might you respond personally to this comment? Would you be comfortable with praying with Maryann? Would you be comfortable listening to her as she discussed her spiritual beliefs? Why or why not? If not, how might you respond to her needs in this regard?

d. What signs of spiritual distress are evident in the excerpt of the case study on p. 162? Use the defining characteristics of spiritual distress in Table 3 (p. 162) to assist you in determining if Maryann is in spiritual distress. Other than referral, how might a nurse address this issue?

4. Read the case study of a 56-year-old woman (pp. 161–162) and also of a 72-year-old man (p. 162) in Jenko and colleagues (2007).

a. A question that the nurse asked in a meeting with the woman and her son was: "What part of yourself would you like to leave with the ones who love you?" (p. 161). Appraise this question in terms of its use as an opening for assisting a client with life review.

b. How prepared would you be to initiate and continue the process of life review for both clients discussed in the article?

c. What was the impact of the life review on the woman and her son? On the man's wife? Why might it be important for family members to be present when a client is working through a life review?

d. Compare and contrast the process of life review for both the woman and the man.

e. Conduct a life review with a client who is terminally ill, perhaps using the prompts provided by Jenko and colleagues (Table 1, p. 163). What benefits do you note for the client and for any family members who may be present during the life review?

f. From the information in this article and from your own clinical experience, write a guide for nurses in conducting a life review with terminally ill clients.

5. Read the case study of Mary Lamont in Griffie and colleagues (2004, pp. 48–49).

   a. How would you respond to Mrs. Lamont's comments on p. 49 in order to encourage her to further discuss death/dying?

   b. Appraise Mrs. Lamont's comments on p. 49 with respect to any feelings that might be underlying such comments; and also with respect to any spiritual needs that might be suggested.

   c. Would you begin a conversation with Mrs. Lamont after her comments on p. 49 by focusing on her feelings? If so, why would you do this? Where might you proceed from there and how would you proceed?

   d. Do you find it difficult to initiate conversations with clients about death and dying? Why or why not?

   e. Reflect on the metaphor of death as "the elephant in the room" (p. 49). What are the implications of such a metaphor for nurses in terms of how death and dying are addressed with clients/families?

   f. How can the nurse create an environment conducive to conversing with Mrs. Lamont? Make a list of suggestions and compare your list with those on pp. 50–51.

   g. How might Mr. Lamont be included in the conversation?

   h. Read the information about a family conference (p. 54). What is the potential for such a conference in terms of family-focused care in palliative care?

   i. What is your appraisal of the overall care of Mrs. Lamont and her family? What spiritual needs were discussed and how? What were the outcomes?

6. Read the case study of Michael Cantos in Mazanec and Tyler (2003, pp. 52, 54, 55, 57).

   a. What generational conflicts related to culture are operant in this case scenario? How might nurses deal with such situations?

   b. What spiritual struggles had Michael encountered prior to his illness? How might his developmental stage have contributed to such struggles?

   c. What were the spiritual issues of Michael's grandmother? Appraise how the health care team dealt with these issues. What was the outcome for both the grandmother and Michael?

   d. Reflect on the possible outcomes if a family-focused approach had not occurred in this scenario.

   e. Reflect on the need for nurses to not only know various cultural beliefs regarding illness and death/dying, but also cultural beliefs regarding the hereafter. Also, reflect on treating each client as an individual. Why are both important?

   f. Does this case scenario raise any questions for you regarding the relationship between culture and spirituality/religion in end-of-life care? What are these questions and how might you address them?

g. What ethical conflicts arise for you in terms of beliefs that you have about death/dying and the hereafter compared to those of Michael's and that of his family members? If you have any, how might you, as a nurse, resolve such conflicts?

h. Reflect on how ethnicity, age, and spirituality impact decisions when death is imminent, not only in the context of this case scenario, but more broadly.

7. Read the case study of James in Friedemann, Mouch, and Racey (2002, pp. 329–330).

a. How is this case study an illustration of nursing the spirit of a terminally ill client?

b. Read the explanation of the Framework of Systematic Organization (Friedemann, 1995) provided in the article by Friedemann and colleagues (2002, pp. 327–329). How does the case study illustrate this framework as an approach to meeting clients' spiritual needs? What is your appraisal of the potential of this framework in your own care of terminally ill clients?

c. What information is given in the case study that relate to James's spiritual needs? What needs are suggested?

d. What spiritual struggles are suggested in this case study? How were they dealt with?

e. What is your personal reaction to this case study? Imagine that you were a nurse caring for James at the end of his life. How comfortable would you feel initiating and maintaining discussions with James about his spiritual issues?

f. How does the case study illustrate the importance of developing a trusting relationship with the client who is dying? And the importance of family-focused care in palliative care?

g. A comment is made in the article regarding James that "the need for spirituality lay dormant until his situation became desperate" (p. 330). What is your personal reaction to this statement? Have you encountered this situation in your own life or in the lives of clients in your clinical practice? How can nurses respond to such a situation?

8. Read the case study of Lynne in Taylor (2001, pp. 398–399)—read only to the end of Lynne's comments before proceeding with the following directives.

a. What are the indicators of spiritual needs in this case study?

b. What signs of resilience can you identify in Lynne?

c. Imagine that you are a nurse listening to Lynne's comments. What, in her comments, would you explore further and why? What might you say to her (in actual words)?

d. On what spiritual/religious resources does Lynne draw? Are there additional spiritual/religious resources that a nurse could encourage to help Lynne further? If so, what might these be?

e. Read the information on Fitchett's 7×7 Model for Spiritual Assessment (Fitchett, 1993) in Taylor (2001, p. 398). Then read the information regarding the application of this model to the case study (after Lynne's comments on p. 399). Compare your responses to (a–d) with the assessment according to Fitchett's model.

f. Appraise the potential for Fitchett's model of spiritual assessment for the spiritual assessment of terminally ill clients.

g. Review the other spiritual assessment tools/models described in this article. What is your appraisal of their potential for use in a palliative care context?

9. Read the case study in Buck (2006, p. 288).

a. If you were the nurse standing by the bedside of the client in this scenario, how would his statement "So this is it." (p. 288) make you feel? How might you have responded (in actual words)?

b. Considering the client's previous comment to the nurse about the fact that he had a strong faith, what might the nurse want to explore further in this regard? How might this statement impact nursing care of this client?

c. At one point in the conversation, the nurse used silence. Why do you think she did this? Was her use of silence therapeutic and, if so, how do you know this? How comfortable are you with silence? When is silence therapeutic? And when is it more akin to "I don't know what to say, so I will remain silent?"

d. Would you have initiated further conversation with this client about spiritual matters? Why or why not? If you would continue the conversation, how might you focus it? What might you say (in actual words)?

10. Read the case studies of Ms. Arcenaux (p. 368), Ms. Bourgeois (pp. 368–369), and Mr. Bordelon (pp. 369–370) in Mitchell, Bennett, and Manfrin-Ledet (2006).

a. Read the information on care mapping on pp. 367–368. Develop a care map for Ms. Arcenaux, Ms. Bourgeois, and Mr. Bordelon. Compare your nursing care maps with the care maps given in the article for each client (Mrs. Arcenaux, p. 367; Ms. Bourgeois, p. 368; and Mr. Bordelon, p. 369).

b. Appraise the value of nursing care maps for clients in a palliative care context. What would be the strengths of such an approach to documenting nursing care? What would be some of the challenges?

c. Develop your own care map for a terminally ill client you encounter in your nursing practice. (Use a spiritual assessment tool of your own choice to assess the spiritual impact of the client's illness.) What client outcomes did you observe? Reflect on how planning care in this format ensures a holistic approach to care.

d. Reflect on how nursing care maps can contribute to your own competency in spiritual assessment and spiritual care.

e. Could a modified version of a nursing care map be shared with a client/family? What might be some of the potential benefits in terms of the overall care of the client?

11. Read the case study of Anna in O'Connor (2001, p. 38).

   a. If you were the nurse encountering Anna in the emergency room, what thoughts would you have had? How might you have responded to Anna and the two people who accompanied her? What might you have said (in actual words) and what actions, if any, might you have employed?

   b. How did the nurse's question "Where did the tears go?" (p. 38) facilitate Anna's healing?

   c. What is the difference between "grieving" and "grieving with hope?" Knowing that Anna was a "woman of faith" (p. 38), presumably Christian based on the case study, what further information might you want to obtain from Anna? What questions might you ask that would elicit this information?

   d. What is the "hope" that was the topic of conversation with the nurse and Anna? Research the concept of hope from a Christian worldview if necessary. How did this hope impact Anna's grief response?

12. Read the three case studies of Mr. Santana (pp. 24–25), Lisa and her mother (p. 25), and Mr. Arthur (pp. 25–26) in Van Dover and Bacon (2001).

   a. To which of these clients do you most relate in terms of your own clinical practice?

   b. What cues (verbal and nonverbal) suggest that each of these clients may have a spiritual need? Which cues were more evident, and which more subtle? Which cues clearly point to a spiritual need, and which might have been "missed" as a spiritual need?

   c. What interventions were employed in each of these case studies? What were the outcomes for both the clients and the nurses?

   d. What communication skills were used in each case study (e.g., probes, self-disclosure, empathetic statements) and what was the impact from the use of such skills?

   e. Which interventions might you feel comfortable with/competent in with respect to working with terminally ill clients? How would you deal with spiritual issues that you do not feel comfortable with/competent in addressing with clients?

   f. When the nurse reflects on Mr. Arthur's care, she makes the following statement:

   > A very spiritual day. It's still a very emotional, from-the-soul experience. It is not a physical reaction. And you could feel the energy in the whole room—it was like we were elevated for just a few moments, in a whole different realm. (p. 26)

Have you had a similar experience to this nurse in terms of caring for a client? If so, under what conditions did this occur? How did it impact your nursing practice?

REFERENCES

Anandarajah, G., & Hight, E. (2001). Spirituality and medical practice: Using the HOPE questions as a practical tool for spiritual assessment. *American Family Physician, 63*(1), 81–89.

Bailey, M. E., Moran, S., & Graham, M. M. (2009). Creating a spiritual tapestry: Nurses' experiences of delivering spiritual care to patients in an Irish hospice. *International Journal of Palliative Care, 15*(1), 42–48. doi:10.12968/ijpn.2009.15.1.37952

Beckman, S., Boxley-Harges, S., Bruick-Sorge, C., & Salmon, B. (2007). Five strategies that heighten nurses' awareness of spirituality to impact client care. *Holistic Nursing Practice, 21*(3), 135–139. doi:10.1097/01.HNP.0000269150.80978.c3

Bjarnason, D. (2010). Nurse religiosity and end-of-life care. *Journal of Research in Nursing, 17*(1), 78–91. doi:10.1177/1744987110372046

Bolmsjo, I. (2000). Existential issues in palliative care: Interviews with cancer patients. *Journal of Palliative Care, 16*(2), 20–24.

Bonura, D., Fender, M., Roesler, M., & Pacquiao, D. F. (2001). Culturally congruent end-of-life care to Jewish patients and their families. *Journal of Transcultural Nursing, 12*(3), 211–220. doi:10.1177/104365960101200305

Boston, P., Bruce, A., & Schreiber, R. (2011). Existential suffering in the palliative care setting: An integrated literature review. *Journal of Pain and Symptom Management, 41*(3), 604–618. doi:10.1016/j.jpainsymman.2010.05.010

Brown, A. E., Whitney, S. N., & Duffy, J. D. (2006). The physician's role in the assessment and treatment of spiritual distress at the end of life. *Palliative and Supportive Care, 4*(1), 81–86. doi:10.1017/S1478951506060093

Buck, H. G. (2006). Spirituality: Concept analysis and model development. *Holistic Nursing Practice, 20*(6), 288–292.

Buck, H. G., & McMillan, S. C. (2012). A psychometric analysis of the Spiritual Needs Inventory in informal caregivers of patients with cancer in hospice home care. *Oncology Nursing Forum, 39*(4), E332–E339. doi:10.1188/12.ONF.E332-E339

Carr, T. (2008). Mapping the processes and qualities of spiritual nursing care. *Qualitative Health Research, 18*(5), 686–700. doi:10.1177/1049732307308979

Cheraghi, M. A., Payne, S., & Salsali, M. (2005). Spiritual aspects of end-of-life care for Muslim patients: Experiences from Iran. *International Journal of Palliative Nursing, 11*(9), 468–474. doi:10.12968/ijpn.2005.11.9.19781

Christopher, S. A. (2010). The relationship between nurses' religiosity and willingness to let patients control the conversation about end-of-life care. *Patient Education and Counseling, 78*(2), 250–255. doi:10.1016/j.pec.2009.05.018

Clarke, E. B., Curtis, J. R., Luce, J. M., Levy, M., Danis, M., Nelson, J., & Solomon, M. Z. (2003). Quality indicators for end-of-life care in the intensive care unit. *Critical Care Medicine, 31*(9), 2255–2262. doi:10.1097/01.ccm.0000084849.96385.85

Cockell, N., & McSherry, W. (2012). Spiritual care in nursing: An overview of published international research. *Journal of Nursing Management, 20*(8), 958–969. doi:10.1111/j.1365-2834.2012.01450.x

Conrad, N. L. (1985). Spiritual support for the dying. *Nursing Clinics of North America, 20*(2), 415–426.

Cutcliffe, J. R. (1995). How do nurses inspire and instil hope in terminally ill HIV patients? *Journal of Advanced Nursing, 22*(5), 888–895. doi:10.1111/j.1365-2648.1995.tb02639.x

Cutcliffe, J. R. (2006). The principles and processes of inspiring hope in bereavement counselling: A modified grounded theory study—part two. *Journal of Psychiatric and Mental Health Nursing, 13*(5), 604–610. doi:10.1111/j.1365-2850.2006.01020.x

Davies, B., Brenner, P., Orloff, S., Sumner, L., & Worden, W. (2002). Addressing spirituality in pediatric hospice and palliative care. *Journal of Palliative Care, 18*(1), 59–67.

DeLima, L., Bennett, M. I., Murray, S. A., Hudson, P., Doyle, D., Bruera, E., . . . Wenk, R. (2012). International Association for Hospice and Palliative Care (IAHPC) list of essential practices in palliative care. *Journal of Pain and Palliative Care Pharmacotherapy, 26*(12), 118–122.

Department of Health. (2011). *Spiritual care at the end of life: A systematic review of the literature.* Retrieved from http://www.gov.uk/government/uploads/system/uploads/attachment_data/file/215798/dh_123804.pdf

Dobratz, M. C. (2005). A comparative study of life-closing spirituality in home hospice patients. *Research and Theory for Nursing Practice: An International Journal, 19*(3), 243–256.

Doorenbos, A. Z., Wilson, S. A., & Coenen, A. (2006). A cross-cultural analysis of dignified dying. *Journal of Nursing Scholarship, 38*(4), 352–357. doi:10.1111/j.1547-5069.2006.00126.x

Dudley, J. R., Smith, C., & Millison, M. B. (1995). Unfinished business: Assessing the spiritual needs of hospice clients. *American Journal of Hospice and Palliative Care, 12*(2), 30–37.

Ekedahl, M. A., & Wengstrom, Y. (2010). Caritas, spirituality, and religiosity in nurses' coping. *European Journal of Cancer Care, 19*(4), 530–537. doi:10.1111/j.1365-2354.2009.01089.x

Fast, J. D. (2003). After Columbine: How people mourn sudden death. *Social Work, 48*(4), 484–491. doi:10.1093/sw/48.4.484

Fillion, L., Dupuis, R., Tremblay, I., De Grace, G. R., & Breitbart, W. (2006). Enhancing meaning in palliative care practice: A meaning-centered intervention to promote job satisfaction. *Palliative and Supportive Care, 4*(4), 333–344. doi:10.1017/S1478951506060445

Fitchett, G. (1993). *Assessing spiritual needs: A guide for caregivers.* Minneapolis, MN: Augsburg.

Foster, T. L., Bell, C. J., & Gilmer, M. J. (2012). Symptom management of spiritual suffering in pediatric palliative care. *Journal of Hospice & Palliative Care, 14*(2), 109–115. doi:10.1097/NJH.0b013e3182491f4b

Friedemann, M., Mouch, J., & Racey, T. (2002). Nursing the spirit: The framework of systematic organization. *Journal of Advanced Nursing, 39*(4), 325–332. doi:10.1046/j.1365-2648-2002.02293.x

Friedemann, M. L. (1995). *The framework of systemic organization: A conceptual approach to families and nursing.* Thousand Oaks, CA: Sage.

Galek, K., Flannelly, K. J., Vane, A., & Galek, R. M. (2005). Assessing a patient's spiritual needs: A comprehensive instrument. *Holistic Nursing Practice, 19*(2), 62–69. doi:10.1097/00004650-200503000-00006

Gijsberts, M. H. E. (2015). Spirituality and spiritual palliative care for older people. In L. van den Block, G. Albers, S. M. Pereira, B. Onwuteaka-Philipsen, R. Pasman, & L. Deliens (Eds.), *Palliative care for older people: A public health perspective* (pp. 169–175). Oxford, England: Oxford University Press.

Gijsberts, M. H. E., Echteld, M. A., van der Steen, J. T., Muller, M. T., Otten, R. H. J., Ribbe, M. W., & Deliens, L. (2011). Spirituality at the end of life: Conceptualization of measurable aspects—a systematic review. *Journal of Palliative Medicine, 14*(7), 852–863. doi:10.1089/jpm.2010.0356

Greenstein, M., & Breitbart, W. (2000). Cancer and the experience of meaning: A group psychotherapy program for people with cancer. *American Journal of Psychotherapy, 54*(4), 486–501.

Griffie, J., Nelson-Marten, P., & Muchka, S. (2004). Acknowledging the "elephant": Communication in palliative care: Speaking the unspeakable when death is imminent. *American Journal of Nursing, 104*(1), 48–57.

Hayden, D. (2011). Spirituality in end-of-life care: Attending the person on their journey. *British Journal of Community Nursing, 16*(11), 546, 548–551. doi:10.12968/bjcn.2011.16.11.546

Heilferty, C. M. (2004). Spiritual development and the dying child: The pediatric nurse practitioner's role. *Journal of Pediatric Health Care, 18*(6), 271–275. doi:10.1016/j.pedhc.2004.03.007

Hendriks, M. P., van Laarhoven, H. W. M., van de Sande, R., van Weel-Baumgarten, E., Verhagen, C. A., & Vissers, K. C. (2012). Palliative care for an Islamic patient: Changing frameworks. *Journal of Palliative Medicine, 15*(10), 1053–1055. doi:10.1089/jpm.2012.0190

Hermann, C. P. (2001). Spiritual needs of dying patients: A qualitative study. *Oncology Nursing Forum, 28*(1), 67–72.

Hermann, C. P. (2007). The degree to which spiritual needs of patients near the end of life are met. *Oncology Nursing Forum, 34*(1), 70–78. doi:10.1188/07.ONF.70-78

Hills, J., Paice, J. A., Cameron, J. R., & Shott, S. (2005). Spirituality and distress in palliative care consultation. *Journal of Palliative Medicine, 8*(4), 782–788. doi:10.1089/jpm.2015.8.782

Hills, M., & Watson, J. (2011). *Creating a caring science curriculum: An emancipatory pedagogy for nursing*. New York, NY: Springer Publishing Company.

Hogan, N. S., Greenfield, D. B., & Schmidt, L. A. (2001). Development and validation of the Hogan grief reaction checklist. *Death Studies, 25*(1), 1–32. doi:10.1080/07481180125831

Holland, J. M., & Neimeyer, R. A. (2005). Reducing the risk of burnout in end-of-life care settings: The role of daily spiritual experiences and training. *Palliative & Supportive Care, 3*(3), 173–181. doi:10.1017/S1478951505050297

Holloway, M. (2006). Death the great leveller? Towards a transcultural spirituality of dying and bereavement. *Journal of Clinical Nursing, 15*(7), 833–839. doi:10.1111/j.1365-2702.2006.01662.x

Hospice Foundation of America. (2014). *What is hospice?* Retrieved from http://www.hospicefoundation .org/End-of-Life-Support-and-Resources/Coping-with-Terminal-Illness/Hospice-Services

Iversen, A., & Sessanna, L. (2012). Utilizing Watson's Theory of Human Caring and Hills and Watson's Emancipatory Pedagogy to educate hospital-based multidisciplinary healthcare providers about hospice. *International Journal for Human Caring, 16*(4), 42–48.

Jackson, J. (2004). The challenge of providing spiritual care. *Professional Nurse, 20*(3), 24–26.

Jenko, M., Gonzalez, L., & Alley, P. (2010). Life review in critical care: Possibilities at the end of life. *Critical Care Nurse, 30*(1), 17–27. doi:10.4037/ccn2010122

Jenko, M., Gonzalez, L., & Seymour, M. J. (2007). Life review with the terminally ill. *Journal of Hospice & Palliative Care, 9*(3), 159–167. doi:10.1097/01.NJH.0000269995.98377.4d

Kao, C., Hu, W., Chiu, T., & Chen, C. (2014). Effects of the hospital-based palliative care team on the care for cancer patients: An evaluation study. *International Journal of Nursing Studies, 51*(2), 226–235. doi:10.1016/j.ijnurstu.2013.05.008

Kendall, M. L. (1999). A holistic model for spiritual care of the terminally ill. *American Journal of Hospice & Palliative Care, 16*(2), 473–476. doi:10.1177/104990919901600210

Kissane, D. W. (2000). Psychospiritual and existential distress: The challenge for palliative care. *Australian Family Physician, 29*(11), 1022–1025.

Kisvetrova, H., Klugar, M., & Kabelka, L. (2013). Spiritual support interventions in nursing care for patients suffering death anxiety in the final phase of life. *International Journal of Palliative Nursing, 19*(12), 599–605.

Kloss, W. E. (1988). Spirituality: The will to wellness. *Harding Journal of Religion and Psychiatry, 7*, 3–8.

Kruse, B. G., Ruder, S., & Martin, L. (2007). Spirituality and coping at the end of life. *Journal of Hospice and Palliative Nursing, 9*(6), 296–304. doi:10.1097/01.NJH.0000299317.52880.ca

Kuuppelomaki, M. (2001). Spiritual support for terminally ill patients: Nursing staff assessments. *Journal of Clinical Nursing, 10*(5), 660–670. doi:10.1046/j.1365-2702-2001.00534.x

MacKinlay, E. (2001). Understanding the ageing process: A developmental perspective of the psychosocial and spiritual dimensions. In E. MacKinlay, J. W. Ellor, & S. Pickard (Eds.), *Aging, spirituality, and pastoral care: A multi-national perspective* (pp. 111–122). Binghamton, NY: Haworth Pastoral Press.

Maloney, H. N. (1993). Making a religious diagnosis: The use of religious assessment in pastoral care and counseling. *Pastoral Psychology, 41*(4), 237–246. doi:10.1007/BF01080455

Mazanec, P., & Tyler, M. K. (2003). Cultural considerations in end-of-life care: How ethnicity, age, and spirituality affect decisions when death is imminent. *American Journal of Nursing, 103*(3), 50–58. doi:10.1097/00000446-200303000-00019

Meraviglia, M., Sutter, R., & Gaskamp, C. D. (2008). Providing spiritual care to terminally ill older adults. *Journal of Gerontological Nursing, 34*(7), 8–14. doi:10.3928/00989134-20080701-08

Milligan, S. (2011). Addressing the spiritual care needs of people near the end of life. *Nursing Standard, 26*(4), 47–56. doi:10.7748/ns2011.09.26.4.47.c8730

Mitchell, D. (2011). Spiritual and cultural issues at the end of life. *Medicine, 39*(11), 678–679. doi:10.1016/j .mpmed.2011.08.009

Mitchell, D. L., Bennett, M. J., & Manfrin-Ledet, L. (2006). Spiritual development of nursing students: Developing competency to provide spiritual care to patients at the end of life. *Journal of Nursing Education, 45*(9), 365–370.

Mok, E., Wong, F., & Wong, D. (2010). The meaning of spirituality and spiritual care among the Hong Kong Chinese terminally ill. *Journal of Advanced Nursing, 66*(2), 360–370. doi:10.1111/j.1365-2648.2009.05193.x

Morita, T., Murata, M. A., Hirai, K., Tamura, K., Kataoka, J., Ohnishi, H., . . . Uchitomi, Y. (2007). Meaninglessness in terminally ill cancer patients: A validation study and nurse education intervention study. *Journal of Pain and Symptom Management, 34*(2), 160–170. doi:10.1016/j.jpainsymman.2006.10.021

Murphy, N. M. (1999). *The wisdom of dying: Practices for living.* Boston, MA: Element Books.

National Consensus Project for Quality Palliative Care. (2009). *Clinical Practice Guidelines for Quality Palliative Care, Second Edition.* Retrieved from http://www.nationalconsensusproject.org/guideline.pdf

O'Connor, C. I. (2001). Characteristics of spirituality, assessment, and prayer in holistic nursing. *Nursing Clinics of North America, 36*(1), 33–46.

O'Shea, E. R., & Kanarek, R. B. (2013). Understanding pediatric palliative care: What it is and what it should be. *Journal of Pediatric Oncology Nursing, 30*(1), 34–44. doi:10.1177/1043454212471725

Otis-Green, S., Ferrell, B., Borneman, T., Puchalski, C., Uman, G., & Garcia, A. (2012). Integrating spiritual care within palliative care: An overview of nine demonstration projects. *Journal of Palliative Medicine, 15*(2), 154–162. doi:10.1089/jpm.2011.0211

Paterson, J. G., & Zderad, L. T. (1988). *Humanistic nursing.* New York, NY: National League for Nursing.

Pattison, N. A., & Lee, C. (2011). Hope against hope in cancer at the end of life. *Journal of Religion & Health, 50*(3), 731–742. doi:10.1007/s10943-009-9265-7

Penman, J., Oliver, M., & Harrington, A. (2013). The relational model of spiritual engagement depicted by palliative care clients and caregivers. *International Journal of Nursing Practice, 19*(1), 39–46. doi:10.1111/ijn.12035

Peterson, C. L. (2014). Spiritual care of the child with cancer at the end of life: A concept analysis. *Journal of Advanced Nursing, 70*(6), 1243–1253. doi:10.1111/jan.12257

Pittroff, G. E. (2013). The humbled expert: An exploration of spiritual care expertise. *Journal of Christian Nursing, 30*(3), 164–169. doi:10.1097/cnj.0b013e318294e8d3

Planalp, S., Trost, M. R., & Berry, P. H. (2011). Spiritual feasts: Meaningful conversations between hospice volunteers and patients. *American Journal of Hospice & Palliative Medicine, 28*(7), 483–486. doi:10.1177/1049909111398238

Prebendary, R., & Speck, P. (1999). Book Review: Sharing the journey: Spiritual assessment and pastoral response to persons with incurable illnesses. *Journal of Medical Ethics, 25*(3), 286. doi:10.1136/jme.25.3.286

Price, J. L., Stevens, H. O., & LaBarre, M. C. (1995). Spiritual caregiving in nursing practice. *Journal of Psychosocial Nursing, 33*(12), 5–9.

Pruyser, P. W. (1976). *The minister as diagnostician.* Philadelphia, PA: Westminster.

Puchalski, C. (2004). Spirituality in health: The role of spirituality in critical care. *Critical Care Clinics, 20*(3), 487–504. doi:10.1016/j.ccc.2004.03.007

Puchalski, C., & Ferrell, B. (2010). *Making health care whole: Integrating spirituality into patient care.* West Conshohocken, PA: Templeton Press.

Puchalski, C., Ferrell, B., Virani, R., Otis-Green, S., Baird, P., Bull, J., . . . Sulmasy, D. (2009). Improving the quality of spiritual care as a dimension of palliative care: The report of the census conference. *Journal of Palliative Care, 12*(10), 885–904. doi:10.1089/jpm.2009.0142

Puchalski, C., & Romer, A. L. (2000). Taking a spiritual history allows clinicians to understand patients more fully. *Journal of Palliative Medicine, 3*(1), 129–137. doi:10.1089/jpm.2000.3.129

Puchalski, C. M., Lumford, B., Harris, M. H., & Miller, R. T. (2006). Interdisciplinary spiritual care for seriously ill and dying patients: A collaborative model. *Cancer Journal, 12*(5), 398–416.

Ronaldson, S., Hayes, L., Aggar, C., Green, J., & Carey, M. (2012). Spirituality and spiritual care: Nurses' perspectives and practice in palliative and acute care environments. *Journal of Clinical Nursing, 21*(15–16), 2126–2135. doi:10.1111/j.1365-2702-2012.04180.x

Rosenbaum, J. L., Smith, J. R., & Zollfrank, R. (2011). Neonatal end-of-life spiritual support care. *Journal of Perinatal & Neonatal Nursing, 25*(1), 61–69. doi:10.1097/JPN.0b013e318209e1d2

Ross, L., & Austin, J. (2015). Spiritual needs and spiritual support preferences of people with end-stage heart failure and their carers: Implications for nurse managers. *Journal of Nursing Management, 23*(1) 87–95. doi:10.1111/jonm.12087

Ruder, S. (2008). Incorporating spirituality into home care at the end of life. *Home Healthcare Nurse, 26*(3), 158–163. doi:10.1097/01.NHH.0000313346.01228.1f

Ruder, S. (2013). Spirituality in nursing: Nurses' perceptions about providing spiritual care. *Home Healthcare Now, 31*(7), 356–367. doi:10.1097/NHH.0b013e3182976135

Satterly, L. (2001). Guilt, shame, and religious and spiritual pain. *Holistic Nursing Practice, 15*(2), 30–39. doi:10.1097/00004650-200101000-00006

Saunders, C. (2000). The evolution of palliative care. *Patient Education and Counseling, 41*(1), 7–13. doi:10.1016/S0738-3391(00)00110-5

Steed, M. (2012). Palliative care: Are you asking the right questions? *Nursing 2012, 42*(10), 59–61. doi:10.1097/01.NURSE.0000418787.36065.c7

Steinhauser, K. E., Christakis, N. A., Clipp, E. C., McNeilly, M., McIntyre, L., & Tulsky, J. A. (2000). Factors considered important at the end of life by patients, family, physicians, and other care providers. *The Journal of the American Medical Association, 284*(19), 2476–2482. doi:10.1001/jama.284.19.2476

Tamburro, R. F., Shaffer, M. L., Hahnlen, N. C., Felker, P., & Ceneviva, G. D. (2011). Care goals and decisions for children referred to a pediatric palliative care program. *Journal of Palliative Care, 14*(5), 607–613. doi:10.1089/jpm.2010.0450

Tan, H. M., Wilson, A., Olver, I., & Barton, C. (2011). The experience of palliative patients and their families of a family meeting utilized as an instrument for spiritual and psychosocial care: A qualitative study. *BMC Palliative Care, 10*(7), 1–12. doi:10.1186/1472-684X-10-7

Taylor, E. J. (2000). Spiritual and ethical end-of-life concerns. In C. H. Yarbro, M. H. Frogge, M. Goodman, & S. L. Groenwald (Eds.), *Cancer nursing: Principles and practice* (5th ed., pp. 1565–1578). Sudbury, MA: Jones & Bartlett.

Taylor, E. J. (2001). Spiritual assessment. In B. Ferrell & N. Coyle (Eds.), *Textbook of palliative nursing* (pp. 397–406). New York, NY: Oxford University Press.

Taylor, E. J. (2013). New Zealand hospice nurses' self-rated comfort in conducting spiritual assessment. *International Journal of Palliative Care, 19*(4), 178–185.

Taylor, E. J., & Brander, P. (2013). Hospice patient and family carer perspectives on nurse spiritual assessment. *Journal of Hospice & Palliative Nursing, 15*(6), 347–354. doi:10.1097/NJH.0b013e3182979695

Tiew, L. H., Kwee, J. H., Creedy, D. K., & Chan, M. F. (2013). Hospice nurses' perspectives of spirituality. *Journal of Clinical Nursing, 22*(19–20), 2923–2933. doi:10.1111/jocn.12358

Vachon, M., Fillon, L., & Achille, M. (2009). A conceptual analysis of spirituality at the end of life. *Journal of Palliative Medicine, 12*(1), 53–59. doi:10.1089/jpm.2008.0189

Vachon, M., Fillion, L., & Achille, M. (2012). Death confrontation, spiritual-existential experience and caring attitudes in palliative care nurses: An interpretive phenomenological analysis. *Qualitative Research in Psychology, 9*(2), 151–172. doi:10.1080/14780881003663424

Vachon, M., Fillion, L., Achille, M., Duval, S., & Leung, D. (2011). An awakening experience: An interpretative phenomenological analysis of the effects of a meaning-centered intervention shared among palliative care nurses. *Qualitative Research in Psychology, 8*(1), 66–80. doi:10.1080/14780880903551564

van der Poel, C. J. (1998). *Sharing the journey: Spiritual assessment and pastoral response to persons with incurable illnesses.* Collegeville, MN: Liturgical Press.

Van Dover, L. J., & Bacon, J. M. (2001). Spiritual care in practice: A close-up view. *Nursing Forum, 36*(3), 18–28. doi:10.1111/j.1744-6198.2001.tb00245.x

Vassallo, B. M. (2001). The spiritual aspects of dying at home. *Holistic Nursing Practice, 15*(2), 17–29. doi:10.1097/00004650-200101000-00005

Waldrop, D. P., Milch, R. A., & Skretny, J. A. (2005). Understanding family responses to life-limiting illness: In-depth interviews with hospice patients and their family members. *Journal of Palliative Care, 21*(2), 88–96.

Wasner, M., Longaker, C., Fegg, M. J., & Borasio, G. D. (2005). Effects of spiritual care training for palliative care professionals. *Palliative Medicine, 19*(2), 99–104. doi:10.1191/0269216305pm995oa

Watson, J. (2012). *Human caring science: A theory of nursing* (2nd ed.). Sudbury, MA: Jones & Bartlett.

Weidner, N. J., Cameron, M., Lee, R. C., McBride, J., Mathias, E. J., & Byczkowski, T. L. (2011). End-of-life care for the dying child: What matters most to parents. *Journal of Palliative Care, 27*(4), 279–286.

West, R. (1996). Nursing the spirit. *Australian Nursing Journal, 4*(1), 34–35.

World Health Organization. (2007). *Definition of palliative care.* Retrieved from http://www.who.int/cancer/palliative/definition/en

Wynne, L. (2013). Spiritual care at the end of life. *Nursing Standard, 28*(2), 41–45. doi:10.7748/ns2013.09.28.2.41.e7977

Yardley, S. J., Walshe, C. E., & Parr, A. (2009). Improving training in spiritual care: A qualitative study exploring patient perceptions of professional education requirements. *Palliative Medicine, 23*(7), 601–607. doi:10.1177/0269216309105726

Appendix A:

Boutell's Inventory for Identifying the Nurses' Assessment of Patients' Spiritual Needs

If you work only with patients who are 17 years of age or younger, STOP HERE and return the questionnaire.
If you presently work with ANY patients who are 18 years of age or older, please complete the questionnaire.

PART I. ABOUT YOURSELF

Please check the appropriate space for the following information about <u>YOURSELF</u>. Do not leave any question unanswered.

A. General Information

1. Your gender: male _____, female _____.

2. Your age: 0–19 _____, 20–29 _____, 30–39 _____, 40–49 _____, 50–59 _____, 60–above _____.

B. Present R.N. Work Status

3. Your present place of work: hospital _____, nursing home _____, school of nursing _____, private duty _____, community health _____, school nurse _____, industrial nurse _____, office nurse _____, other, specify _____.

(continued)

4. Your present position: administrator or assistant _____, consultant _____, supervisor or assistant _____, instructor _____, head nurse or assistant _____, general duty or staff _____, other, specify _____.

5. Your present number of working hours per week: 8 _____, 16 _____, 24 _____, 32 _____, 40 _____, other, specify _____.

6. Your average number of hours per 8 hours of working time excluding meals and breaks that you presently have DIRECT patient contact (e.g., giving baths, making patient rounds, counseling, teaching, assessing patient needs, etc.): 0 _____, 1 _____ 2 _____, 3 _____, 4 _____, 5 _____, 6 _____, 7 _____, 8 _____.

7. Type of patient you presently have DIRECT contact with: medical _____, surgical _____, psychiatric _____, obstetrical _____, pediatric _____, other, specify _____.

8. Your TOTAL number of years as an R.N. during which you have had DIRECT patient contact: 0–2 _____, 3–4 _____, 5–9 _____, 10–14 _____, 15–19 _____, other, specify _____.

C. Educational Preparation

9. Your level of education completed. Check ALL that apply: Diploma _____, Associate degree _____, Baccalaureate in Nursing _____, Baccalaureate in other field _____, Master's in Nursing _____, Master's in other field _____, Doctorate in Nursing _____, Doctorate in other field _____.

D. Present Religious Status

10. Your religious affiliation: Protestant _____, Catholic _____, Jewish _____, none _____, other, specify _____.

11. Your frequency of attending church/synagogue services: daily _____, more than once a week _____, weekly _____, monthly _____, once a year _____, twice a year _____, only for events such as weddings, funerals, etc. _____, never _____, other, specify _____.

12. Your practicing religious status: active _____, inactive _____, other, specify _____.

E. Personal Beliefs

13. Your belief about people's spiritual dimension: it exists _____, it does not exist _____, don't know _____.

14. Do you know your own philosophy of life? Yes _____, No _____, Not sure _____.

15. Does your philosophy of life include a spiritual dimension? Yes _____, No _____, Not sure _____.

(continued)

PART II. ABOUT YOU AND YOUR PATIENTS

Please circle ONE answer per item which best describes what you do with <u>PATIENTS</u> who are 18 years of age or older. Do not leave any question unanswered.

	Never	Seldom	Occasionally	Often	Always	Not Applicable
A. I determine my patients' SPIRITUAL NEEDS by the following:						
16. Listening in report	0	1	2	3	4	5
17. Reading the patient's Kardex	0	1	2	3	4	5
18. Reading the patient's care plan	0	1	2	3	4	5
19. Reading the nursing history	0	1	2	3	4	5
20. Reading the nurses' notes	0	1	2	3	4	5
21. Reading the patient's medical history	0	1	2	3	4	5
22. Reading the patient's name band	0	1	2	3	4	5
23. Asking the patient	0	1	2	3	4	5
24. Taking a nursing history that includes spiritual assessment	0	1	2	3	4	5
25. Asking the patient's family	0	1	2	3	4	5
26. Asking a patient's significant other (other than the family)	0	1	2	3	4	5
27. Observing clues from the patient (e.g., jokes about death, asks "Why me?" etc.)	0	1	2	3	4	5
28. Observing clues from the patient's environment (e.g., rosary in bed, has a religious station on the radio or TV, etc.)	0	1	2	3	4	5
29. Listening to the patient	0	1	2	3	4	5
30. Discussing patient's needs with other nurses	0	1	2	3	4	5
31. Discussing patient's needs with the clergy	0	1	2	3	4	5
32. Other, specify_____						

(*continued*)

	Never	Seldom	Occasionally	Often	Always	Not Applicable
B. I determine my patients' RELIGIOUS PRACTICES related to:						
33. Special diet (e.g., no pork products, fasting, etc.)	0	1	2	3	4	5
34. Surgery (e.g., blood administration, etc.)	0	1	2	3	4	5
35. Birth (e.g., circumcision, infant baptism, etc.)	0	1	2	3	4	5
36. Death (e.g., last rites, communion, etc.)	0	1	2	3	4	5
37. Other, specify _____						
C. I determine my patient's need for:						
38. Visiting a chapel or church	0	1	2	3	4	5
39. Seeing clergy	0	1	2	3	4	5
40. Receiving sacraments (e.g., communion, confession, etc.)	0	1	2	3	4	5
41. Having religious artifacts in environment (e.g., Bible, Torah, cross, religious pictures, appropriate reading materials, etc.)	0	1	2	3	4	5
42. Prayer (e.g., someone to pray with them, etc.)	0	1	2	3	4	5
43. Other, specify _____						
D. I talk with my patients about their:						
44. Feeling a sense of forgiveness (e.g., able to forgive self or others for past mistakes, etc.)	0	1	2	3	4	5
45. Fear of death	0	1	2	3	4	5
46. Understanding of meaning and purpose <u>of</u> life (e.g., to grow in ability to love, life is absurd—has no meaning or purpose, etc.)	0	1	2	3	4	5
47. Meaning and purpose <u>in</u> life (e.g., support my family, achieve goals that may be focused on career, etc.)	0	1	2	3	4	5

(continued)

	Never	Seldom	Occasionally	Often	Always	Not Applicable
48. Belief in a Supreme Being (e.g., that a Supreme Being exists, etc.)	0	1	2	3	4	5
49. Ability to rise above the worldly and material values of life (e.g., through prayer, meditation, etc.)	0	1	2	3	4	5
50. Giving love to God (e.g., prayer, hymns, good works, etc.)	0	1	2	3	4	5
51. Work status	0	1	2	3	4	5
52. Receiving love from God (e.g., in church, in sacraments, in the gift of life itself, etc.)	0	1	2	3	4	5
53. Belief in life after death	0	1	2	3	4	5
54. Being at peace with the future	0	1	2	3	4	5
55. Feeling of being helped in a time of need	0	1	2	3	4	5
56. Faith in God (e.g., that God loves us, etc.)	0	1	2	3	4	5
57. Creative self-expression (e.g., reading, painting, listening to music, etc.)	0	1	2	3	4	5
58. Being at peace with the present	0	1	2	3	4	5
59. Meaning in suffering	0	1	2	3	4	5
60. Feeling love about yourself (e.g., self-acceptance, etc.)	0	1	2	3	4	5
61. Chance to re-examine life's priorities	0	1	2	3	4	5
62. Being at peace with the past	0	1	2	3	4	5
63. Unifying force in self (e.g., what most makes you whole, etc.)	0	1	2	3	4	5
64. Appreciation of nature (e.g., cares for pets, plants, garden, enjoys sunsets, parks, etc.)	0	1	2	3	4	5
65. Receiving love from others (e.g., in kindnesses experienced in friendships and others, etc.)	0	1	2	3	4	5

(continued)

	Never	Seldom	Occasionally	Often	Always	Not Applicable
66. Giving love to others (e.g., acts of kindness in relationships with others, etc.)	0	1	2	3	4	5
67. Future goals	0	1	2	3	4	5
68. Fear of medical procedures (e.g., surgery, biopsy, etc.)	0	1	2	3	4	5
69. Source of personal strength (e.g., self, spouse, significant others, clergy, work or social contacts, etc.)	0	1	2	3	4	5
70. Feeling a sense of hope (e.g., in outcome of life events, etc.)	0	1	2	3	4	5
71. Feeling abandoned in a time of need	0	1	2	3	4	5

E. My general approach to patients with whom I have direct contact:

	Never	Seldom	Occasionally	Often	Always	Not Applicable
72. I talk with my patients about their spiritual needs	0	1	2	3	4	5
73. I am not very comfortable talking about God or spirituality with patients	0	1	2	3	4	5
74. I treat my patients holistically	0	1	2	3	4	5

75. Additional comments about how you assess your patients' spiritual needs:

76. Any additional comments:

When you finish, please look over the entire questionnaire to be certain that you have answered every question.

Reprinted with permission from Karen Boutell.

Appendix B

Wellness Spirituality Protocol

I. Clinical Presentation

A. The extent and direction of the wellness spirituality assessment and spiritual wellness care is directed by how aging clients are responding to conditions in life or illness. These responses are, overtly or covertly, identified early on in the interview process as the clinician inquires about an aging client's chief complaint, present problem, and data about his or her personal and social history other than spirituality.
    1. Actively involved in life
    2. Heightened awareness of aging changes
    3. Separation from religious and cultural ties
    4. Challenges in beliefs and value system
    5. Disfigurement or altered body image
    6. Disability or loss of function
    7. Chronic pain
    8. Anger toward others or God
    9. Change in meaningful relationships
    10. Limitations imposed by situations or others
    11. Hospitalization or institutionalization
    12. Isolation or confinement
    13. Opposition or interference by caregivers or family caregiver
    14. Cognitive regression

II. Diagnosis/Evaluation [12,15,19,34–36]

A. History: Self-Actualization Activities
    1. What are the good things about growing older?
    2. What are the difficult things about growing older?
    3. On a scale of 0 to 10 (0 = very closely related; 10 = only slightly related), how do you feel about your life at the present time?

| Boring | Rewarding | Hopeless |
| Lonely | Useless | Many friends |

(continued)

II. Diagnosis/Evaluation [12,15,19,34–36] (continued)

Hopeful   Interesting   Disappointing
Filled with guilt   Free from guilt
Filled with worry   Free from worry
Brings out the best in me—the worst in me

4. What are your plans for the future?
5. Tell me about some of your personal achievements and other significant life experiences.
6. What were the achievements that make (made) you feel proud?
7. What is your role in the family now?
8. What bothers you most about your present circumstances?
9. What are you doing to cope with your present circumstances?

B. History: Connectedness Activities
1. What helps you keep in touch with nature and the world?
2. What do you hope to leave to your family or this world?
3. Who or what do you turn to for help?
4. Have you had the opportunity to help a family member, close relative, or disabled or elderly person in the past 12 months?
5. Have you had the opportunity to visit a sick or shut-in person who is not a family member?

C. History: Healing and New Life Activities
1. What else is going on in your life?
2. What about being sick has been most troublesome?
3. Have you found a meaning for your life? How does it make you feel?
4. Is there anything particularly frightening or meaningful to you now?
5. What are some of the things you look forward to each day?
6. In what way do you enjoy the people in your life?
7. What do you like about being alone?
8. In what way do others show they care for you?
9. What do you do to show you care for them?
10. Do you have a role in saving our environment?
11. What are some of the things that give you a strong sense of fulfillment?
12. What in your daily life brings you a sense of closeness to God or a sense of relationship with a higher power?
13. What is God's role in all of this?

D. History: Religious or Humanistic Activities
1. In what or whom do you find hope and strength?
2. Who or what brings you joy and laughter?
3. Who or what gives you a sense of peace and harmony?
4. How would you describe your current relationship with a church or spiritual community?
5. In what way is prayer, Scripture, meditation, religious reading, or music helpful to you?
6. Does your relationship with God or a higher power contribute to your sense of well-being?
7. Do religious rituals or sacraments improve your well-being?
8. Is God or your religion helpful to you at this time in your life?

(continued)

III. *Plan/Management* [12,18,22]

A. Consult or refer when clinician recognizes that the activities or work of the spirit would be served better through contact with clergy, a spiritual leader, or a parish nurse.

B. Treatment to support or restore self-actualization
   1. Listen, encourage, affirm, and support.
   2. Respect habits of personal hygiene or attire that have special significance.
   3. Discuss anxieties and concerns about the future.
   4. Obtain life history to assist creative expression of aging clients' experiences.
   5. Arrange visits from those who appreciate them.
   6. Recommend assistive mobility aids to support independence.
   7. Arrange for guidance in taping their memories and autobiography.
   8. Review life accomplishments through reminiscence.
   9. Teach and practice methods of visual imagery of life accomplishments.

C. Treatment to support or restore connectedness
   1. Suggest ways for sharing self with others (e.g., a meal with another).
   2. Promote awareness of the world around them (e.g., sitting and observing traffic or pigeons on the roof carrying on their wooing).
   3. Arrange for mentorships, bartering activities, and sharing their talents.
   4. Encourage reminiscence through music, pictures, and religious symbols (e.g., crosses, rosaries, and menorahs).
   5. Encourage storytelling with adults and children.
   6. Suggest letter "writing" by tape to grandchildren and friends.
   7. Facilitate regular contacts with nearby neighbors, clubs, and social groups.
   8. Recommend calling others who need help.
   9. Arrange for converting a legacy into some tangible form (i.e., photograph albums, taped memories, and so forth).
   10. Stimulate interest in writing letters to politicians.
   11. Advise serving in volunteer capacities.

D. Treatment to support or restore healing and new life
   1. Encourage dialogue and sharing painful memories and events with another.
   2. Perform or arrange for therapeutic touch.
   3. Encourage discussion of anxieties and uncertainties.
   4. Inquire about future plans.
   5. Foster anticipation of enjoyment from everyday events.

E. Treatment to support or restore religious and humanistic activities orientation
   1. Promote the possibility of gardening with what is available to them (i.e., garden spot, windowsill, and flowerpot).
   2. Identify avenues for them to participate in recycling.
   3. Support prayer or meditation.
   4. Advise journal keeping.
   5. Advocate time alone.
   6. Arrange for access to religious or spiritual articles and religious ceremonies.

Reprinted with permission from Mary Leetun.

Index

Printed in the United States
By Bookmasters